Fundamentals
of Musculoskeletal
Assessment Techniques

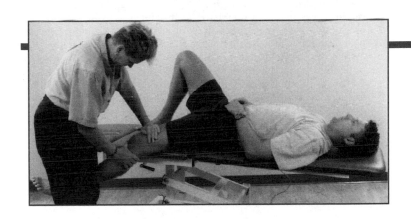

Fundamentals of Musculoskeletal Assessment Techniques

Second Edition

M. Lynn Palmer, PhD, PT
Professor Emeritus—Simmons College
Lecturer—Harvard Medical School
Boston, Massachusetts

Marcia E. Epler, PhD, PT, ATC
Assistant Professor
Department of Physical Therapy
Philadelphia College of Pharmacy and Science
Philadelphia, Pennsylvania

With Two Contributors

Illustrations by Michael Adams

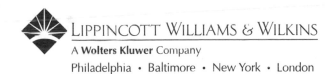

LIPPINCOTT WILLIAMS & WILKINS
A **Wolters Kluwer** Company
Philadelphia · Baltimore · New York · London
Buenos Aires · Hong Kong · Sydney · Tokyo

Acquisitions Editor: Margaret Biblis
Coordinating Editorial Assistant: Patricia Moore
Project Editor: Erika Kors
Senior Production Manager: Helen Ewan
Production Coordinator: Patricia McCloskey
Design Coordinator: Nicholas Rook

2nd Edition

9 8 7 6

Library of Congress Cataloging-in-Publications Data

Palmer, M. Lynn.
    Fundamentals of musculoskeletal assessment techniques/ M. Lynn Palmer, Marcia F. Epler ; illustrations by Michael Adams.—2nd ed.
        p.   cm.
    Includes bibliographical references and index.
    ISBN 0-7817-1007-3 (alk. paper)
    1. Musculoskeletal system—Examination.   2. Physical Therapy.
I. Epler, Marcia F.   II. Title.
RC925.7.P24   1998
616.7'075—DC21   97-48521
                                                        CIP

Care has been taken to confirm the accuracy of the information presented and to describe generally accepted practices. However, the authors, editors, and publisher are not responsible for errors or omissions or for any consequences from application of the information in this book and make no warranty, express or implied, with respect to the contents of the publication.

The authors, editors and publisher have exerted every effort to ensure that drug selection and dosage set forth in this text are in accordance with current recommendations and practice at the time of publication. However, in view of ongoing research, changes in government regulations, and the constant flow of information relating to drug therapy and drug reactions, the reader is urged to check the package insert for each drug for any change in indications and dosage and for added warnings and precautions. This is particularly important when the recommended agent is a new or infrequently employed drug.

Some drugs and medical devices presented in this publication have Food and Drug Administration (FDA) clearance for limited use in restricted research settings. It is the responsibility of the health care provider to ascertain the FDA status of each drug or device planned for use in their clinical practice.

▲ The rehabilitation practioner in a managed care environment must efficiently evaluate and develop a focused treatment plan based on evaluation findings. Consequently, all instruction in rehabilitation professional education programs must be well structured and precise. In this manner, students will learn to perform precise evaluation skills with a higher degree of reliability and validity.

Clinical Assessment Procedures in Physical Therapy comprehensively presents musculoskeletal assessment procedures. Drs. Palmer and Epler begin their textbook with a general overview of evaluation, principles of evaluation, pain quantification, and posture screening. The text guides the reader by region through goniometry, muscle length, manual muscle testing, special clinical tests, and accessory movement examinations. The extensive illustrations complement the easy-to-read text. Since all basic evaluation procedures are contained in this one textbook, it can serve as a clinical reference for experienced therapists as well as a structured instructional text for students.

As a clinician and academician, I am pleased to promote this text as an asset to physical therapy education. It will serve as a foundation to the scope of practice of the clinician of today—a clinician who is well organized, precise, and poised to give patients quality, efficient care.

Z. Annette Iglarsh, PhD, PT
Director of Physical Therapy
Philadelphia College of Pharmacy
  and Science
Philadelphia, Pennsylvania

▲ The second edition of this text was written as a way of continuing to provide a single integrated source of the comprehensive approach to evaluating and assessing musculoskeletal structures. Based on input from clinicians, faculty, and students, the authors and publisher recognize the need for a text such as this to continue to be available for clinical use. In addition to updating the topics covered in the first edition, the authors have added a chapter on the quantitative assessment of pain. Furthermore, information on muscle length testing and on gross observation and screening have been incorporated into Chapter 2 "Principles of Examination Techniques" and the subsequent regional chapters. Surface anatomy introduced in each chapter should also enhance the reader's ability to palpate more effectively in a patient care situation.

▲ This clinical text has been designed to teach entry-level physical therapy students techniques for assessing persons who have neuromuscular or musculoskeletal disorders, according to standardized criteria. The book stresses that consistency of technique provides consistency of results. While intended for use by students, this book is also a well-illustrated reference for the practicing physical therapist.

The book begins by describing screening examinations and gross evaluations that enable students to determine the need for more definitive physical therapy examinations. Chapter 2 describes the principles of specific clinical assessments. Chapter 4 is devoted entirely to posture and muscle imbalance. Subsequent chapters focus on specific regions of the body, and their format follows the normal sequence of clinical assessment of those specific regions.

The appendices at the end of the book are in two parts. Appendix A contains recording forms that have been developed as guidelines for examiners as they assess their patients. The objective of an assessment procedure is to establish baseline data on the patient from which a treatment plan is developed. The examples of assessment forms included in Appendix A can be used for recording initial patient evaluations and for periodic reevaluation of patient progress.

Appendix B contains multiple-choice objective examination questions for readers to assess their knowledge of clinical assessment procedures. The questions are organized by chapter.

An outstanding feature of this book is the number of quality photographs and illustrations. They do not serve merely to support text, rather, they tell their own story and join with the text to form a total information package.

The material covering goniometry, functional muscle testing, and manual muscle testing was written by Dr. Palmer. Dr. Epler wrote the sections covering orthopedic examination, clinical tests, and joint play.

Acknowledgments

▲ The authors would like to thank the following people for their contributions to the development and publication of this text:

Jill S. Galper, PT, MEd (President, Rehabilitation and Fitness Services, Philadelphia, PA and New Castle, DE) and Vincent W. Verno, PT (Partner and Center Coordinator of Clinical Education, Rehabilitation and Fitness Services, Philadelphia, PA and New Castle, DE) for researching and writing Chapter 3 of this edition.

Barbara Bourbon, PhD, PT, for her help in the preparation of Chapter 8.

Michael Adams, whose illustrative talent is apparent in the accuracy and detailed complexity of his work.

Jan Buhler Callahan, MEd, PT, EMT, for researching and writing for the first edition of this textbook the orthopedic clinical assessment portions of Chapters 9, 10, and 11.

Gail Baker, Kathy Hensley, Stephanie Homan, Barbara Proud, and J. Julian Washington, whose expertise in photography is evident in the professional quality of the numerous photographs used throughout this textbook.

Danny DiSabatino, PT, for providing his time and expertise in composing the biomechanics of the ankle and foot section of Chapter 14 for the first edition of this textbook.

Kevin Coloton, John Fields, Beth Gallagher, Al Jette, Rachel Lafarge, Jean Marchant, Linda Miller, Efrain Paz, Rauf Rashid, John Stemm, and Janice E. Toms for contributing their time to pose for the photographs contained in this book.

Finally, thank you to our colleagues, friends, and family who, in their own ways, have helped us become the individuals and professionals that we are today.

Contents

1

Gross Evaluations

Cognitive and psychomotor skills are necessary for mastery of patient assessment. This process involves identifying the appropriate procedures, which are usually determined from the patient's chart, history, and other sources of information. Careful selection of assessment procedures is important and depends on the patient's condition. Only assessments that contribute to the development of treatment strategies should be performed. Unless accurate use of technical skills during evaluation produces concrete information, the results will be meaningless, and time will be wasted.[1]

Standardized criteria have been developed to establish a range of normal performance or functional mobility. Patients' results are compared with the established norms. The desirable level of function may depend on the patient's physical build, age, and previous activity level. The patient's performance is tested at intervals to monitor response to treatment. These assessments must also adhere to normative criteria and be conducted in a reliable manner.

Because the results of clinical assessment are used to develop a plan of care, to determine the appropriate treatment techniques, and to monitor the patient's functional and physiological changes, the consistency of technique cannot be overemphasized. When therapists evaluate the efficacy of a treatment, they rely heavily on the quality of the measurements of the patients. Thorough and accurate patient assessment is necessary to prevent functional disability, to improve impaired function, and to maintain a given level of function.

PURPOSE

The purpose of assessment procedures is to gather data on the status of the patient at specific times. Assessments are performed to accomplish the following:

1. Develop a database to establish the patient's level of function, identify the patient's problem, and determine why the problem exists.
2. Plan a treatment program based on the results. The therapist analyzes the results, lists strengths and weaknesses, ranks the problems, develops treatment goals, and establishes the patient's outcomes. Prioritizing problems is important. For example, a patient needs to learn bed mobility activities before learning wheelchair transfers; joint range of motion is evaluated before muscle strength is determined.
3. Evaluate the results of the treatment program to know how treatments are affecting the patient.
4. Modify treatment to suit the patient or to terminate the treatment.

Assessments are the basis of all therapy treatment. A complete and accurate evaluation allows therapists to establish a database against which to assess progress. It allows them to determine a level of function so that an appropriate treatment program can be developed and adapted to the changing status of the patient. At times, it also allows therapists to identify the cause of the patient's problem.

For every type of assessment, there is a set of criteria for performing the evaluation and a specific method of recording the results.

RELIABILITY, OBJECTIVITY, AND VALIDITY

Assessments must be reliable and objective, and the results must be valid. Reliability is the extent to which comparable results are achieved every time a test is repeated. If a muscle test is repeated by one or more therapists who obtain the same grade every time, then the test is reliable. The key to reliability for manual muscle testing is to follow the standard procedure, performing the test in the same way each time and in the same way that other therapists perform it. Reliability is increased if the therapist gives clear instructions to the patient.

Evaluation procedures should exhibit intertester (interrater) and intratester (intrarater) reliability. Interrater reliability means that another person who performs the test should arrive at the same results. Intrarater reliability means that one person should come up with the same results on every repetition of the test. D.L. Riddle performed an intratester-reliable test by examining the effects of goniometer size on the reliability of passive shoulder joint measurements. He concluded that goniometric passive measurement of the range of shoulder joint motion can be highly reliable when taken by a single therapist (intratester reliability), regardless of the size of the goniometer. The degree of *intertester* reliability for those measurements appeared to be specific to the range of motion.[2]

Assessment procedure objectivity means that the findings are reported without distortion by personal opinion or feelings. Therapists should not let concern for the patient influence the results of an evaluation procedure. In manual muscle testing, the most difficult area in which to be objective is deciding whether the resistance the patient can tolerate is minimal, moderate, or maximal. If the patient's weakness is unilateral, the therapist should test the opposite side and use the result as the baseline for normal. If the patient has bilateral involvement, the therapist must rely on experience in testing other patients to know what is normal for a particular muscle in a person of a given age, sex, size, and occupation.

Objectivity is of prime importance when third-party payers are involved. These systems allow patients to receive many therapy services and require accurate and comprehensive documentation of treatments and outcomes.

Validity means that a test actually measures what it is supposed to measure. In muscle testing, therapists are testing the strength of a specific muscle. For a muscle test to be valid, the therapist must know the location and function of the muscle being tested and the location and function of surrounding muscles. Validity of assessments means that therapists evaluate exactly what they say they are going to and that the results are correct, or true.

GROSS MUSCLE SCREENING

A quick screening evaluation of a patient is an important component of the entire evaluative process; it gives a picture of the patient's status and is a basis for planning effective treatments. Seeing a patient for the first time, the therapist performs subjective and objective assessments. The therapist takes a history and hears the patient's complaints. The therapist then performs a general evaluation to determine which specific evaluation procedures are indicated.

The purpose of a muscle screening test is to determine quickly a level of muscle strength. If the therapist finds weakness during the muscle screening test, a specific manual muscle test is then performed to focus on such factors as resistance, positions, grades, palpations, and substitutions. Muscle screening is not a detailed determination of strength; it simply classifies levels of strength as either normal or weak. The results of the evaluation provide therapy practitioners with sufficient information to devise a plan of care or to proceed with a definitive muscle test for areas found to be weak.

Following are some general considerations for the technique of a muscle screening test that will assist the therapist.

- Simple observation of the patient prior to the assessment may give a general idea of his or her strength.
- Explanation of the purpose and procedure of the test must be given in terms that the patient can understand.

- As many tests as possible should be performed with the patient in one position to avoid unnecessary fatigue and discomfort.
- The assessment is based on movements usually performed in less than the full range of motion and tests groups of muscles performing a specific activity. Not all muscle groups need to be tested.
- A muscle screening test of the entire body should take no longer than 5 minutes.

The following are guidelines for a muscle screening test that may be altered to suit the patient and circumstances. The therapist should also keep these in mind when administering the test.

- The patient is directed to complete the test motion before the therapist provides resistance.
- The command, "Hold," to the patient precedes the application of resistance when using the "break test."
- Resistance is applied and released gradually, not quickly. Resistance is usually applied distally to the joint tested, unless otherwise indicated.
- The patient should perform most motions bilaterally simultaneously, except for motions of the hands. Bilateral motion provides the therapist the opportunity to compare one side with the other.
- Palpation is not usually done during a gross muscle test.
- Test positions may vary to allow for patient comfort: Upper limb motions, for example, may be performed with the patient sitting in a wheelchair.
- Adequate stabilization is usually accomplished if the patient resists motions bilaterally. If testing is performed unilaterally, the patient must be stabilized.
- If a recording form does not exist, a summary of results should be entered in the patient's medical record, even if all muscles are found to be within normal limits.

Table 1-1 outlines the evaluation procedures for muscle screening tests.

RANGE-OF-MOTION SCREENING

The purpose of a screening evaluation for range of motion is to determine whether and where a specific goniometric assessment is necessary. The motions are performed actively. The patient should be comfortably positioned and stable; tight or binding clothing should be removed. General considerations for performing any assessment should be followed.

TABLE 1.1 Evaluation Procedures for Muscle Screening Tests

Position of Patient	Muscle Group Tested	Instruction to Patient	Therapist's Actions
Supine	1. Neck and trunk flexors	1. Hold arms straight in front of body. Raise head and shoulders off table. Hold.	1. None
	2. Hip flexors	2. Keep legs straight. Raise both legs off table simultaneously. Hold.	2. None
	3. Hip abductors	3. Abduct legs to each side. Hold.	3. Attempt to bring legs together.
	4. Hip adductors	4. Keep legs together. Hold.	4. Attempt to separate legs.
	5. Hip extensors	5. Flex hips and knees, keeping soles of feet on table. Raise hips from table.	5. None
	6. Shoulder adductors	6. Bring hands together in front of chest, elbows straight. Hold.	6. Attempt to separate arms into horizontal abduction.
	7. Shoulder flexors and scapular upward rotators	7. Flex shoulder to 90 degrees, elbows straight. Hold.	7. Attempt to push arms into extension.
	8. Shoulder extensors and scapular downward rotators	8. Same as 7.	8. Attempt to push arms into flexion.
	9. Shoulder horizontal abductors	9. Same as 7.	9. Attempt to push arms into horizontal adductions.
Supine or sitting	10. Shoulder abductors	10. Abduct shoulder to the side to shoulder level, elbows straight. Hold.	10. Attempt to push arms down to sides into shoulder adduction.
	11. Shoulder adductors	11. Same as 10.	11. Attempt to push arms over head into shoulder abduction.
	12. Shoulder medial rotators	12. Hold arms at sides, elbows bent, forearms in neutral position. Hold.	12. Attempt to push arms outward into lateral rotation.
	13. Shoulder lateral rotators	13. Same as 12.	13. Attempt to push arms in toward body into medial rotation.
	14. Elbow flexors	14. Bend elbows to 90° and hold.	14. Attempt to push forearms toward table into elbow extension.
	15. Elbow extensors	15. Same as 14.	15. Attempt to push forearms toward shoulders into elbow flexion.
	16. Supinators	16. Turn palms up and hold.	16. Attempt to turn palms down into pronation.
	17. Pronators	17. Turn palms down and hold	17. Attempt to turn palms up into supination.
	18. Wrist extensors	18. Bring hand up and hold.	18. Attempt to flex the wrists.
	19. Wrist flexors	19. Bring hand down and hold.	19. Attempt to push palms away from body into wrist extension.
	20. Finger flexors	20. Squeeze my fingers. Hold.	20. Place index and middle fingers in patient's hands; attempt to pull fingers out.
	21. Finger extensors	21. Straighten fingers. Hold.	21. Attempt to push fingers into flexion.
	22. Palmar interossei	22. Adduct fingers. Hold.	22. Attempt to pull fingers into abduction.

continued on page 6

TABLE 1.1 *(Continued)*

Position of Patient	Muscle Group Tested	Instruction to Patient	Therapist's Actions
	23. Dorsal interossei	23. Abduct fingers. Hold.	23. Attempt to push fingers into adduction.
	24. Opponens pollicis	24. Pinch my finger. Hold.	24. Place index finger between patient's thumb and each finger, one at a time.
Sitting	25. Latissimus dorsi and triceps	25. Place hands on treatment table next to hips, elbows straight, shoulders shrugged. Depress scapula by lifting buttocks off table.	25. None
	26. Upper trapezius and levator scapulae	26. Shrug shoulder toward ears. Hold.	26. Push shoulders down into depression.
	27. Medial rotators of the hips and everters of the feet	27. Evert feet. Hold.	27. Push on lateral borders of each foot, into inversion and lateral rotation.
	28. Lateral rotators of the hips and inverters of the feet	28. Invert feet. Hold.	28. Push on medial border of each foot into eversion and medial rotation.
Prone	29. Rhomboids, middle trapezius, and posterior deltoid	29. Bend elbows level with shoulders; pinch or adduct scapulae together, raising arms from table. Hold.	29. Attempt to push arms down.
	30. Elbow and shoulder extensors	30. Begin with arms at sides, elbows straight. Raise arms off table. Hold.	30. Attempt to push arms down.
	31. Extensors of the hips, back, neck, and shoulders	31. Begin with arms at sides. Arch back, raising head, shoulders, arms, and legs off table simultaneously. Hold.	31. None
Prone or sitting	32. Hamstrings	32. Flex knees. Hold.	32. Attempt to pull knees into extension.
	33. Quadriceps	33. Same as 32.	33. Attempt to push knees into further flexion.
Standing	34. Gastrocnemius soleus	34. Stand on one leg. Rest fingers lightly on table. Rise up on tiptoes; repeat 10 times. Repeat with other leg.	34. None
	35. Dorsiflexors	35. Walk on heels for 10 steps.	35. None
	36. Hip and knee extensors	36. Do five partial deep knee bends.	36. None

TABLE 1.2 **Range-of-Motion Screening Test**

Position of Patient	Motion Being Tested	Instructions to Patient
Sitting	1. Shoulder abduction and lateral rotation	1. Reach behind head and touch opposite scapula, or place hands behind neck and push elbows posteriorly.
	2. Shoulder adduction and medial rotation	2. Reach to opposite shoulder or touch the inferior angle or opposite scapula, or place both hands behind back as high as possible.

continued on page 7

TABLE 1.2 *(Continued)*

POSITION OF PATIENT	MOTION BEING TESTED	INSTRUCTIONS TO PATIENT
	3. Shoulder flexion and extension	3. Raise arms in front of body overhead and reverse to behind back.
	4. Elbow flexion and extension	4. Bend and straighten elbows.
	5. Radioulnar supination and pronation	5. With elbows flexed 90 degrees, supinate and pronate.
	6. Wrist flexion and extension	6. Flex and extend wrists.
	7. Radial and ulnar deviation	7. Move wrist laterally and medially.
	8. Finger abduction and adduction	8. Spread fingers apart and bring them together.
	9. Finger flexion and extension	9. Make a tight fist and open fingers wide.
	10. Thumb flexion and extension	10. Bend thumb across the palm and out to the side.
	11. Neck flexion and extension	11. Place chin on chest, tilt head back.
	12. Neck rotation	12. Turn head to the right and left.
	13. Hip flexion and adduction	13. Sitting, cross one thigh over the other.
	14. Hip flexion, abduction, and lateral rotation	14. Uncross thighs and place the lateral side of foot on opposite knee.
	15. Ankle inversion	15. Turn foot in.
	16. Ankle eversion	16. Turn foot out.
Supine	17. Hip abduction and adduction	17. Spread legs apart and bring them together.
Supine or sitting	18. Hip extension	18. Flex hips and knees; lift buttocks as in bridging. Rise to standing from sitting position.
	19. Knee flexion and extension	19. Pull knees to chest, heels toward buttocks, and return.
Standing	20. Trunk flexion	20. Bend forward and reach for toes with knees straight.
	21. Trunk extension	21. Bend backward (the pelvis is stabilized by the therapist).
	22. Trunk lateral bending	22. Lean to the left, then right (the pelvis is stabilized by the therapist).
	23. Trunk rotation	23. Turn to the right and to the left (the pelvis is stabilized by the therapist).
	24. Ankle plantar flexion and toe extension	24. Stand on tiptoes.
	25. Ankle dorsiflexion	25. Stand on heels.

The quick and easy evaluation of a patient's range of motion is also an important component of the entire evaluation process. It gives a quick picture of the patient's willingness to move.

If limitations in joint range of motion are identified, a specific goniometric test should be performed to obtain a detailed account of the restrictions in range of motion. A specific range of motion test is then performed to focus on such factors as position, stabilization, alignment of the goniometer, and recording of the limitations (Table 1-2).

REFERENCES

1. Campbell SK: Measurement and technical skills: Neglected aspect of research education. Phys Ther 61:523, 1981
2. Riddle DL, Rothstein JM, Lamb RL: The reliability of shoulder joint range of motion measurements in a clinical setting. Presented at the annual meeting of the American Physical Therapy Association, Chicago, 1986

2

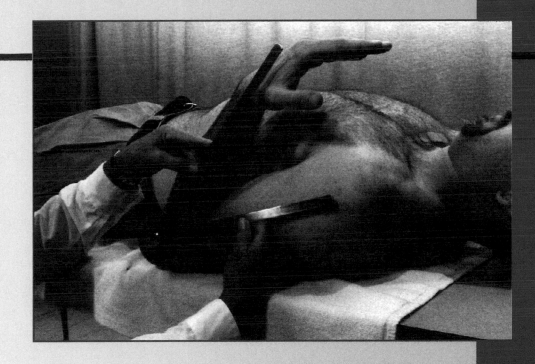

Principles of Examination Techniques

OVERVIEW OF A MUSCULOSKELETAL ASSESSMENT

A thorough and accurate assessment of a subject's musculoskeletal system is essential for correct diagnosis and treatment. It is appropriate to begin an examination by taking a history, followed by a physical assessment. Correct diagnosis and treatment depend on an accurate history, observation during movements, and a thorough assessment of the musculoskeletal system and its related structures.

The main purpose of a history is to gather all information that is pertinent to the problem that brought the subject in for an assessment. The history is geared to the social, economic, and cultural factors that affect the subject. A detailed history of the mechanism for the trauma or insult may be necessary for complex problems. A subject with a localized or single-joint injury may not need an extensive interview to obtain the history. The questions asked must always be easily understood and directed to the subject's level of sophistication. A cardinal principle of interviewing is to permit subjects to express the mechanism of injury in their own words. Listening without interruption is important and requires skill on the part of the examiner. Another important point to remember is to always treat the subject with respect. The subject is usually in pain and needs comforting and has to maintain confidence in the examiner. Even if the diagnosis is obvious, the history will give valuable information about the problem, the prognosis, and the appropriate treatment approach.

History taking is based on open-ended questions asked by the examiner. An open-ended question allows the subject to tell the story spontaneously. Examples of open-ended questions follow:

What kind of problem are you having?
Tell me about the pain in your ankle.
How was your health before your injury?

Following the period of open-ended questions, the interviewer should direct attention to specific facts learned during the open-ended questioning. The direct questions clarify the areas and add detail to the story, as in the following examples:

Where does it hurt?
What movements increase the discomfort?
What does the discomfort feel like?

The answers to these questions will help to establish an organized and thorough assessment of the subject. The use of "SOAP" notes forms the problem-oriented medical record. SOAP is the four-part system for documenting an assessment—S, subjective; O, objective; A, assessment; and P, plan—that is helpful in organizing the medical record for developing a treatment plan. This method of documentation helps the examiner solve a problem.

The format of the history may be subdivided into logical categories, such as the following:

- Chief complaint
- History of the injury
- Past medical history
- Occupation
- Family history
- Psychological history (includes information on education, life experiences, knowledge of injury)

Details in this area of the assessment should be left to qualified personnel if the information obtained goes beyond the physical complaints.

Once the pertinent data have been obtained, the physical assessment of the injury should begin. Symptoms are considered in the classic seven dimensions, which include *body location, quality, quantity, chronology, setting, aggravating (or alleviating) factors,* and *associated manifestations.*[43] The dimensions are considered with each subject who is evaluated. Four cardinal principles of a physical assessment have been identified:

- Inspection and observation
- Palpation
- Percussion
- Auscultation[43]

The examiner should establish a logical, sequential method to ensure that nothing is overlooked during the assessment. The inspection, observation, and palpation are most appropriate for assessment of the musculoskeletal system; however, percussion and auscultation may be used occasionally.

This textbook has been developed to help guide students and clinicians in specific assessment procedures for musculoskeletal disorders. This is a comprehensive text that includes descriptions for assessment of joint range of motion (ROM), muscle length (flexibility), peripheral nervous integrity, muscle strength, joint play, and special orthopedic tests.

Clinical evaluation procedures have been developed to measure the function of joints, muscles, and soft tissues of people who require the services of a therapist. The application of these techniques requires basic knowledge of the human body and well-developed practical skills. An understanding of the evaluation techniques and of the principles of application is required if reliable and valid results are to be obtained. The therapist assesses the results of the measurements and uses them to develop a plan of care.

This chapter is divided into sections dealing with goniometry, muscle length testing, specific manual muscle testing, and peripheral joint assessment. Each section contains information on the purpose, techniques, and recording of measurements and on factors that influence the assessment.

GONIOMETRY

Goniometry is the most commonly used evaluation technique in physical therapy practice.[5] Therapists have used it since the 1920s to assess joint ROM. The range, or amount, of motion a joint can move is a function of joint morphology, capsule, and ligaments and of the muscles or tendons that cross the joint.

Joints are described as having degrees of freedom of movement. If the motion occurs in only one plane and around one axis, the joint is said to have one degree of freedom. A joint that allows movement in two planes and around two axes has two degrees of freedom. A joint that moves in three planes and around three axes has three degrees of freedom—the most that occur in any anatomical joint. Joints are physiologically "designed" to allow more motion at the end of the range as a protective mechanism. The "end feel" provides a passive ROM that is obtained by the examiner at the end of each joint motion. The end feel allows a joint to possess some elasticity to protect the joint in the extreme end range.

Purposes of Joint Range-of-Motion Evaluation

1. To establish the existing ROM available in a joint and to compare it with the normal range for that subject or the noninvolved side. The information will permit a therapist to establish a database for the subject. This information is used to develop goals and a treatment plan to increase or decrease the ROM.
2. To aid in diagnosing and determining the subject's joint function. Goniometry reveals joint limitations in the arc of motion but does not identify the dysfunction. It does, however, provide information regarding limitations if joint disease is suspected.

    Hypomobility or hypermobility of joints affects a subject's function in activities of daily living. Hypermobility—laxity in the joint or structures surrounding the joint—allows motion to exceed the normal range. Hypomobility is joint tightness or a less than normal ROM. An example of joint hypomobility interfering with a person's daily living activities would be

an inability to perform stair climbing because of an inability to flex the knee joint to 70 to 80 degrees of flexion.
3. To reassess the subject's status after treatment and compare it with that at the time of the initial evaluation. Goniometric measurements are used to evaluate the effectiveness of treatment programs. If the ROM is not increasing, the treatment program may need to be changed to obtain effective clinical results.
4. To develop the subject's interest in and motivation and enthusiasm for the treatment program. Most subjects are aware of changes in joint motion and usually are motivated by these improvements to participate in the treatment.
5. To document results from treatment regimens for medicolegal reasons and to communicate with other medical personnel, third-party payers, and workmen's compensation companies.
6. To participate in vital research to improve function. Research has contributed, for example, to the design of chairs and desks and placement of pedals in cars that are ergonomically ideal for the average driver.

Several factors that influence ROM must be considered to ensure that goniometry is an objective assessment.

Reliability of Joint Angle Measurements. Reliability of measurement of joint angles refers to the degree of consistency between goniometric measurements. An article by Stratford discusses the various methodologies used to establish the reliability of joint measurements.[41] Measurement of joint angles is one of the most common assessments performed by therapists, and the measurements are the basis for decisions regarding treatment. The following table, developed by Stratford, summarizes the design, reliability coefficients, and conclusions for five reliability goniometric studies. There is general agreement that intratester variations are usually smaller than intertester variations and that measurement error may differ for different joints.[5,18,28] (Table 2-1).

Reliability studies have been performed since the 1940s. It may be difficult to compare many of the studies because of different research designs and instrumentation. The universal goniometer as the measurement tool of choice for the joints of the limbs has generally been found to have good to excellent reliability. ROM measurements for the upper limbs have been found to be slightly more reliable than the studies with the lower limbs.[5,35] Studies using the universal goniometer to measure trunk ROM report low reliability.[12,46,51] Many devices and techniques

TABLE 2.1 Five Reliability Studies on Goniometry Compared and Contrasted

INVESTIGATOR	DESIGN	RELIABILITY COEFFICIENT	CONCLUSIONS
Hellebrandt, Duvall, Moore (1949)	"Gold standard" observer versus eight others All measured 30 patients Estimates of intraobserver and interobserver error "Same" angle	Comparison of mean values	Well-trained observer can measure with a high degree of accuracy. Different observers (therapists) should not be used interchangeably among cases unless their reliability has been established. Some evidence to suggest that the reliability may vary for different joints and different movements within the same joint.
Baldwin & Cunningham (1974)	Five groups: one "gold standard" observer per group Five normal ranges—5 restricted ranges Estimates of interobserver error "Same" angle within groups Estimated and measured joint angle	Mean error Paired t-test	A wide range of error existed (up to 50 degrees). In subjects with normal range, observer estimates were more accurate than goniometric measurement. In the restricted range group, the opposite was true.
Low (1976)	One normal subject 50 observers all measured "same" angle Five observers made 10 repeat measures each Estimated both intra-observer and interobserver error	Mean Standard deviation Mean error	Reliability can be enhanced when all observers use the same measurement strategy and several measurements are taken. Intraobserver error is less than interobserver error. Error estimates may differ for different joints.
Boone et al (1978)	Six normal subjects Four observers measured all subjects 3 times each session Four sessions Estimates of intraobserver and interobserver error "Same" angle	Standard deviation % variation due to observer Reliability coefficient (Product moment?)	Intraobserver error is less than interobserver error. One measurement per session is as reliable as the average of several measurements. When more than one observer is responsible for evaluating a patient, changes of 5 degrees for the upper limb and 6 degrees for the lower limb should be taken into account prior to declaration of improvement.
Ekstrand (1982)	22 normal subjects One pair of observers Estimates of intra-assay and interassay error "Same" angle	Standard deviation Coefficient of variation	Range-of-motion measurements can be reproduced accurately by the same observer. Intra-assay error is less than interassay error.

have been developed to improve trunk measurements. In the study by Southwick and associates, which used a plurimeter (gravity-activated angle finder) as the assessment tool, clinical measurements of lumbar lordosis were highly reliable if taken by the same examiner.[42]

Many goniometric studies have found intratester reliability to be higher than intertester reliability.[5,16,17,18,28,35,46] A few have found that intertester is higher than intratester reliability.[2,6,11] Many studies have compared the reliability of different types of measuring devices used to assess ROM. Devices compared in the studies were the pendulum goniometer, gravity-activated devices (inclometer, plurimeter), tape measures, and the universal goniometer. Many of the studies found no difference in reliability, and others reported poor reliability.[6,10,11,15–18,27,30,37–40,46,47,49,51] To have the most reliable goniometric measurement, the examiner should use consistent test positions and anatomical landmarks with which to align the arms and axis of the goniometer. The same manual force should be applied to the joint when passive ROM is used to determine the end feel of each joint. Using the same measuring device when repeating measurements will aid in reliability of measurement. Examiners with little experience may choose to take several measurements and record the mean of the measurements. It is advisable to use the same examiner for repeat measurement rather than a different examiner for higher reliability of measurement.

Although Moore and associates showed that experienced therapists were reliable in taking goniometric measurements,[31] there is still some concern about the clinical reliability of goniometry. Miller states, "Although the inferences that can be made from measuring joint motion are limited (validity), the measurement itself is invaluable as a basic indicator of patient status."[5]

When measuring, the therapist must try to rule out as many of the factors as possible that decrease reliability. Some of these factors that will improve reliability include removal of tight and restrictive clothing, duplications of positions used, and measuring at the same time of day.

Validity of Joint Measurements. Rothstein defines validity as "evidence that a test measures what it is supposed to measure." Does the goniometer accurately measure the angle of a joint between the two body segments that form the angle? Studies have been performed comparing radiographs and goniometric measurements.[40] A valid goniometric measurement is a measurement that truly represents the joint position or the joint ROM. A study by Gogia and colleagues[40] measured knee joints on 30 subjects at various angles and compared the goniometric results with radiographs. There was a high correlation between the two types of measurements. Another study by Ahlbach and Lindahl[40] found close agreement with radiographs compared with goniometric measurements of hip joint flexion and extension movements.

The goniometer is considered to be the "gold standard" by which other tools of joint measurements are compared.

Age. Generally, the younger the subject, the greater the ROM. Bell and Hoshizak found that there was a decline in ROM in most subjects between age 20 and 30 years, followed by a plateau until the age of 60 years, after which a decline again occurred.[4]

Gender. Many studies have been performed to determine the difference in ROM between men and women. Overall, it has been found that women tend to have greater ranges than men, but not all studies confirm that finding.[4] During pregnancy, women may have an increase in ROM due to hormonal changes.

Occupation or Pattern of Activity. Occupation or activity patterns may cause more or less ROM (ie, gymnasts display an increased ROM in the hips and lower trunk, weight lifters or boxers generally have a decreased ROM in their trunk).

Joint Structures. Some people, because of genetics or posture, normally have hypermobile or hypomobile joints. Body type can influence joint mobility, as can flexibility of the tendons and ligaments crossing the joint.

Joints are structured so that motion is limited by the capsule, ligaments, and tendons or by the bony configuration. Some motions are limited by soft-tissue bulk of the segments and not by a limitation associated with the joint. For instance, elbow flexion is usually limited by the muscle bulk of the arm against the forearm.

Soft tissues, such as ligaments, tendons, and capsules, are dense, regular connective tissues with inherent elastic properties; they may become tight or loose and affect the motion available at joints. Muscles associated with the joints may become stretched or contracted, thereby affecting the joint motion. The shape of the joint surfaces is designed to allow motion in particular directions. These surfaces may be altered by such factors as posture, disease, or trauma to allow more or less motion than normal at a joint.

Normally, each joint has a small amount of motion at the end of the range that is not under voluntary control. These accessory motions are not assessed during active range evaluation but are included under the realm of passive measurement. Accessory motions help protect the joint structures by absorbing extrinsic forces.

Examiners performing goniometric measurements should consider the end feel of each joint when determining passive ROM. The structure or structures that limit the ROM at a joint have a characteristic feel at the end of the motion. The feel is a subjective measurement of the resistance encountered at the end of the ROM and is part of the ROM evaluation.[32] A description of end feel is found on page 34.

Dominance. Most researchers have found that there is essentially no difference for corresponding joints between the left and right sides of the body.[31]

Comparative goniometry is done when a joint is involved unilaterally; the contralateral limb can then be used as the standard for normal ROM for that subject.

Type of Motion. Active ROM testing provides limited information regarding joint motion. Assuming that the subject has complete passive motion, an inability to move the segment actively completely through the motion must be attributed to muscle weakness. Active range grossly evaluates coordination of movement and functional ability and provides information about muscle strength.

Passive ROM is usually evaluated in goniometry and is the amount of motion possible when the examiner moves a body part with no assistance from the subject. It is usually greater than active ROM because the integrity of the soft tissue structures may in themselves dictate the limits of movement. A passive ROM test gives the examiner information about the integrity of the joint but provides no information about the capabilities of the contractile tissues, muscles.

Norkin and White state, "Comparisons between the passive and active ranges of motion provide information about the amount of motion permitted by the joint structure relative to the person's ability to produce motion at a joint."[32] A comparison may be an advantage in developing a subject's treatment plan or aiding in a diagnosis.

Instruments

The instruments practitioners use for measuring joint ROM are called goniometers, or arthrometers. The tools, although varying in size, shape, and appearance, all possess the capabilities to provide specific information regarding joint motion. The widely used universal goniometer is durable, washable, and can be applied to almost all joints.

The goniometer is basically a protractor with two long arms. One arm is considered movable and the other stationary, and both are attached to the body of the protractor by a rivet or tension knob (Fig. 2-1).

A variety of goniometers have been developed to conform to specific joints. There are goniometers with short arms for short anatomical segments, such as the digits. Such tools can be made easily by cutting down the arms of a plastic goniometer to about 1 in (Fig. 2-2). The arms on finger goniometers are placed on the dorsal or ventral aspect of the joint being measured rather than on the lateral aspect of the joints (lateral placement is standard procedure for sagittal plane motions and anterior-posterior for frontal plane).

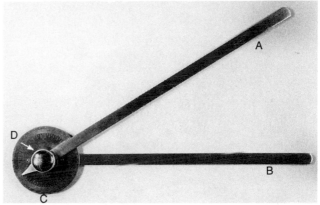

▲ **Figure 2.1** A metal goniometer showing a moving arm (**A**), stationary arm (**B**), body, or protractor (**C**), and axis (**D**).

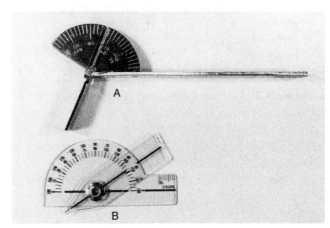

▲ **Figure 2.2** Two goniometers designed for measuring digits. (**A**) The first is constructed of metal and is placed on the dorsal or ventral surface for measurement at the joint. (**B**) The other is constructed of plastic, and the stationary and moving arms have been shortened to conform easily to the digits. They may be placed on the lateral, ventral, or dorsal side of the digits.

Another type of goniometer, which works like a carpenter's level, relies on the effects of gravity. The gravity-activated or fluid (bubble) goniometer has a 360-degree scale (Fig. 2-3).

Another type is designed with a needle or pointer instead of being fluid filled (Fig. 2-4). The device is strapped to or held firmly on the limb segment. This type of device is easy and quick to use because it is not aligned with bony landmarks; however, reliability suffers as a result of a lack of landmark orientation.[15] In many instances, the armless goniometer is better than the universal (two-armed) goniometer because it does not have to conform to body segments. It is particularly useful for measuring joint rotation and axioskeletal motion.

In 1959, the electric goniometer was developed by Karpovich and Karpovich.[22] This device is attached to an electromyograph machine. The two arms of the goniometer are attached to a potentiometer and are

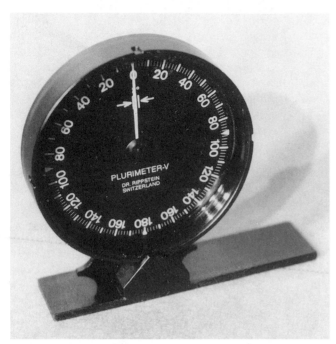

▲ **Figure 2.3** Fluid goniometer, which is activated by the effects of gravity.

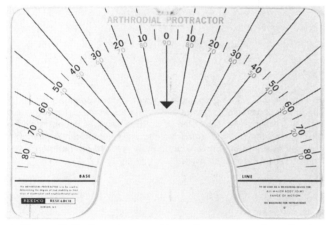

▲ **Figure 2.4** A goniometer without alignment arms has a level on the straight edge to indicate that the protractor is level.

strapped to the proximal and distal body segments. Movement from arms of the device causes resistance in the potentiometer, which measures dynamic joint motion. Aligning the arms of the electrogoniometer is difficult and time consuming.

Clinically, the most commonly used instrument is the universal goniometer, which has not changed in design in over 30 years. One type of instrument is the transparent plastic goniometer, which was developed by Wainerdi in 1952 to allow greater accuracy of alignment with the body segments.[46] A line on the goniometer along the stationary and moving arms facilitates alignment with body parts. Other

universal goniometers are constructed of light-weight metals.

The goniometer's protractor has a full or a half circle. It is marked in increments of 1, 2, or 5 degrees. The degrees on the protractor are usually numbered in both directions from 0 to 180 degrees and 180 to 0 degrees. Full-circle protractors indicate 360 degrees in both directions. The half-circle goniometer has an advantage over the full-circle type in that it can be applied easily to joints when the subject is supine or prone.

The stationary arm of the goniometer is aligned with the fixed body segment, and the moving arm, with the moving body segment. When a half-circle goniometer is used, the two arms are interchangeable.

The rivet or fulcrum of the goniometer should be free to move without being too loose. Some metal goniometers are equipped with a knob to adjust the tension of the arms.

Large goniometers have 12- to 16-in arms for use on the large joints of the body with long limb segments. Intermediate sizes developed primarily for the wrists and ankles have arms approximately 6 to 8 in long. The intermediate-size goniometer is convenient because it fits easily into a pocket and can be used for most joint measurements. The fingers and toes are usually measured with a special goniometer or one whose arms have been shortened to ½ to 1 in.[53]

Other devices, such as tape measures and rulers, may be used to assess trunk and scapular mobility. The tape should be made from a durable fabric that withstands washing and does not stretch.

X-rays may be made of joints, which then are measured with a ruler or goniometer. Tracings can be taken of motions to compare initial measurements with subsequent ones. Tracings are used most commonly with the fingers: the shape of each finger is drawn on a piece of paper (Fig. 2-5). Motion analysis with videotaping can be used. Markers are placed over bony landmarks, and the motion can be analyzed by computer programs.

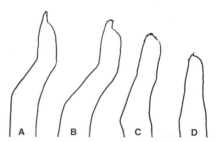

▲ **Figure 2.5** A starting position tracing for the (**A**) index, (**B**) middle, (**C**) ring, and (**D**) little fingers.

General Principles for Measuring Joint Range of Motion

Passive Range. Passive ROM measurement is used whenever possible to assess the extent of structural limitation to the available joint ROM.

The therapist estimates available ROM before actually placing the goniometer. Having a mental idea of the starting or ending ROM helps the therapist minimize faulty readings from the instrument.

Starting Position. The anatomical position of 0 degrees is the starting position for all measurements except rotation at the shoulder and hip and pronation/supination of the radioulnar joints. These exceptions are explained under the specific test motions (see Chaps. 5, 6, and 12). In the starting position (preferred position), it is easy to isolate the movement, place the goniometer, stabilize the subject, and see the motions being performed. Tension in the muscles passing over adjacent joints and in the soft tissues surrounding the joint is lessened or eliminated. For example, the measurement of knee flexion is performed with the hip flexed to eliminate tension in the rectus femoris muscle.

The end of the range is assisted by the weight of the limb, so the effects of movement against gravity are minimal. The subject usually lies supine on a firm, comfortable surface. The examiner should be comfortable and in a position to read the goniometer at eye level to avoid errors in visual perception (Fig. 2-6). The sitting position is also used, which provides for proper stabilization and accessibility for the subject and examiner.

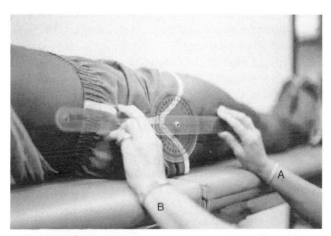

▲ **Figure 2.6** The examiner reads the goniometer from the same horizontal level as the protractor. Hip extension is measured with the axis aligned with the greater trochanter, **(A)** the moving arm aligned with the midline of the femur in line with the lateral femoral epicondyle, and **(B)** the stationary arm aligned with the midline of the trunk.

Alignment. For most sagittal plane measurements, the goniometer is aligned on the lateral side of the test joint. This placement enables the examiner to see the protractor and to align the goniometer arms properly with the bony landmarks of the body. Frontal plane motions are usually measured either anteriorly or posteriorly. The alignment should be convenient for both the subject and the examiner.

Axis. The axis of the goniometer is the intersection of the two arms and should coincide with the axis of the joint being tested. The axis of the joint will shift during the motion; therefore, it is important to adjust the axes of the goniometer accordingly.

If the moving arm is placed parallel to the long axis of the moving body segment and the stationary arm is parallel to the long axis of the fixed segment of the joint, then the axis of motion will fall where the two intersect.

Moving Arm. The moving arm of the goniometer is aligned parallel and lateral to the long axis of the moving body segment. The therapist palpates the specific bony landmarks before aligning the moving arm of the goniometer. The moving segment of the body along which the moving arm is aligned is the segment distal to the test joint. The proximal portion of the movable arm near the fulcrum is either pointed, has a line through to the end, or is notched to enable the examiner to read the goniometer with ease.

Stationary Arm. The stationary arm of the goniometer is aligned parallel and lateral to the long axis of the fixed body segment. As with the moving arm, the therapist palpates the specific landmarks before aligning the stationary arm. The fixed segment is the proximal body segment and does not change position during the testing.

NUMERICAL EXPRESSION OF JOINT RANGE OF MOTION

Most therapists use a system of measurement based on 0 to 180 degrees that was proposed in 1923 by Silver and is the method of the American Academy of Orthopedic Surgeons.[44] The subject is placed in the starting, or anatomical, position that represents the 0 position on the measuring device (rotation and forearm measurements are an exception). The arc of motion produced by the subject and the goniometer is based on 180 degrees. For instance, the starting position for measuring the elbow joint ROM is 0 degrees of elbow extension. The elbow joint is then passively flexed through an arc of motion, followed by the goniometric arc of motion, through approximately a normal range of 145 degrees. As the joint

TABLE 2.2	**Hip Range of Motion Represented by Three Different Notation Systems**		
	0–180	180–0	360
Flexion	0–125	180–55	0–55
Extension	0–15	180–165	0–195
Abduction	0–45	180–45	0–135
Adduction	0–45	180–15	0–195
Internal rotation	0–45	180–135	0–45
External rotation	0–45	180–135	0–45

(Using "normal" values taken from Gerhardt JJ, Russe OA: International SFTR Method of Measuring and Recording Joint Motion. Bern, Huber, 1975. From Rothstein JM: Measurement in Physical Therapy, p. 118. New York, Churchill Livingstone, 1985)

increases in motion, the numbers on the goniometer scale increase and are positive.

Other methods of expressing ROM have been developed, but they are not widely used because they are more difficult to interpret than the 0-to-180-degree method. Another method of measuring ROM is based on a 360-degree arc to test motions of extension or adduction that go beyond the anatomical position. This method is also useful for measurements that are performed from a starting position of 180 degrees. The numerical values of abduction and flexion motions would decrease toward 0 degrees (Table 2-2).

RECORDING MEASUREMENTS

Examples of recording forms appear in Appendix A.

The methods of recording ROM have ranged from tables, charts, and graphs to tracings. The most common recording method is based on a 0-to-180-degree scale. The starting and ending ranges of each motion are identified separately. The goniometer is aligned in the starting position or anatomical position at 0 degrees, except for rotation and ankle movements, in which cases the moving arm starts at 90 degrees.

A calculation must be done for motions in which the goniometer placement begins at 90 degrees to attain the starting and ending degrees to record the appropriate ROM. For instance, to examine ankle dorsiflexion, the goniometer is aligned at 90 degrees in the preferred position and recorded as 0 degrees. Following the dorsiflexion motion, the arc produced by the goniometer may show 100 degrees. It is recorded as 10 degrees of ankle dorsiflexion motion. If a subject lacks motion and is unable to assume the starting position, the goniometer is aligned as close to 0 degrees as possible.

For accuracy in measuring and recording limitation of joint motion, the therapist must be sure to use the preferred position or an alternate position and specific placement of the goniometer. Use of an alternate position is noted by an asterisk in the recording space, and reasons for use of the alternate position are explained in the Remarks column. If neither the preferred nor an alternate position is used, the position and the reason for that choice of position are described in the Remarks column. Any deviation from the key, such as use of active range, presence of pain, or other limiting factors, should be also noted and explained in the Remarks column.

The goniometer is aligned, and readings are made at the beginning and at the completion of each movement. The goniometer is removed from the subject during the motion and realigned at the completion of the motion. If the examiner is interested in the end of the ROM, only that measurement needs to be taken. It would be assumed that the starting point was zero. The number of degrees of motion away from zero is recorded. If limited range prevents the subject from starting the motion at the preferred position, the amount of limitation is measured and recorded in degrees.

The range and date are recorded, and the therapist initials the test form.

Whenever possible, the subject's normal range is determined by measuring the uninvolved limb.

PROCEDURE FOR MEASUREMENT

Using the proper sequence and techniques for goniometry ensures reliability, validity, and objectivity:

1. Place the subject in correct body alignment, which should correspond as nearly as possible to the anatomical position. Rotations at the shoulder and hip joints and forearm motion are exceptions. The segment to be examined should be exposed and unrestricted in the "preferred position."
2. Explain and demonstrate the desired motion to the subject.
3. Perform the motion passively two or three times to eliminate substitutions and tightness due to inactivity.
4. Stabilize the proximal body segment.
5. Locate the approximate center of motion (axis) actively or passively by palpating the appropriate bony landmark on the lateral aspect of the joint.
6. Place the stationary arm of the goniometer parallel to the longitudinal axis of the midline of the fixed segment in line with the designated bony landmark.
7. Place the movable arm parallel to the longitudinal axis of the moving segment, in line with the designated bony landmark.

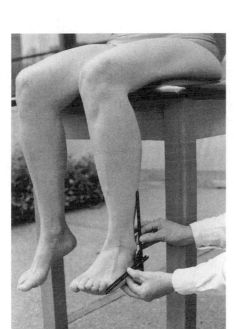

▲ **Figure 2.7** The arms of the goniometer are placed at a 90-degree angle, indicating the starting position for ankle dorsiflexion measurements.

8. Determine the axis of motion by the intersection of the midline of the two segments. Hold the goniometer between your fingers and thumb. Place it loosely against the subject so as not to compress soft tissues, possibly resulting in an erroneous reading or limitation of the ROM. If you are unable to hold the goniometer steady, rest your forearms against the treatment table.

9. Align the goniometer, and take readings at the beginning and at the completion of each movement. Remove the goniometer from the subject during the motion, and realign it at the end of the motion. If you are interested only in the end ROM, then the starting measurement need not be taken. It would be assumed that the starting point is 0 degrees (Fig. 2-7). Record the number of degrees of motion away from zero. If limitation in the range prevents the subject from starting the motion at the preferred position, measure the amount of limitation and record it in degrees.

PRINCIPLES OF MUSCLE LENGTH TESTING

Muscles cross joints and effect the action that occurs at those joints. Muscles have an important role in supporting and moving the skeletal structures. A muscle must be short enough to provide stability of a joint and long enough to allow normal mobility. If muscle tightness limits ROM, then elongation or stretching must be achieved. If the muscles are too long and the joint is hypermobile, demonstrating excessive ROM, allowing a muscle to shorten would be a treatment of choice.

The purpose of assessment of muscle length (flexibility) is to determine whether the ROM occurring at a joint is limited or excessive by the intrinsic joint structures or by the muscles crossing the joint. One example of this situation is ankle dorsiflexion. When the knee joint is extended, the gastrocnemius muscle is stretched or "tight," which may lead to a limitation in dorsiflexion, compared with the situation in which the knee joint is flexed. The stretch is off the gastrocnemius muscle with knee joint flexion allowing a greater ROM in dorsiflexion. Muscle length is determined by the distance between the proximal and distal ends of the muscle and is measured by its effect on the joint's ROM.

Joint ROM is the number of degrees of motion allowed by the joint with minimal influence from any muscles crossing the joint surfaces. Specific details on joint ROM have been discussed previously in this chapter under the topic of goniometry. Muscle length also is expressed in degrees that a joint is permitted to move when a muscle crossing the joint has influenced the movement.

One classification of muscles is by the number of joints over which the muscle passes. Muscles may be identified as one-joint muscles, those that cross only one joint; two-joint muscles, those that cross two different joints; and multijoint muscles, those that cross more than two joints. Muscles that cross more than one joint generally are more efficient than one-joint muscles. They produce motions at more than one joint. The two-joint and multijoint muscles are also more susceptible to the loss of tension or may develop active insufficiency. Muscles that cross more than one joint are more efficient because they can maintain torque while the muscle is performing a contraction. If both ends of the muscle shorten at the same time, the muscle loses torque and will develop active insufficiency. Active insufficiency is the inability of a muscle to produce or maintain active tension while the muscle is shortening during contraction. Active insufficiency produces a weak contractile force when both muscle attachments are coming closer together. Other muscles associated with the joint will help prevent active insufficiency by ensuring that two joint muscles maintain their optimal length. Usually, two-joint or multijoint muscles are able to function most effectively when they are shortened over one joint and lengthened over the other joint. Physiologically, two-joint or multijoint muscles can retain a favorable length through a larger ROM with the length of shortening being less.[25] An example would be the hamstring muscles that cross the hip and knee joints posteriorly. If both hip joint extension and knee joint flexion occur simultaneously, the muscle loses torque (power) and is not effective at either joint. The two-joint or multijoint muscles can also be stretched over more than one joint at the same time and may exert tension without shortening.

When muscles are elongated or stretched over two or more joints, passive insufficiency may develop. Passive insufficiency occurs when an inactive antagonist muscle is of insufficient length to allow a full ROM at the joints crossed.[25] Using the hamstring muscle example, when the hip joint is flexed and the knee joint is extended (straight leg raise), the hamstring muscles become tight or less extensible crossing the hip and knee joints. The human body is well designed in that muscles contract within a functional ROM to maintain an appropriate length-tension relationship. One-joint muscles are rarely passively insufficient. Two or more joint muscles are often of insufficient length or flexibility to permit a full ROM at the joints they cross. When maximum passive flexibility has been reached, these muscles become passively insufficient and passive tension develops. This tension is often acknowledged by a painful sensation in the area of the muscle being passively elongated. Muscles that pass over one joint demonstrate that the range of joint motion and the range of muscle length are identical. The ranges may be limited, normal, or excessive. Muscles that cross over more than one joint demonstrate often that the range at the joint will be less that the total ROM of the joint due to tightness of the muscle.

When assessing range of joint motion in which muscles cross more than one joint, one end of the muscle should remain in a slack position. This position will allow the degrees of motion at a joint to be truly an assessment of the joint and associated structures and not the length of the muscle crossing that joint. The hamstring example shows that when assessing hip flexion, the knee joint must be flexed to assess only the motion at the hip joint. If the knee joint is extended, then the degrees of motion for hip flexion would be determined by the length of the hamstring muscles and not a true measurement of hip joint flexion but the muscle length under tension crossing the hip joint posteriorly.

Hypermobility at a joint is demonstrated when the joint has excessive ROM beyond a functional length. Excessive ROM at a joint usually will not be a stable joint. Both excessive elongation of muscle, looseness of joint capsular structures, and laxity of supporting ligaments are evident in hypermobility at a joint. Excessive muscle length would be deter-

mined only when a muscle is placed in its lengthened position, elongated over each joint it crosses.

The more knowledge one may gather during an assessment of a subject, the more accurate and successful will be the treatment plan. Identification of a limitation or hypermobility of the joint resulting from muscular problems rather than bony or capsular problems would influence the treatment goals and success. The test position for assessment of muscle length is also a position for increasing the length or stretching the muscles. A faulty posture may be one cause for a decrease in muscle length. Correction of the posture may be sufficient to gain appropriate muscle length.[23]

Principles of Muscle Length

1. Range of muscle length is usually expressed in degrees of motion across a joint and is usually measured by using a goniometer, ruler, or an instrument such as a plurimeter. The assessment technique is based on the principles of goniometric measurements.
2. One-joint muscles usually do not limit joint ROM due to their ability to have sufficient flexibility to allow full ROM across a joint.
3. Two-joint or multijoint muscles may not have sufficient flexibility to allow full ROM, and the muscle develops passive insufficiency.
4. When a muscle that spans two or more joints is elongated over one joint and slack over the other joint, then full joint ROM can be achieved.
5. Muscle length assessment is performed when a muscle is passively elongated over its joints. The result is usually limitation of joint ROM but may show hypermobility.
6. Age is a factor to be considered in muscle length. According to Florence Kendall, flexibility decreases as one ages.[23] Children younger than 3 years have extreme flexibility; they can touch their forehead to their toes. Gradually as the lower limbs become proportionately longer in relation to the trunk, limitations in muscle flexibility become apparent. A 6-year-old may be able to touch the fingers to the toes, a teenager or an adult may not be able to touch the toes because of limitations in muscle length.

PRINCIPLES OF MANUAL MUSCLE TESTING

Manual muscle testing (MMT) is one method by which muscle strength is defined and measured.[24] A manual muscle test is an attempt to determine the subject's ability to contract a muscle or muscle group voluntarily. Standard manual muscle tests as a measurement of strength are not suitable for people who cannot actively or voluntarily control the tension developed in their muscles. As a result, patients with disorders of the central nervous system who demonstrate spasticity are not appropriate candidates for muscle testing. Also, factors that activate the stretch reflex, such as gravity or manual resistance, will produce an inaccurate assessment of a patient's voluntary control of muscle activity. MMT is not as reliable, valid, and objective as other physical therapy testing procedures.

For MMT, reliability means that the test can be repeated by any examiner with results that vary by no more than one half of a grade. The measurement technique for determining strength of muscles is subjective, particularly in the area of manual resistance, and requires refinement. A half-grade intertester difference is acceptable. If the test is repeated by several therapists and the same grades are obtained, then the muscle test is said to be reliable. The key to reliable MMT is to follow the procedures that have been developed and used for the past 70 years. Reliability is increased by giving clear instructions to the subject. The therapist may help the subject understand the procedure by passively moving the joints through the motions, testing the opposite side, and demonstrating and explaining the movement.

Frese, Brown, and Norton tested intertester reliability by having 11 physical therapists test the middle trapezius and gluteus medius bilaterally on 100 subjects.[13] They found that practitioners are reliable within one muscle testing grade of each other. They also found poor intertester reliability in grades below "fair," a finding that agrees with Beasley's findings of poor differentiation in grades below "fair."[3] Another study performed by Williams in the mid-1950s found that two examiners agreed on the muscle testing grade 60% to 75% of the time.[48]

Few reliability studies have been performed to establish the reliability of MMT as an assessment tool. There have been some genuine concerns about the reliability of muscle testing results, particularly for the grades of "good minus" to "normal." There seems to be better discrimination between the grades from "zero" to "fair plus." Can the grades be reproduced on subjects? Is there true intratester and intertester reliability for MMT? A few reliability studies were performed during the poliomyelitis era.[9,50,52] The studies were based on establishing muscle strength grades. The overall results demonstrated that approximately 50% of time, there was complete agreement, 66% of the time they agreed within a plus or minus of a grade, and 90% of the time they agreed

within one full grade.[19] The agreement among examiners for manual muscle strength exact grades is relatively low.

A standardized method of MMT is needed so that comparable results can be obtained by different examiners. The resistance given for muscle testing grades of "fair plus" and above is subjective and needs standardization. The hand-held dynamometer developed by Smidt shows some potential for establishing reliability among therapists.[33]

Muscle strength testing should be a valid procedure—it must test the specific muscles that it purports to test. Validity can best be maintained by palpating each muscle, stabilizing the proximal segment, and preventing substitution of muscles or patterns.

Lamb states the following:

Manual muscle testing is hypothesized as a valuable tool for the clinical assessment of patients with neuromuscular problems. Information relevant to its reliability is sparse. More research must be done in today's clinical environment using appropriate research design. MMT appears to have content validity, however, there is no published evidence that gives credence to the degree to which an examiner can generalize the results of MMT to immediate and future behavior of patients.[24]

According to Payton, MMT has face and content validity.[35] Both face and content validity are based on the anatomical and physiological knowledge the examiner has about each muscle. The test of strength does not consider all the types of muscle contraction; rate of tension produced, however, does measure the torque produced by individual muscles.[24] Can the results be generalized to functional ability? A functional muscle test does not exist that has been validated and shown to be reliable. More clinical studies need to be performed to validate the use of MMT.

Presently, specific muscle testing is used in a clinical setting to develop a program to increase strength for weakness detected in skeletal muscle. Other uses of muscle testing may aid in planning for surgery to transfer a strong muscle to an area of prolonged weakness or to determine if a patient may require an assistive device.

Objectivity means reporting the facts without distortion by personal opinion or bias. Following the standardized procedure and giving clear instructions help to make a muscle test objective. The most difficult variable to gauge objectively in muscle testing is the resistance the patient can take: Is it minimal, moderate, or maximal?

The muscle test based on gravitational effects was developed by Dr. Robert Lovett, professor of orthopedic surgery at Harvard Medical School.[13] He developed this method of measuring specific muscle strength because of his involvement in the treatment of patients with poliomyelitis. In the 1940s and 1950s, during the poliomyelitis epidemic in the United States, physical therapists developed skill in evaluating manual muscle strength. MMT continues to be useful for assessing muscle integrity for peripheral nerve lesions or musculoskeletal disorders. Even though the types of patients treated by physical therapists have changed over the past 30 years, the techniques developed continue to be useful for assessing strength of voluntary muscle contractions.

Manual muscle strength testing is usually performed by clinicians in a qualitative rather than a quantitative manner. The MMT method in use clinically is not sensitive enough to reveal and quantify subtle deficiencies in strength.

Uses of Manual Muscle Testing

1. To establish a basis for muscle reeducation and exercise. The therapist uses the data to develop a plan of care and to determine the patient's progress. Because it shows the effectiveness of the treatment, it evaluates the treatment program. MMT provides additional information before muscle transfer surgery. A muscle's strength should be rated "good" or grade 4 before it is transferred because its strength will decrease one grade increment after the transfer.
2. To determine how functional a patient can be.
3. To determine a patient's needs for supportive apparatus, such as orthoses, splints, and assistive devices for ambulation.
4. To help determine a diagnosis. Some diseases affect only certain muscle groups. Peripheral nerve or nerve root lesions may affect all muscles served by that nerve or the cutaneous distribution. For example, muscular dystrophies and myopathies affect proximal muscle groups, and ulnar nerve lesions affect the intrinsic muscles of the hand.
5. To determine a patient's prognosis. A plateau in the progression of strength attained by the patient during treatment will be indicative of that patient's maximal level of function.

Factors That Contribute to the Effectiveness of Muscle Contraction

Muscle strength testing involves anatomical, physiological, and mechanical factors that influence muscle contractions.

The length of a muscle at the time of activation markedly affects the tension developed in that muscle. How much tension a muscle produces depends on its length in contraction. For some muscles, the lengthened position is more favorable than the shortened position. Each muscle has its own optimal length to produce its optimal tension. Skeletal muscles cross and affect one joint, two joints, or multiple joints in the body. One-joint muscles act only at one joint and can be shortened or lengthened over one joint. Muscles that cross two or more joints can act on each joint. The muscle can be stretched at one joint while shortening at another. Two-joint and multijoint muscles functionally can be more efficient torque producers than one-joint muscles. The multijoint type of muscle has an advantage over one-joint muscles in that they can maintain a constant tension while an active concentric contraction occurs. The advantage is due to the ability of the muscle to maintain an optimal length at one joint while it shortens over another. Refer to the previous section on muscle length for more details.

As a one-joint muscle shortens or as the distal and proximal attachments of a two-joint muscle approach each other during a concentric contraction, the tension diminishes, and the muscle may become actively insufficient. The patient may complain of pain and cramping in the tested muscle if it is in an actively insufficient position.

Physiologically, a muscle is capable of generating its greatest tension during an eccentric contraction. A muscle will generate less tension isometrically and even less when contracting concentrically.[3] Maximum isometric strength at any joint angle is always greater than the strength of a dynamic concentric contraction at the same angle. Maximum strength at a given joint angle is greatest when the muscle is lengthening eccentrically (as it attempts to overcome too great a load) than when it is contracting concentrically or isometrically.[3]

Skeletal muscles are composed of individual muscle fiber types that react differently to an action potential. Muscles classified as type I have a predominance of slow-twitch muscle fibers, which increase and decrease their tension slowly and are considered fatigue resistant. Muscles classified as type II have a predominance of fast-twitch muscle fibers, which increase and decrease their tension rapidly and fatigue quickly. All skeletal muscles have a mixture of both fiber types. Clinically, the speed of contraction and the resistance applied during the evaluation of strength must be considered. Much less resistance must be applied to muscles with a predominance of type II fibers to obtain a "normal" grade than to those that are predominantly type I fibers. An example that demonstrates a remarkable difference in natural strength is the amount of resistance applied to the sternocleidomastoid muscle, a type II muscle. The resistance used is much less than that applied to the soleus muscle (type I), yet the identical strength grade is obtained. The speed of muscle contraction is an important consideration when evaluating muscle strength. The rate and type of muscle contraction influence muscle strength and are determined by MMT. For the results of the test to be reliable, rate and speed of contraction must be consistent. If a concentric muscle contraction is the method of choice, a moderate speed is used. With an isometric muscle contraction, the muscle holds at the end of the test range, and no motion occurs; the strength test result will be a whole grade higher than with the concentric muscle contraction.

If the test muscle is performing an eccentric contraction against resistance, the test results will be greater than with the isometric muscle contraction. The faster the eccentric contraction, the greater will be the tension that develops in the muscle. For a concentric muscle contraction, the opposite is true: Less tension will develop as the velocity of the muscle contraction increases. Isometric and concentric types of muscle contractions are used most commonly in specific MMT.

The rate of shortening substantially affects the force a muscle can develop. The faster a muscle produces a concentric contraction, the less ability the muscle has to generate tension. Therefore, as velocity increases, tension decreases. During an eccentric muscle contraction, the tension initially increases, then tapers off as velocity increases. This increase in tension associated with an increased velocity may help to provide protection from structural damage exceeding tissue limitations as muscle lengthening occurs. Isokinetic muscle contractions occur when

the velocity of movement remains constant and the resistance accommodates to the external force with changing joint angle. The muscle can therefore maintain maximal output throughout the full ROM.

Mechanical devices such as a dynamometer have been developed that control the velocity of movement (Fig. 2-8). Dynamometers are used extensively for evaluating and exercising muscles, but they do not replace MMT. Practitioners may apply manual resistance in an attempt to simulate the function of the mechanical dynamometer. With practice, the therapist can continuously adjust the amount of resistance being offered so that the motion produced is approximately constant throughout the range, thereby approaching an isokinetic condition.

Anatomically, many factors are involved in objectively assessing the strength of any given muscle. Factors that affect muscle strength include the number of motor units per muscle, functional excursion, cross-sectional area, line of pull of muscle fibers, number of joints crossed, sensory receptors, attachments to bone and the relationship of the muscle to the joint axis, and the age and sex of the subject. These factors cannot be changed clinically; however, the literature has information on differences in strength for sex, age, and some occupations. In men, muscle strength tends to increase from 2 to 19 years of age; then it plateaus until age 30, after which it starts to decline unless resisted exercises continue as one ages. In women, muscle strength increases uniformly until age 20 and remains level for approximately 10 years, then begins to decrease. Criteria for grading are being developed on the basis of age, sex, and occupation of the population.

Lehmkuhl and Smith state that biomechanical leverage in a muscle is an important consideration for muscle contraction.[25] As muscles go through

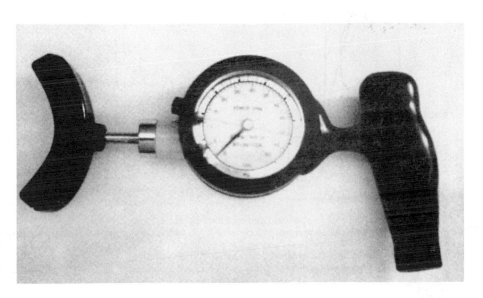

▲ **Figure 2.8** A hand-held dynamometer designed by G. Smidt (Spark Instruments and Academics Inc., P.O. Box 5123, Coraville, IA 52241) for measuring muscle strength.

their ROM, the torque generated varies with the length of the moment arm (the distance from the axis of rotation). For example, as the elbow moves from full extension in flexion, the moment arm increases, reaching its maximum at 90 degrees of flexion, then decreases through the remainder of the ROM (Fig. 2-9).

Direct measurement of active voluntary tension developed in a muscle is not clinically practical. Muscle tension developed by a patient can be resolved into forces. One force is along the longitudinal axis of the segment on which the muscle attaches, and the other is at a right angle to the axis of motion. The component that is perpendicular to the body segment is called the rotary component; the component that is parallel to the body segment is the tension component when the direction of the force is away from the joint involved. It is called the compression component, or stabilizing force, when the direction of the force is toward the joint.[25] The rotatory force around an axis is the torque, which also can be expressed as muscle strength. Torque equals the product of the force and the perpendicular distance from the joint axis. The internal torque of muscle forces changes throughout the ROM. Changes in the angle of attachment, which occur throughout the ROM, produce changes in leverage and torque. The leverage of a muscle is greatest when the angle of insertion is 90 degrees.

Gravity (the weight of the body segment) also has a rotational component. It can be resolved in the same manner as muscle tension and acts in a direction opposite to that of muscle torque. The force of gravity has the greatest leverage and therefore is able to produce the greatest torque on a body seg-

ment when the segment is horizontal. External resistance applied to the moving segment must change as the body segment changes its position. Muscle torque must overcome applied external force and the weight of the limb to move or maintain a body segment in a specific position.

There are several mechanical methods of assessing muscle strength using instruments such as Kin Com, Lido, and Cybex dynamometers. The inherent properties of the instrument may dictate the mechanical factors relevant to the measurement, torque output. These factors include the capability of maintaining a constant moment arm, assessing strength of different types of muscle contractions, and maintaining a constant limb velocity. The segment to be tested can be positioned and the resistance applied where, biomechanically and physiologically, the muscle is at its best advantage to generate torque.

General Principles for Evaluating Skeletal Muscle Strength

In MMT, the muscle grades express the examiner's objective evaluation of the functional strength of the muscle. Manual muscle tests are used to determine the degrees of muscle weakness resulting from disease, injury, or disuse. The aim in muscle testing is to administer the test as accurately as possible. Knowledge of human anatomy and kinesiology is critical to success. The following factors are essential for therapists to make an accurate evaluation of muscle strength.

1. Anatomical, physiological, and biomechanical knowledge of skeletal muscle positions and stabilization
2. Elimination of substitution motions
3. Skill in palpation and application of resistance
4. Careful direction for each movement that is easily understood by the patient
5. Adherence to a standard method of grading muscle strength
6. Experience testing many individuals with normal muscle strength and varying degrees of weakness

Basic considerations in the technique of MMT are worthy of mention prior to an explanation of the procedure for evaluating muscle strength. MMT is preceded by a general review of the subject's medical history, an interview, introduction to the subject and family, and a generalized or gross assessment of muscle strength. If the gross muscle evaluation shows specific muscle weakness, then those muscles are evaluated with specific MMT techniques. Sel-

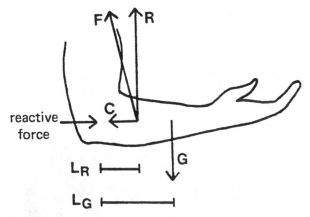

▲ **Figure 2.9** Resolution of muscle force demonstrated on forearm. The drawing shows the resolution of flexor muscle force F into two vectors at right angles to each other, one perpendicular to the forearm because *rotary force* must act at right angles to the segment that it is moving. In this drawing, R represents the vector of a *rotary force*. The one at a right angle to it, C, along the forearm is a *compression* force.

dom is an entire-body MMT performed; only muscles that have been identified previously warrant specific evaluation.

The examiner must explain the purpose of the test and give the directions in understandable terms. If the contralateral limb or segment is uninvolved, it is often useful to test that side first. Not only does it make the subject aware of the movement desired, but it also provides a valuable standard for comparison.

The body area or segment to be evaluated is exposed, and the subject is properly draped. Each muscle to be tested must be palpated, and palpation through a hospital gown or clothing must be avoided because it will render the muscle test invalid. When possible, the subject is evaluated in a quiet area free of distractions. The therapist requires the subject's cooperation and undivided attention to make an accurate determination of strength.

Results from the gross muscle evaluation will provide a general knowledge of total body muscle strength and enable the examiner to test all of the appropriate muscles in one position before having the subject change to another position, thus avoiding unnecessary fatigue and discomfort.

GRADING

The examiner must be aware of variables that affect the grading of muscle strength. These variables are important if MMT is to be clinically significant. The grading systems used in the practice of physical therapy are rather simple and easy to apply. Three basic factors are considered in MMT:

1. The weight of the limb or distal segment with a minimal effect of gravity on the moving segment. The muscle contracts in a plane horizontal to the effects of gravity. The test segment is supported on a smooth surface so that the frictional force is minimized during movement.
2. The weight of the limb plus the effects of gravity on the limb or segment. The motion occurs in a plane perpendicular to the effects of gravity.
3. The weight of the limb or segment plus the effects of gravity plus manual resistance. Practitioners must be consistent with respect to the point of application of resistance. Resistance is always applied at right angles to the long axis of the segment. The magnitude and direction of the resistance are opposite to that of the contracting muscle (Fig. 2-10).

The grading system for muscle strength is based on specific factors:

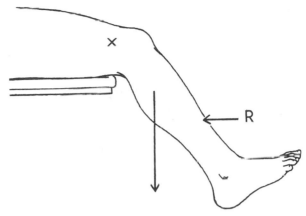

▲ **Figure 2.10** Illustration of resistance or rotational influence for knee extension. *X* is axis of knee joint, ↓ is gravitational force for leg and foot, *R* is external force applied to leg.

1. The amount of resistance given manually to a contracted muscle or muscle group determines strength. The force is applied by the tester in a direction opposite to the torque exerted by the muscle being tested.
2. The ability of a muscle or muscle group to move a part through a complete test ROM is a measure of muscle strength.
3. Evidence of the presence or absence of a muscle contraction as determined by palpation and observation is critical to muscle strength evaluation.
4. Grades are obtained on the basis of the effects of gravity and manual resistance. Gravity affects movement, depending on the position of the subject. When a muscle contracts parallel to the gravitational force, the position is referred to as gravity minimized (GM). When a muscle contracts against the downward gravitational force, the position is referred to as against gravity (AG). The AG position may also involve the application of manual resistance.

The standard muscle testing grades are applicable to the adult population and may need to be adjusted for older or younger subjects. Grading criteria depend on the subject's body build, age, sex, and occupation. For example, a "good" (4) grade for a professional football linebacker is not the same as the "good" grade for a 75-year-old woman or a 3-year-old child. Some muscles within the body normally are not capable of exerting significant amounts of torque, for example, the finger flexors versus the quadriceps muscles. The examiner must be aware of the variability of normal muscle function to avoid incorrectly assigning a weak grade to a normal-functioning muscle.

Table 2-3 describes various grading systems that have been used in clinical practice over the past 60 years.

There are some basic differences between Lovett's (Daniels and Worthingham) and Kendall's methods of grading.[23] Overall, because Daniels and Worthingham's method tests a motion that uses all agonists and synergists involved in the motion, it is a more functional approach. Kendall's approach tests a specific muscle rather than a motion and requires selective muscle performance on the part of the subject.[23] Specific muscle testing requires a greater knowledge of anatomy and kinesiology than testing voluntary motions. It gives accurate results of a muscle's function but is more time consuming for the examiner.

Kendall's method tests muscles isometrically in which the segment is aligned in the direction of the muscle fibers in a midrange position, and the subject is asked to hold against resistance.[23] Kendall's technique maintains the subject in the same antigravity position and uses assistance to determine which grades the subject is unable to attain moving AG.[23] In Lovett's technique the subject moves through the full test range, a concentric contraction, or holds at the end of the range while the muscle is in its shortened position. Although Lovett's is a more subjective test, it will identify where in the range weakness exists. Daniels and Worthingham place the subject in the GM position when the subject is unable to move AG.[9] Both Lovett's and Daniels and Worthingham's techniques have an inherent subjectivity in the area of applied resistance.

Most physicians use the Medical Research Council scale, which is based on numbers that are easy to remember and to interpret.[14] The grades of 0, 1, and 2 are tested in the GM position. All others are tested AG. Resistance is applied as an isometric hold at the end of the test range to determine AG grades. Another infrequently used grading system is based on a

TABLE 2.3 **Comparison of Gravity-Resisted Muscle Grading Criteria**		
LOVETT AND DANIELS AND WORTHINGHAM	KENDALL AND MCCREARY	MEDICAL RESEARCH COUNCIL
N (Normal): Subject completes range of motion against gravity, against maximal resistance.	100%: Subject moves into and holds test position against gravity, against maximal resistance.	5
G+ (Good Plus): Subject completes range of motion against gravity, against nearly maximal resistance.		4+
G (Good): Subject completes range of motion against gravity, against moderate resistance.	80%: Subject moves into and holds test position against gravity, against less than maximal resistance.	4
G– (Good Minus): Subject completes range of motion against gravity, against less than moderate resistance.		4–
F+ (Fair Plus): Subject completes range of motion against gravity, against minimal resistance.		3+
F (Fair): Subject completes range of motion against gravity with no manual resistance.	50%: Subject moves into and holds a test position against gravity.	3
F– (Fair Minus): Subject does not complete range against gravity but does complete more than half the range.		3–
P+ (Poor Plus): Subject initiates range of motion against gravity or completes range with gravity minimized against slight resistance.		2+
P (Poor): Subject completes range of motion with gravity minimized.	20%: Subject moves through small motion with gravity minimized.	2
P– (Poor Minus): Subject does not complete range of motion with gravity minimized.		2–
T (Trace): Subject's muscle can be palpated, but there is no joint motion.	5%: Contraction is palpable with no joint motion.	1
0 (Zero): Subject exhibits no palpable contraction.	0%: No contraction is palpable.	0

numerical scale that ranges from 5 to 1, 5 indicating a trace of muscle strength and 1 indicating normal.

Body segments that have short lever arms are not significantly influenced by gravity. Their grades are determined by manual resistance or no resistance. The fingers and toes are short segments, and the effect of gravity on them is insignificant. Physical therapists in different areas of the country determine grades variously by means of palpation alone or by gravity assistance of the muscle. When a subject is unable to change testing positions or when the subject demonstrates weakness in the AG position and cannot be appropriately positioned in the GM position, other grading methods may be used.

When a subject is unable to assume standard test positions, grades may be determined by palpation. This type of grading is one for which considerable experience in palpating normal and weak muscle contractions is necessary.

Grading by Palpation Criteria

N (normal, 5): The muscle is well delineated and the contraction feels hard.

G (good, 4): The muscle is well delineated and the contraction feels firm.

F (fair, 3): The muscle outline is well delineated, but the contraction feels soft.

P (poor, 2): The muscle is not well delineated, and a slight, mushy contraction is felt.

T (trace, 1): A flicker or mere tension or relaxation after contraction is felt.

0 (zero, 0): No muscle contraction is palpated.

Grades also may be determined by the assistance to the segment or body part when positions or other factors may prevent the subject from assuming the standard positions. The subject is positioned to allow the effects of gravity to assist the contraction of the muscle, and a determination of strength is made by estimating the amount of assistance given to a weak muscle. The subject relaxes the part to be tested so the examiner can feel the weight of the test segment. As the subject moves through the ROM, the examiner attempts to measure the decreased weight of the part. The examiner should guide the movement and give assistance but not precede the motion.

Grading by Assistance Criteria

0 (zero): 100% of the weight of the segment is supported by the examiner throughout the test range.

T (trace): 100% of the weight of the segment is supported by the examiner throughout the test range, but a contraction is felt or observed.

P− (poor minus): 75% of the maximal weight of the segment is supported by the examiner.

P (poor): 50% or moderate assistance is required to move the part through the test range.

P+ (poor plus): 30% or minimal assistance is required to move the part through the test range.

Higher muscle strength grades would be against the effects of gravity, as indicated previously.

As stated previously, grades obtained by experienced examiners should not vary more than half a grade when half grades are used (ie, a grade difference of 3 versus 3+ ["fair" and "fair plus"] is permissible, because MMT has not been professionally validated). If the examiner is undecided between two grades, it is best to record the lower one to establish a treatment plan that is appropriate for the subject. Recording the lower grade may also motivate the subject by demonstrating gains in strength between sessions.

Factors Affecting Manual Muscle Testing Results

The examiner must be aware that some musculoskeletal disorders or weaknesses cause muscles to fatigue more easily and rapidly than normal. Fatigue is a reason to test various areas of the body during one evaluation session rather than several muscles around a single joint or limb. For example, test a few hand muscles, then move to the lower limb, then come back to the upper limb.

Some subjects are unable to complete the test ROM because of joint limitation rather than muscle weakness. A person with rheumatoid arthritis may have limited range in the wrist or knee joints. The test ROM is determined by the amount of passive ROM available in the joint. In such a situation, a range grade–strength grade is used to determine strength and record the measurements. The purpose is to assign a grade of strength to a muscle in which the passive test range is incomplete. Range grade–strength grade is used to evaluate muscles that are incapable of contracting through a complete test range because of joint limitations but that can complete the available range and can hold against resistance. For example, tightness of a muscle or lack of joint stability may give such a grade. The limited range should be measured before muscle strength is evaluated. Range grade–strength grade is recorded as a fraction in which the numerator is the number of degrees completed through the available passive limited ROM and the denominator is the strength. If knee extension is lacking 20 degrees and the strength of the quadriceps muscle is "good" (4), the range grade–strength grade is stated as "−20 degrees / 4 good."

The numerator of range–strength grades also may be stated as F− or P+. F− means that the test range is not complete, but the motion is more than one-half the standard test ROM. P+ means that the test range is less than one-half the test range.

A question mark in MMT is used when the validity of the strength is in doubt. For instance, if the subject has a painful joint that limits the muscle's contractile force, one may use the question mark or write on the form "pain—unable to test."

Sliding grades have been recorded when muscle strength ranges between two grades. For instance, T to P− ("trace" to "poor minus") indicates the grade is better than a trace but does not demonstrate sufficient strength to be assigned a grade of "poor minus." There can be only a half-grade difference when using the sliding grade scale.

Subjectivity becomes a factor in determining muscle grades any time one uses manual resistance, assistance, or palpation to determine muscle strength.

Grades obtained during MMT do not represent the absolute amount of muscle tension developed during contraction. A muscle grade of 4 ("good," 75%) is not equivalent to 75% of the strength represented by a grade of 5 ("normal," 100%). It is a natural grade determined by the effect of gravity, manual resistance, subject's age, degree of disability, and so forth. Absolute muscle strength is determined by the physiological cross-sectional area of the muscle and is an indication of the muscle's functional capacity. The larger the cross-sectional area, the more tension can be produced. The cross-section alone, however, does not determine how much work the muscle is able to produce. To determine the muscle's work capacity, the distance a muscle can shorten must be known. Rudolph Fick computed work capacity of individual muscles by multiplying 3 to 4 kg of force per square centimeter (cm^2) by the cross-sectional area.[25] Tables have been developed and published for individual muscles. It is obvious that absolute muscle strength is not a practical criterion for evaluating muscle strength in the clinical setting.

POSITIONS

Positioning a subject for testing varies with the muscle tested, its strength, and the subject's overall condition. The subject and the part to be tested should be positioned comfortably on a firm surface. The body part must be exposed and the individual properly draped. Not all subjects can be examined using the standard test positions. Subjects may be on frames or may be medically unable to tolerate certain positions. In these situations, grades may be determined by palpation or by allowing gravity to assist the motion.

Two test positions (GM and AG) are used as standard positions to determine the strength of muscles based on the effects of gravity.

GM (Gravity Minimized). The test segment is positioned to minimize or diminish the effects of gravity for a specific muscle. The term "gravity eliminated" is used by Daniels and Worthingham to describe this position,[9] although gravitational effects are eliminated only in a weightless environment. Movements are not assisted or resisted by gravity. The testing surface is free of friction. A powder board is often used to reduce friction from the patient's skin and the supporting surface. It is usually constructed of wood or lightweight plastic (Fig. 2-11A and B).

Muscles tested that flex and extend while one is seated AG are tested GM with the subject in a sidelying position. There are no gravitational effects on the contracting muscle.

Muscles that produce motions AG in the coronal plane are tested in the transverse plane with the subject in a prone or supine position. To test in the GM position for abductor and adductor muscles, the

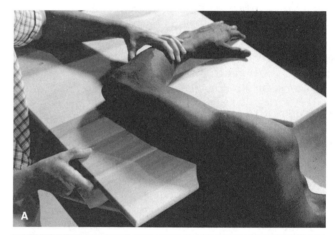

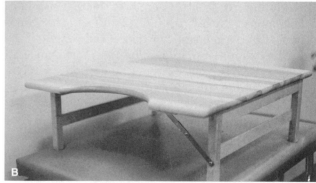

▲ **Figure 2.11** **(A)** A powder board, made of wood and treated to permit movement on a smooth, frictionless surface. The board is lightly covered with powder to reduce friction on the test segment during gravity-minimized muscle strength testing. **(B)** Placement of the powder board with the subject in a sidelying position. A pillow may be placed under the board if it rests on the subject.

subject is usually in the sitting position. The body segments for the rotator muscle groups tested in the GM position are positioned parallel to gravity.

AG (Against Gravity). The subject is positioned so that the effects of gravity are working against the test segment, and the body segment contracts against the downward gravitational force.

The list of Positions for Testing Against Gravity, later in this chapter, contains a summary of test positions. Positioning details for specific muscles are presented in subsequent chapters.

Test Position or Range. The test position is the ROM a joint completes by contraction of the test muscle. The ROM for specific muscle testing is not necessarily the complete ROM that the muscle can produce at that joint. For instance, the muscles involved with shoulder flexion are able to contract through an ROM of 180 degrees, but the MMT position is only to 90 degrees. A muscle contracts through a full ROM or through a test range to obtain a strength grade. The position of complete or test range for muscle contraction is based on the influence of gravity on the movement. The effect of gravity is based on the length of the lever arm being tested. A segment or limb that is at a right angle to its proximal segment has the longest lever arm, resulting in a maximal effect from gravity. A segment that moves toward a right angle to its proximal segment is increasing its lever length and gravitational affect. A segment that moves beyond a right angle toward 180 degrees decreases its lever length, and the effect from gravity is lessening. Therefore, muscle strength testing AG is usually performed in a test position with maximal resistance from gravity.

The ROM testing is initially performed passively to determine any limitation within the joint that the muscle to be evaluated is going to move. The practitioner assesses the test position before making a judgment on the strength of a muscle.

If the test position is limited by a joint problem, manual muscle strength can still be tested and graded (see range grade–strength grade, previously).

Palpation. Palpation should be done to assess the contraction of the muscle being tested. The number of fingers used depends on the size of the muscle or tendon being palpated. If the muscle is small, the middle finger is the most sensitive to tension in muscle contraction. Every muscle evaluated must be palpated to make MMT a valid assessment tool. Palpation is necessary to determine exactly which muscle is being contracted and to allow the examiner to detect substitutions by adjacent muscles.

Resistance. Resistance is the force applied at the end of the test range (break method) or throughout the test range (make method) in a direction opposite the muscle's rotatory component. Manual resistance is applied at right angles to the long axis of the segment. Resistance may be applied at the end of the test range, with the muscle providing an isometric hold as described by Daniels and Worthingham or throughout the test range while the muscle is performing a concentric type of contraction.

The results in the assessment of muscle strength differ depending on the method used. The isometric hold, or the break test, shows the muscle to have a higher test grade than the resistance given throughout the range in the make test. In either method, manual resistance is applied gradually and released gradually, giving the subject time to contract the muscle and then relax it before the resistance has been removed.

The skill and consistency with which the examiner applies the manual resistance to the segment are important. The force should be applied gradually in a direction opposite the muscle's rotatory component and at a consistent location—distally without crossing another joint—on the moving segment.

The effect of manual resistance on muscle torque is a function of the distance of its application from the joint axis. The tester who changes the point at which resistance is applied to the body segment will find that the muscle torque exerted will also change. This inconsistency in technique will prevent the examiner from developing an appreciation for what is "normal strength" relative to an individual's sex, age, body type, and lifestyle.

The proper location for the application of resistance is as far distal as possible from one joint axis of movement on the moving segment without crossing another joint. There are a few exceptions, such as testing the hip and shoulder rotator muscles. Resistance should never cross an intervening joint unless the integrity of the joint has been assessed and is considered normal.

The MMT developed for this book allows the examiner to apply resistance using either the isometric muscle contraction (break test) or the concentric muscle contraction (make test). The important factor is consistency for each patient and among the coworkers who may be evaluating and treating the patient.

STABILIZATION

Extrinsic stabilization, or fixation, is counterpressure to resistance that provides support for the subject and helps prevent substitute motions. Manually or with an external support, the tester stabilizes the proximal segment while contraction of the muscle moves the distal segment. Stabilization adds validity to the muscle test. To evaluate the strength of the quadriceps, for example, the therapist would stabilize the thigh. If the proximal attachment of a muscle is unstable, the rotatory component of the contracting muscle will not have an adequate advantage.

Intrinsic methods of stabilization are achieved by structures or factors found inherently within the body. For example, the importance of the scapula in providing stability for shoulder and upper limb function is widely accepted.

SUBSTITUTION

Substitute motions occur when muscles are weak or movement is uncoordinated. Synergistic muscles contract to produce the desired motion with or without the action of the agonist muscle.

Subjects typically use any muscle to produce a desired motion when the muscle being tested is too weak to perform the action. Substitution movements by synergist muscles are common in normal people. When the therapist applies too much resistance, the subject is tempted to use substitute muscles to do the desired motion. In evaluating wrist flexion, for instance, if too much manual resistance is applied, the subject substitutes with the finger flexors.

Substitutions can be minimized by careful and appropriate positioning and stabilizing. Detection of substitutions is obvious when the examiner palpates the muscle being evaluated.

RECORDING MEASUREMENTS

Refer to Appendix A for an example of the MMT recording form. Recording forms vary in format from clinical facility to clinical facility. Forms are designed to record muscle strength grades by peripheral nerve innervation, specific muscle, or muscle group actions. The grades that are recorded on the forms also vary by the method chosen.

At the bottom of the MMT form is an area in which to record any comments about the subject. For example, the subject may experience pain on motion, a variation from the standard position may have been used, or the subject may have appeared confused or disoriented during the evaluation. All are events that should be noted in the Comment section of the recording form. It is important to record muscle strength status as part of the medical record to develop a treatment plan, for documentation, and for reimbursement of medical services.

The form is designed for recording three to four measurements on subsequent evaluations. The records are dated and written on the designated side, right or left, with the muscle grade written on the inside column and subsequent recordings added

to the outside columns. If all the muscles test "good" to "normal" in strength, it is not necessary to record the finding for each muscle on the form. It is suggested that a recording of within functional limits (WFL) or within normal limits (WNL) is used to complete the form. It is necessary, however, to record the findings and include them in the medical record.

GENERAL PROCEDURE FOR SPECIFIC MANUAL MUSCLE TESTING

Performing the test in the prescribed sequence benefits subject and examiner. When the sequence is followed, the test is performed without omissions, and the results should be valid and reliable.

1. Following the gross muscle test, the first step is to position the subject in the AG position, unless that is contraindicated. The subject should be positioned so that the muscle contracting and the motion being performed can be observed easily. If muscle weakness is evident in more than one area, all muscles that can be tested in one position should be. Changing positions tires the subject and may yield an inaccurate evaluation of muscle strength. The subject should be stabilized and positioned comfortably. It also is important for the examiner to be comfortable while testing.

2. The body part or segment to be tested is exposed, and the rest of the body is well draped.

3. After explaining the test and demonstrating it to the subject, the examiner determines the available ROM associated with the test muscle. Usually the test range is evaluated passively unless the examiner knows that the muscle is functional and can move the part through the entire test range, in which case active motion may be performed. If the subject also requires goniometry of the joint, such measurement should precede the manual muscle evaluation.

4. The body part or segment to be evaluated is aligned according to the direction of the muscle fibers. This alignment allows optimal muscle function.

5. Before the subject contracts the muscle, the therapist provides adequate stabilization to the proximal segment.

6. During proximal segment stabilization, the subject attempts to contract the muscle to move the distal segment throughout the test

ROM. The moving segment may also be placed at the end of the ROM, in which case the subject is asked to hold the contraction. Speed of the contraction is moderate; accuracy is more important.

7. During the active contraction, the examiner observes the movement and the muscle and palpates the tendon or muscle belly. The examiner is positioned to palpate the muscle prior to movement of the segment. Palpation occurs throughout the active motion until relaxation occurs. The therapist can help avoid substitutions by palpating the muscle that should perform the desired movement. Also the examiner may provide simple, clear verbal clues as feedback to the subject to assist in avoiding substitutions. As a rule, the joint is not graded on motion alone—the therapist should *always palpate*.

8. The examiner applies resistance to the muscle that is able to complete the test range AG. Application and release of resistance are firm and smooth. Resistance is applied at the distal end of the segment, without crossing an intervening joint, in a direction as nearly op-posite the line of pull of the muscle fibers as possible. The subject is instructed to establish a maximum contraction before resistance is given. The therapist may apply resistance at the end of the test range, as in the break test, or throughout the range, as in the make test.

The movement is repeated until the muscle strength grade has been determined, but not so many times that the subject becomes fatigued. Muscle testing is designed to test strength, not endurance. The subject should be able to perform three consecutive repetitions at the same grade level. It is advisable to compare the strength with that of the uninvolved muscle, if possible. Fatigue of a muscle may be a diagnostic sign of a neuromuscular disorder. Also, fatigue with repetitions may be an early sign of nerve root compression.

9. The final step in the MMT evaluation is to record the grade and date and initial the test form.

10. The assessment of the subject's performance is derived from the recording form, and the treatment plan is developed therefrom.

Summary of Muscle-Testing Positions

Sitting	Supine	Sidelying	Prone	Standing
Hip—flexors (AG)	Scapula—abductors (AG)	Hip—abductors and adductors (AG)	Hip—extensors (AG)	Ankle—plantarflexors (AG)
Knee—extensors (AG)	Shoulder—flexors (AG)	Ankle/foot—invertors and evertors (AG)	Knee—flexor (AG)	Pelvis—hiking (AG)
Ankle—dorsiflexor and toes (AG)	Elbow—extensors (AG)	Hip—flexors and extensors (GM)	Ankle/foot—plantarflexors (AG)	
Scapula—elevators (AG)	Wrist/hand—all (AG)	Knee—flexors and extensors (GM)	Scapula—adductors and downward rotators (AG)	
Shoulder—flexors and abductors (AG)	Neck/trunk—flexors (AG)	Ankle/foot—dorsi/plantarflexors (GM)	Shoulder—extensors and medial and lateral rotators (AG)	
Elbow and radio/ulnar—flexors and rotators (AG)	Hip—abductors, adductors, and rotators (GM)	Shoulder—flexors and extensors GM	Elbow—extensors (AG)	
Wrist—flexors and extensors (AG)	Ankle/foot—invertor, evertors, and toes (GM)	Neck—flexors and extensors (GM)	Neck—extensors (AG)	
Finger—flexors and extensors (AG)	Scapula—elevators (GM)		Trunk—extensors (AG)	
Scapular—adductors and abductors (GM)	Shoulder—abductors (GM)		Scapula—adductors (GM)	
Shoulder—extensors and flexors (GM)	Wrist/hand—all (GM)		Shoulder—extensors and rotators (GM)	
Elbow/radioulnar—extensors, rotator, and flexors (GM)	Pelvis—hiking (GM)			
Wrist and hand—all (GM)				
Neck and trunk—flexors and extensors (GM)				

ORTHOPEDIC EXAMINATION OF SYNOVIAL JOINTS

Orthopedic assessment of a joint must be carried out systematically. Accurate evaluation and assessment depend on complete information regarding subject history, a thorough examination of clinical signs and symptoms, and a comprehensive medical workup.

Clinicians need to establish their own ways of performing a musculoskeletal assessment. When a systematic approach is followed repeatedly, it is unlikely that any information relative to the correct diagnosis will be overlooked.

This section deals with the components of synovial joint assessment and is divided into the following sections:

1. Patient history
2. Gross observation and palpation
3. Examination of inert and contractile structures
4. Special tests
5. Joint play movements

Patient History

Before examining the subject, the clinician should thoroughly review the medical chart, paying specific attention to parts that are clinically relevant to the diagnosis. The subject must have a complete medical diagnostic workup. Information such as radiology reports, laboratory tests, and electrodiagnostic testing assist in definitively confirming or ruling out orthopedic and neurological pathology.

The therapist next obtains information from the subject; this portion of the examination process may yield the most constructive information. An astute clinician many times is able to arrive at an accurate diagnosis on the basis of a very complete and thorough history related by the subject.

Questioning of the subject should be done in a systematic manner. The examiner must not "lead" the subject in the course of questioning. Questions should be asked that require specific answers. For example, the clinician should not say, "Does this increase your pain?" but instead, "Tell me if this alters your symptoms in any way." The examiner should not accept vague responses that do not specifically answer the question and should persist with a question until a satisfactory response is obtained.

Answers to the following questions should be obtained as part of the subjective examination:

1. The first question should be, "What is the complaint that has brought you here today?" This question not only sets the tone for the rest of the interview, but also allows subjects to describe the problem in their own words.

2. The next question should inquire into the subject's occupation, athletic endeavors, and hobbies. Answers will provide the examiner with information regarding stresses and postures typical of the subject and may suggest the mechanism of injury.

3. "Was the onset of the problem sudden, or did the problem appear gradually over a period of hours, days, or weeks? Were you able to relate it to a specific activity or posture? Was the onset associated with direct trauma in a contact injury or with an indirect, noncontact situation?"

4. "Is this the first time that this particular problem has occurred? If not, how do the symptoms now compare to past experiences? How long did the problem persist in previous episodes? How were you treated for this problem in the past, and was that treatment regimen successful in relieving the symptoms?"

5. "How long have you had your present symptoms?" This information may help the examiner determine the acuteness or chronicity of the problem.

6. "How are your symptoms today as compared with the first day they became apparent?" Response to this question will yield information about the stage of healing or will indicate if the condition is getting worse.

7. "What is the nature of your symptoms?" If the patient expresses pain as the primary complaint, the examiner must delve thoroughly into the nature of the pain. It is important that the subject describe the type of pain. "Is the pain sharp, dull, achy, or throbbing? Is it constant or intermittent? If the pain is intermittent, do certain postures or activities exacerbate or relieve it? Do rest and activity make your pain worse or better, or do they have no effect?" For example, rest usually alleviates a mechanical problem in or around the joint. Pain felt in the morning that diminishes progressively during the day is indicative of a chronic inflammatory process, such as arthritis. Pain and stiffness felt at the beginning of activity that subside as the activity continues may indicate a muscle problem. An increase in pain noted in the morning also may relate to sleeping postures, mattresses, or pillows.

"Can you pinpoint the pain, or is it diffuse or radiating?" Bone pain tends to be very deep and localized, whereas nerve root pain, which is burning and sharp, characteristically radiates following the distribution of specific nerve(s). Dull and achy muscular pain tends to be somewhat diffuse and is aggravated by movements involving contraction or stretching of the affected muscle. Vascular pain is often vague and diffuse, not following any dermatomal or myotomal patterns.

8. "Are you now experiencing or have you experienced sensations other than pain?" These may take the form of pins and needles, tingling, numbness, or anesthesia. These symptoms are usually associated with neurological or vascular involvement.

9. "Do you experience any joint locking or 'giving way'?" Locking may be a result of internal derangement, as in a meniscal tear or the temporary lodging of a loose body between articular surfaces. Giving way is often related to ligamentous instability or reflex muscle inhibition.

10. "Have you experienced any dizziness or fainting spells?" These symptoms may be representative of a more serious underlying neurological disorder.

Gross Observation and Palpation

Observation should begin as the subject enters the department or examination area. The gait pattern may be observed and any gross deviations noted. An antalgic gait pattern may indicate to the examiner which joints are affected and may demonstrate the subject's willingness or reluctance to bear weight on the affected limb. Examination of the subject's facial expression may provide information about the intensity of pain or sleeplessness.

The subject's freedom of movement should also be noted during removal of coats, pullover sweaters, and shoes and socks. The ease or difficulty with which the subject gets on the examining table and assumes various positions should be noted because it may suggest the necessity for more specific regional assessment.

Once the subject has exposed the body part to be examined and is properly draped, the examiner can make the following assessments:

1. Identify any gross postural deformity or abnormality that may be associated with fractures, spinal disorders, congenital abnormalities, or traumatic incidents.

2. Compare the soft-tissue contours between the involved and uninvolved sides, indicating areas of muscular atrophy, hypertrophy, or rupture.

3. Determine the color, texture, and temperature of the part being examined. Temperature elevation usually indicates an active inflammatory state, whereas a cooler temperature usu-

ally reflects vascular compromise. Trophic changes, such as shiny skin, hair loss, and brittle nails, may be evidence of diabetes, vascular problems, or peripheral nerve lesions.

4. Examine for scars, indicating past trauma or surgery. Open or closed sinus tracts are typical of infections such as osteomyelitis.

5. Examine for edema or effusion in or around the problem area.

6. Palpate for pulses and compare the findings to those for the uninvolved limb. The pulses that should be checked as part of this assessment include the brachial, radial, femoral, popliteal, and dorsalis pedis.

7. Palpate for any muscle spasm, indicating an attempt by the musculature to "splint," or immobilize a traumatized or pathological area.

Examination of Inert and Contractile Structures

In the assessment of a synovial joint, it is important to remember that all of the structures comprising the joint, as well the musculature that moves the joint, are stressed when the patient moves actively. In nonsurgical patients, specific examination techniques must be used that isolate inert structures from contractile elements. A systematic approach to the identification of the structures responsible for the subject's complaints follows. The examination procedure outlined below does not apply to post-surgical patients because of the invasion of tissue during surgery. Additionally, the need to delineate pathological structures is eliminated by virtue of the tissues involved being identified or corrected during the surgical procedure.

ACTIVE MOVEMENTS

Little objective information is obtained from active movement, because both contractile and inert structures are moving and are therefore stressed. Active motion, however, does provide information about the subject's willingness to move. As the subject moves, the examiner is able to assess generally whether other joint movements are substituting for the desired movement and where in the available ROM pain is experienced, discern the quality and pattern of the movement, and get an idea of the restriction of the movement.

PASSIVE MOVEMENTS

The examiner passively moves the joint through the available ROM in all directions of movement of which the joint is capable. Passive ROM assesses the integrity of the inert structures of the joint by stressing them at various points in the range. These inert structures, which have no inherent ability to contract, include the capsule, ligament, bursa, cartilage, nerves and nerve sheaths, and dura mater. Objective information regarding the status of the joint may be gained through passive testing. The identification of the sequence of pain and resistance, end feel, and capsular patterns provides invaluable information about the pathological state of the joint. Passive ROM assessment should first be performed on the uninvolved side to provide a baseline "normal" against which the motion of the involved side can be compared. It should be noted that subjects exhibiting joint hypomobility (decreased ROM) may be more susceptible to muscular strains, overuse tendinitis, and nerve entrapment syndromes. Hypermobile joints (excessive ROM) may be predisposed to recurrent injury, joint sprains, early degenerative joint changes, tendinitis resulting from muscular imbalance, joint effusion, and prolonged pain.

Sequence of Pain and Resistance. The sequence of pain and resistance provides the examiner with information about the acuteness or chronicity of joint pathology.

Stage 1. The subject experiences pain before the examiner feels any resistance to the passive ROM. This stage is representative of an acute joint.

Stage 2. The subject feels pain at the same time the examiner feels resistance to the passive ROM. Stage 2 indicates a subacute condition present in the joint. The clinician can be slightly more aggressive with this joint than at the previous stage.

Stage 3. The examiner feels resistance to the passive ROM before the subject experiences pain. This joint has no active inflammatory process and therefore is considered chronic. With this stage, the clinician can treat aggressively.

End Feels. An end feel is the feeling imparted to the examiner's hands as the end point of passive ROM is reached. It can provide information regarding the nature of the restriction responsible for terminating the range of movement. Each synovial joint in the human body has a normal end feel, which is how the resistance feels at the end point of the normal ROM. During pathological restrictions of ROM, the clinician should be concerned with the assessment of end feel.

The types of end feel commonly found include the following:

1. Soft-tissue approximation—the feeling of soft tissue compressing soft tissue. This is normally found in elbow flexion and knee flexion.
2. Bony—the feeling of bone impacting against bone. This is normally found in elbow extension and is pathological if found in other joints of the body or in restricted elbow extension.
3. Springy—the feeling of the joint stopping and then rebounding, normally not found in the body. This is associated with internal derangements, usually in joints with menisci or cartilaginous disks.
4. Capsular—a feeling of a firm but slightly yielding stop, as if two pieces of hard rubber were pressed together. Normally this is found with shoulder and hip joint rotations; it is pathological if found in other joints or in restricted ranges of shoulder and hip joint rotation.
5. Muscle spasm—a sudden, abrupt cessation of movement accompanied by pain. Subjects with active inflammation may exhibit early muscle spasm at or near the beginning of movement. Joint instability or the aggravation produced by joint movement may produce delayed onset muscle spasm at or near the end of the available ROM.
6. Tissue stretch—similar to the capsular end feel, tissue stretch is characterized by a firm yet slightly forgiving stop to movement. Further, a springy resistance may be appreciated at the end of movement. This end feel can be found normally at the end ranges of ankle dorsiflexion and metacarpophalangeal joint extension.
7. Empty—a feeling that there is nothing mechanically restricting the ability to complete passive motion except the subject's considerable pain. Normally not found in the body, this is associated with acute episodes or neoplasms.

Capsular Patterns. When a synovial joint is traumatized, inflamed, or immobilized, the capsule of that joint undergoes a unique pattern of proportional limitation. Each synovial joint in the body has its own pattern of proportional limitation, or capsular pattern. The presence of a capsular pattern is determined through the comparison of passive ROM measurements in a given joint. When a capsular pattern is identified, it is an indication that the capsule is involved in its entirety. However, a capsular pattern need not be present to have hypomobility in certain parts of the capsule.

Table 2-4 lists the common capsular patterns present in joints in the sequence of most to least restricted.

TABLE 2.4 **Capsular Patterns of Joints**

Joints	Capsular Pattern
Glenohumeral	External rotation (ER) > abduction (abd) > internal rotation (IR)
Sternoclavicular	Pain at extremes of range of motion (ROM)
Acromioclavicular	Pain at extremes of ROM
Humeroulnar	Flexion (flex.) > extension (ext.)
Radiohumeral	Flex. > ext.
Proximal radioulnar	Pronation (pro.) = supination (sup.)
Distal radioulnar	Pro. = sup.
Radiocarpal	Equal restriction all motions
Midcarpal	Ext. > flex.
Carpometacarpal (2–5)	Equal restriction all motions
Carpometacarpal (1)	Abd. > ext.
Metacarpophalangeal (2–5)	Flex. > ext.
Interphalangeal (1–5)	Flex. > ext.
Hip	IR > abd. > flex. > ext. > adduction ER
Tibiofemoral	Flex. > ext.
Talocrural	Plantar flexion > dorsiflexion
Subtalar	
Metatarsophalangeal (2–5)	Flex. > ext.
Metatarsophalangeal (1)	Ext. > flex.
Interphalangeal	Flex. > ext.
Atlanto-occipital	Ext. equal to side flex.
Cervical spine	Side flex. = rotation (rot.); ext.
Thoracic spine	Side flex. = rot.; ext.
Lumbar spine	Side flex. = rot.; ext.
Temporomandibular	Limited ability to open mouth

(Adapted from Kaltenborn FM: Mobilization of the Extremity Joints. Oslo, Olaf Norlis Bolchandel, 1980)

CONTRACTILE TESTING

Contractile testing is performed to assess the integrity of the contractile structures about the joint. Structures identified as being contractile include muscles, tendons, and tendinous attachments to bone.

Contractile testing is performed isometrically at a neutral midposition within the ROM to ensure that positioning alone does not stress inert structures. During isometric contraction, compressive forces are transmitted to the joint. These compressive forces may be minimized with proper technique and by applying slight traction before asking for a response.

The results of contractile testing will yield the following descriptions:

- Pain free and strong indicates normal muscle with no lesions.
- Painful and strong indicates a localized minor lesion in the contractile unit (e.g., tendinitis).
- Pain free and weak indicates a peripheral nerve lesion or muscle rupture.
- Painful and weak indicates serious pathology (e.g., fracture, unstable joint, or metastatic lesion). A painful and weak finding may also be found in chronic problems in which weakness may be secondary to disuse or pain.

All painful movements may represent an acute situation, fatigue, or emotional problems. In cases of the subject being too acute to tolerate an objective examination, it is best to treat symptomatically for pain and inflammation and defer the evaluation until valid information can be obtained.

Contractile findings may be positive during inert passive testing, a result of the muscle being stretched while performing passive ROM in the antagonistic direction. Muscles that test weak should be specifically examined with MMT to determine the degree of weakness.

Special Tests

LIGAMENT INSTABILITY

Ligament testing should be performed as part of the joint examination in the assessment of inert structures. Normal end feel or stability is based on and compared with that of the counterparts on the uninvolved side. Joint instability related to ligament laxity is graded on a scale of 0 to 3:

1. Zero instability indicates no difference in joint excursion between the ligament on the uninvolved side and the ligament on the involved side.
2. First-degree instability indicates an excursion of less than 0.5 cm of the involved ligament compared with the uninvolved ligament.
3. Second-degree instability represents an excursion of 0.5 to 1 cm of the involved ligament compared with the uninvolved ligament.
4. Third-degree instability indicates an excursion of more than 1 cm of the involved ligament compared with the uninvolved ligament.

TRACTION (DISTRACTION)

Traction or distraction in this instance is defined as a movement performed passively (by the examiner) that results in separation of joint surfaces. The clinical significance of assessing joint distraction is that it may yield information about the integrity of the joint.

1. If traction relieves pain, joint surfaces may be involved. The relief is probably secondary to the removal of compressive forces.
2. If traction increases pain, a complete or partial tear of connective tissue may be present.
3. If traction reveals limited range, there may be contracture of connective tissue.
4. If traction indicates increased range, the joint may be hypermobile, and supporting structures may be damaged.

COMPRESSION

Compression of the joint is accomplished by the examiner passively pushing the joint surfaces together. The clinical significance of assessing compression is to provide information about the state of the joint surfaces, as noted below:

1. An increase in pain associated with compression may be an indication of possible internal derangement or a loose body.
2. A decrease in pain noted during compression may be related to increased lubrication of the articular cartilage resulting from the compressive forces.

SCREENING EXAMINATIONS

Screening examinations are extremely helpful to the clinician in assessing the location and nature of the subject's complaints. Often it is difficult to determine whether the source of pathology is localized in the periphery or referred from the spinal nerve roots or whether the problem lies somewhere in the nervous system. An upper- or lower-quarter screen should be performed anytime there is a question of unclear involvement. The screening process is a combination of mobility and neurological testing of the cervical spine and upper limbs or lumbosacral spine and lower limbs.

Upper-Quarter Screening Examination. The upper-quarter screening examination begins with an examination of the cervical region. The examiner should do a postural assessment for any deviations, muscle spasm, or limited movement as the subject actively performs ROM movements. If all active ranges appear normal and the subject does not complain of pain, the motions are repeated, and the examiner applies gentle overpressure at the ends of the range. If there are no signs or symptoms during the active motion and overpressure, the cervical spine may be considered "clear." Resisted motions of the cervical regions are assessed next. The subject's cervical spine is held in neutral position while cervical movements are tested isometrically. If no associ-

ated pain or weakness is found during contractile testing, the musculature is considered clear.

Next the upper limbs are assessed for sensation, myotomal integrity, and reflexes. Upper motor neuron testing is also performed to rule out central nervous system involvement. As in the cervical region, active motion is performed at each peripheral joint, with passive overpressure if the patient is symptom free. The results of the screen will indicate whether there is a pattern consistent with a specific nerve root level or a specific localized problem. If there ap-

TABLE 2.5 Upper-Quarter Screening Examination

Cervical postural assessment
Active cervical range of motion
Passive overpressures, if no signs or symptoms are found actively
Contractile testing of cervical spine

Myotomal Testing

MOTION	MYOTOME
Cervical rotation	C1
Shoulder shrug	C2,3,4
Shoulder abduction	C5
Elbow flexion	C5,6
Wrist extension	C6
Wrist flexion	C7
Elbow extension	C7
Thumb extension	C8
Little finger abduction	T1
Finger adduction	T1

Dermatomal Testing

AREA OF SKIN INNERVATED	DERMATOME
No innervation to skin	C1
Posterior aspect of head	C2
Posterior aspect of neck	C3
Acromioclavicular joint	C4
Lateral arm	C5
Lateral forearm and palmar tip thumb	C6
Palmar distal phalanx middle finger	C7
Palmar distal phalanx little finger	C8
Medial forearm	T1
Medial arm	T2

Reflexes

TENDON	SPINAL CORD SEGMENT
Biceps	C5
Brachioradialis	C6
Triceps	C7

Pathological Reflexes
Wrist clonus
Ankle clonus
Babinski

(Adapted from Cyriax J: Textbook of Orthopedic Medicine, 8th ed, Vol 1, Diagnosis of Soft Tissue Lesions. London, Balliere Tindall, 1982)

pears to be nerve root involvement, the examiner must then thoroughly evaluate the musculature and sensory distribution supplied by that nerve root. If the results indicate a localized joint problem, that particular joint should be examined as outlined previously in this chapter. Table 2-5 outlines the sequence of procedures in the upper-quarter screen.

Lower-Quarter Screening Examination. As with the previous screen, active motion of the lumbar spine is assessed. If movement is symptom free, passive overpressure is applied at the ends of the range. The subject is then asked to perform functional muscle tests of heel walking (L5) and toe walking (S1). The lumbar spine is cleared if the active motion with overpressure is symptom free. The lower limbs are examined in the manner stated in the previous screen.

Table 2-6 presents the format for the lower-quarter screen.

TABLE 2.6	**Lower-Quarter Screening Examination**

Postural assessment of lumbar region
Active range of motion of lumbar spine
Passive overpressure if symptom free
Heel walking (L5)
Toe walking (S1)

Myotomal Testing

MOTION	MYOTOME
Hip flexion	L1,2
Knee extension	L3,4
Ankle dorsiflexion	L4,5
Great toe extension	L5
Ankle plantar flexion	S1
Bowel/bladder problems	S2,3,4

Dermatomal Testing

AREA OF SKIN INNERVATED	DERMATOME
Anterior thigh, 2–3 inches below anterior superior iliac spine	L2
Middle third of anterior thigh	L3
Patella and medial malleolus	L4
Fibular head and dorsum of foot	L5
Lateral side and plantar surface of foot	S1
Medial aspect of posterior thigh	S2
Perianal area	S3,4

Reflexes

TENDON	SPINAL CORD SEGMENT
Patellar	L4
Posterior tibial	L5
Achilles	S1

Pathological Reflexes
Babinski
Ankle clonus

(Adapted from Cyriax J: Textbook of Orthopedic Medicine, 8th ed, Vol 1, Diagnosis of Soft Tissue Lesions. London, Balliere Tindall, 1982)

Dermatomal Testing. A dermatome is defined as an area of skin innervated by a single segmental sensory nerve. Examination of the integrity of a dermatomal distribution should be performed in all apparent or suspected cases of peripheral nerve and nerve-root pathology and central nervous system involvement. In addition, thorough sensory testing should be done on subjects who demonstrate sensory abnormalities during an upper- or lower-quarter screening examination.

A chart illustrating the dermatomes of the body is shown in Figure 2-12.

Myotomal Testing. A myotome is defined as a distribution of musculature that is innervated by a given segmental motor nerve. Assessment of myotomes is performed in any pathological condition of nerve or muscle in which muscle weakness is apparent or suspected. Also, a finding of weakness during the upper- or lower-quarter screening examinations should alert the examiner that thorough muscle testing needs to be carried out on all of the muscles innervated by that particular segmental nerve. Myotomal testing should not be performed in musculature where spasticity is evident.

Explanation and illustration of the myotomes of the body are found throughout this text under the headings of Manual Muscle Testing.

Reflex Testing. Assessment of deep tendon reflexes is helpful in determining the integrity of the nerve root supplying a particular reflex. The involved side is compared with the normal, uninvolved side if possible. In cases of bilateral involvement, reflex assessment becomes more difficult, and clinical experience becomes a tremendous asset. Exaggeration of a reflex (hyperreflexia, hypertonic) is commonly associated with upper motor neuron disorders. Lower motor neuron disorders usually produce a diminished (hyporeflexia, hypotonic) or absent (areflexia) reflex response. A numerical grading system may be used to categorize reflex responses:

0 = absent reflex
1 = lessened or diminished reflex
2 = average or normal reflex
3 = exaggerated or excessive reflex
4 = clonus

Joint Play Movements

Joint play testing is performed as part of the testing of inert structures; primarily it assesses the integrity of the capsule. Joint play or accessory move-

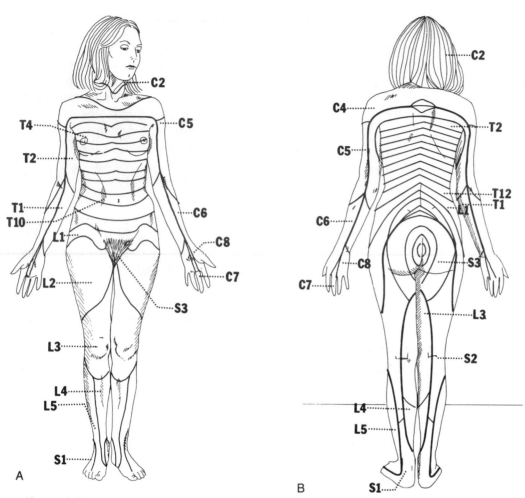

▲ **Figure 2.12** Dermatomal sensory pattern. (**A**) Anterior; (**B**) posterior. (Adapted from Haymaker and Woodhall: Peripheral Nerve Injuries, 2nd ed. Philadelphia, WB Saunders, 1953)

ments are movements that are not under voluntary control but are necessary for full and painless ROM of the joint. The testing techniques presented later in this text may also be used as treatment techniques.

Joint play should always be assessed in the open-packed position in which laxity of capsule and ligaments is greatest and bone contact is least. The greatest amount of joint play is available in the open-packed position. Accessory movements should not be assessed or treated in the closed-packed position, in which the ligaments and capsule are taut and the most bone contact occurs between the articular surfaces. The least joint play is evident in the closed-packed position.

In determining the direction of glide to be performed in restoration of joint play, the type of surface of the moving segment must be considered. The articular surfaces of synovial joints are described as either concave or convex. Arthrokinematically, the direction of gliding that occurs in a joint in which the moving partner is concave is the same as that of the bony movement. For example, when considering the radiohumeral joint to restore elbow extension, the concave superior surface of the radius normally glides dorsally on the convex capitulum of the humerus. This dorsal glide must be replicated if attempts at restoring joint play in extension are to be successful at the radiohumeral joint. Conversely, the direction of gliding that takes place in a joint in which the convex partner is moving is opposite the direction of bone movement. At the glenohumeral joint, the motion of abduction is accompanied by an inferior glide of the convex humeral head on the concave glenoid. Therefore, as the bone movement of abduction is characterized by the limb moving superiorly, the direction of glide of the humeral head will occur opposite to that and move downward. Table 2-7 lists the common open- and closed-packed positions of joints.

TABLE 2.7 Open- and Closed-Packed Positions of Joints

Joint	Open	Closed
Facet of spine	Midway between flexion (flex.)/extension (ext.)	Extension
Temporomandibular	Mouth slightly open	Mouth closed
Glenohumeral	55–70 degrees abduction (abd.); 30 degrees horizontal adduction (add.)	Maximum abd. and external rotation (ER)
Sternoclavicular	Anatomical	Full elevation
Acromioclavicular	Anatomical	Shoulder abd. 90 degrees
Humeroulnar	70 degrees flex.; 10 degrees supination (sup.)	Full ext. and sup.
Radiohumeral	Full ext. and sup.	90 degrees flex. and 5 degrees sup.
Superior radioulnar	70 degrees flex. and 35 degrees sup.	5 degrees sup.
Inferior radioulnar	10 degrees sup.	5 degrees sup.
Radiocarpal	10 degrees flex. and slight ulnar dev.	Max. ext.
Thumb carpometacarpal	Mid flex./ext. and abd./add.	Opposition
2nd–5th metacarpophalangeal (MCP)	Slight flex.	90 degrees flex.
1st MCP	Slight flex.	Max. ext.
1st–5th interphalangeal	Slight flex.	Max. ext.
Hip	30 degrees flex. and abd.; slight ER	IR > ext. > abd. >
Tibiofemoral	25 degrees flex.	Max. ext. and ER
Talocrural	10 degrees PF; mid inversion (inv.)/eversion (ev.)	Max. DF
Subtalar	Mid inv./ev.	Inv.
2nd–5th metatarsophalangeal	Slight flex.	Max. ext.
1st metatarsophalangeal	5–10 ext.	Max. ext.
1st–5th interphalangeal	Slight flex.	Max. ext.

(Adapted from Kaltenborn FM: Mobilization of the Extremity Joints. Oslo, Olaf Norlis Bokhandel, 1980)

REFERENCES

1. Alexander JL, Fuhrer MJ: Functional Assessment of Individuals with Physical Impairments. Baltimore, Paul H Brooks, 1984
2. Balogum JA, et al: Inter- and intratester reliability of measuring neck motions with tape measure and Myrin Gravity-Reference Goniometer. J Orthop Sports Phys Ther 10:248, 1989
3. Beasley WC: Quantitative muscle testing: Principles and application to research and clinical services. Arch Phys Med Rehabil 42:398–425, 1961
4. Bell BD, Hoshizak TB: Relationships of age and sex with range of motion of seventeen joint actions in humans. Can J Appl Sports Sci 6:202, 1981
5. Boone DC, et al: Reliability of goniometric measurements. Phys Ther 58:1355, 1978
6. Capuano-Pucci D, et al: Intratester and intertester reliability of the cervical range of motion. Arch Phys Med Rehabil 72:338, 1991
7. Claper MP, Wolf SL: Comparison of reliability of the ortho-ranger and the standard goniometer for assessing active lower extremity range of motion. Phys Ther 68:214, 1988
8. Cyriax J: Textbook of Orthopedic Medicine, 8th ed, Vol 1, Diagnosis of Soft Tissue Lesions. London, Bailliere Tindall, 1982
9. Daniels K, Worthingham C: Muscle Testing Techniques of Manual Examination, 5th ed. Philadelphia, WB Saunders, 1986
10. Defibaugh JJ: Measurement of head motion. Part 11: An experimental study of head motion in adult males. Phys Ther 44:163, 1964
11. Ellison JB, Rose SJ, Sahrman SA: Patterns of hip rotation: A comparison between healthy subjects and subjects with low back pain. Phys Ther 70:537, 1990
12. Fitzgerald GK, et al: Objective assessment with establishment of normal values for lumbar spine range of motion. Phys Ther 63:1776, 1983
13. Frese E, Brown M, Norton B: Clinical reliability of manual muscle testing: Middle trapezius and gluteus medius muscles. J Phys Ther 67(7):1072–1076, 1987
14. Gill K, et al: Repeatability of four clinical methods of measuring lateral flexion in the thoracolumbar spine. Spine 13:50, 1988
15. Grohmann JEL: Comparison of two methods of goniometry. Phys Ther 63:922, 1983
16. Hamilton GF, Lachenbruch PA: Reliability of goniometers in assessing finger joint angle. Phys Ther 49:465, 1969
17. Hellebrandt FA, Duvall EN, Moore ML: The measurement of joint motion Part 111: Reliability of goniometry. Phys Ther 65:1339, 1985
18. Hicks JH: Mechanics of the foot: 1. The joints. J Anat 87:345, 1953
19. Iddings D, Smith L, Spencer W: Muscle testing. Part 2: Reliability in clinical use. Phys Ther Rev 41:249, 1961
20. Jette AM: State of the art in functional status assessment. In Rothstein JM (ed): Measurement in Physical Therapy, p. 137. New York, Churchill Livingstone, 1985
21. Kaltenborn FM: Mobilization of the Extremity Joints. Oslo, Olaf Norlis Bokhandel, 1980
22. Karpovich PV, Karpovich GP: Electrogoniometer: A new device for study of joints in action. Fed Proc 18:12, 1982
23. Kendall FP, McCreary EK: Muscle Testing and Function, 4th ed. Baltimore, Williams & Wilkins, 1993
24. Lamb R: Manual muscle testing. In Rothstein JM (ed): Measurement in Physical Therapy, pp. 47–102. New York, Churchill Livingstone, 1985
25. Lehmkuhl LD, Smith LK: Brunnstrom's Clinical Kinesiology, 4th ed. Philadelphia, FA Davis, 1983
26. Lindahl O: Determination of the sagittal mobility of the lumbar spine. Acta Orthop Scand 37:241, 1966
27. Low JL: The reliability of joint measurement. Phys Ther 62:227, 1976
28. Manter JT: Movements of the subtalar and transverse tarsal joints. Anat Rec 80:397, 1941

29. Miller MH, et al: Measurement of spinal mobility in the sagittal plane: New skin distraction technique compared with established methods. J Rheum 11:4, 1984

30. Miller PJ: Assessment of joint motion. In Rothstein JM (ed): Measurement in Physical Therapy, pp. 103–136. New York, Churchill Livingstone, 1985

31. Moore ML: The measurement of joint motion. Part 1 Introductory review of literature. Phys Ther Rev 29:195, 1949

32. Norkin CC, White DJ: Measurement of joint motion: A guide for goniometry, 2nd ed. Philadelphia, FA Davis, 1995

33. Pact V, Sirotkin-Roses M, Beatus B: The Muscle Testing Handbook. Boston, Little, Brown, 1984

34. Pandya S, et al: Reliability of goniometric measurement in patients with Duchenne muscular dystrophy. Phys Ther 65:1339, 1985

35. Payton O: Research: The validation of Clinical Practice, p. iii. Philadelphia, FA Davis, 1979

36. Portek I, et al: Correlation between radiographic and clinical measurement of lumbar spine movement. Br J Rheumatol 22:197, 1983

37. Petherick M, et al: Concurrent validity and intertester reliability of universal and fluid-based goniometers for active elbow range of motion. Phys Ther 68:966, 1988

38. Reynolds PMG: Measurement of spinal mobility: A comparison of three methods. Rheum Rehabil 14:180, 1975

39. Rheault W, et al: Intertester reliability and concurrent validity of fluid-based and universal goniometers for active knee flexion. Phys Ther 68:1676, 1988

40. Rothstein JM: Measurement in Physical Therapy. New York, Churchill Livingstone, 1985

41. Stratford P, Agostino V, Brazeau C, Gowitzke BA: Reliability of joint angle measurement: A discussion of methodology issues. Physiology Canada, 36, 1 PP5-9 1984

42. Southwick HY, Keim KE, Flatery SM, Palmer ML: Intratester and intertester reliability of lumbar lordosis measurements in ballet dancers using a plurimeter, unpublished

43. Swartz MH: Textbook of Physical Diagnosis. Philadelphia, WB Saunders, 1989

44. Silver D: Measurement of the range of motion in joints. J Bone Joint Surg 21:569, 1923

45. Tucci SM, et al: Cervical motion assessment: A new, simple and accurate method. Arch Phys Med Rehabil 67:225, 1986

46. Wainerdi HR: An improved goniometer for arthometry. JAMA 149:661, 1952

47. White DJ, et al: Reliability of three methods of measuring cervical motion (abstract). Phys Ther 66:771, 1986

48. Williams M: Manual muscle testing: Development and current use. Phys Ther Rev 36:797–805, 1956

49. Williams R, et al: Reliability of the modified-modified Schober and double inclinometer methods for measuring lumbar flexion and extension. Phys Ther 73:26, 1993

50. Wintz M: Variations in current manual muscle testing. Phys Ther Rev 39:466, 1959

51. Youdas JW, Carey JR, Garrett TR: Reliability of measurements of cervical spine range of motion: Comparison of three methods. Phys Ther 71:2, 1991

52. Zimny N, Kirk C: A comparison of methods of manual muscle testing. Clin Management Phys Ther 7(2):6–11, 1987

3

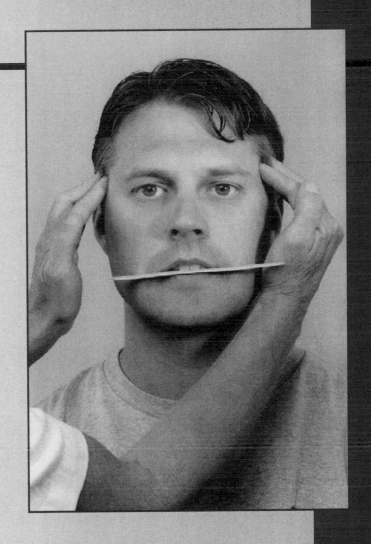

Pain

Jill Galper and Vincent Verno

INTRODUCTION

Pain is one of the most frequently cited reasons a patient is referred for treatment, yet it is elusive to evaluate objectively in clinical practice. A reason for this difficulty is that pain is a subjective experience, with multiple factors influencing the perception and expression of pain. Patients will often state that "you don't know the pain I'm in." This is correct because pain is clinically defined as "an unpleasant sensory and emotional experience associated with actual or potential tissue damage."[3]

Factors that influence an individual's present pain experience include the intensity of the stimulus and, to a greater extent, the interpretation of the stimulus.[7] Interpretation of pain is influenced by age, gender, ethnicity, culture, religious background, attention and distraction levels, environment, and the response of others to the pain behavior.[7] Additional factors affecting pain perception include previous experience with pain, responses learned from others, and perception of control over the cause of pain.[4,14]

Adding to the difficulty in pain management is that the transmission of pain is not fully understood. Two commonly proposed theories include the Melzack and Wall gate control theory and the theory of stimulation-produced analgesia.[14] These theories are reviewed in detail elsewhere, and further discussion here is beyond the scope of this chapter. Between the multiple factors influencing pain perception and the lack of understanding regarding the physical mechanism of pain transmission, it is no wonder that evaluating and treating pain can be so puzzling to the new and the experienced clinician. Both the pain and disability questionnaires will allow pain and function to be quantified so the therapist can monitor these aspects more accurately, comprehensively, and easily during treatment.

Reduction of pain is a common treatment goal, but only rarely is the patient's pain experience adequately quantified in an objective manner to ascertain if this treatment goal is being met. Because pain often impacts on function, any functional deficits should also be evaluated and monitored during the course of a treatment regimen. By doing this, the effectiveness and subsequent success of a treatment program can be clearly demonstrated. The documentation of functional deficits provides justification to insurance carriers and referral sources regarding the reasonableness and necessity for ongoing treatment, which is critical in this growing environment of managed care.

Pain and disability questionnaires can also identify patients displaying signs of inappropriate illness behavior (defined as "a behavior that is out of proportion to the impairment").[11] Identification of this behavior is important in the successful management of the patient, whose response to treatment may be otherwise frustrating and confusing to the clinician. The role of the clinician in case management is emphasized more now than in prior years of clinical practice, because of the focus on cost containment in health care. Clinicians are in an excellent position to assist in case management because of the consistent exposure to their patients on an ongoing basis. The battery of pain and disability questionnaires available offers the clinician tools to function more effectively as a multifaceted member of the health care system. It is therefore prudent to understand what tools are available and how to use them.

THE QUESTIONNAIRES

The following list of pain and disability questionnaires is not intended to be exhaustive, but rather representative of frequently used tools that have been shown to be valid and reliable. The purpose, administration, and scoring of each type of questionnaire are discussed in the text that follows. The instruments are divided into two groups, the basic questionnaires administered to all patients and questionnaires for those with low back pain.

Basic Questionnaires

NUMERIC PAIN SCALE[5,8,9]

Purpose. The purpose of the numeric pain scale is to obtain a subjective rating of pain intensity from the patient. This scale allows a relatively quick "measurement" to be obtained. The 10-point numeric scale has been shown to be more reliable than the 5-point simple descriptive scale.

Administration. The patient is asked to rate his or her current level of pain on a 0-to-10 scale. Zero represents a pain free state and 10 the worst pain imag-

---

▼ Types of Pain and Disability Questionnaires
The Basic Questionnaires
Numeric Pain Scale Visual Analogue Scale McGill Pain Questionnaire Pain Drawing
Low Back Pain Questionnaires
Dallas Pain Questionnaire Oswestry Low Back Pain Disability Questionnaire Inappropriate Symptoms Questionnaire

---

INSTRUCTIONS

Rate your major area of pain on the 0-10+ Pain Rating Scale. Write the number of your pain at the present time and your best day and your worst day over the past 30 days. Remember, the numbers refer to your pain, not how strong or weak you feel. For example: No. 1 is Very Weak Pain and No. 7 is Very Strong Pain.

10+	-- Maximal
10	-- Very, very strong
9	--
8	--
7	-- Very strong
6	--
5	-- Strong
4	-- Somewhat strong
3	-- Moderate
2	-- Weak
1	-- Very weak
0.5	-- Very, very weak
0	-- Nothing at all

YOUR PAIN RATING

Pain now _____

OVER PAST 30 DAYS { Best day _____
Worst day _____

▲ **Figure 3.1** The Borg Scale.

INSTRUCTIONS

Make a mark (—) across the line to indicate how bad your pain is between the extremes of "No Pain At All" on the bottom of the line and "Pain As Bad As It Could Be" on the top of the line. Make a mark across the line to indicate your <u>Pain Today</u> in your major area of injury.

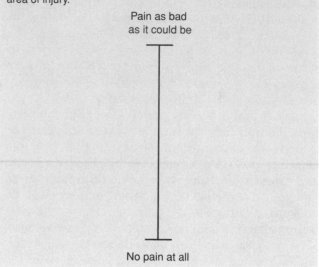

Pain as bad as it could be

No pain at all

▲ **Figure 3.2** Visual Analogue Scale.

---

inable. They are also asked to rate their best and worst levels of pain experienced over the past 30 days or since the onset of pain. This can either be performed verbally or by showing the patient the scale displayed with the additional descriptive words indicated (The Borg scale, Fig. 3-1).[2] Whichever method is chosen initially should be used during subsequent reassessments to ensure consistency.

Scoring. Scoring consists simply of recording the number identified by the patient.

Based on a 10-point scale, a score of 0 to 2 is considered a low pain level; 3 to 5, a moderate pain level; and 6 to 10+, a high pain level.[1] In general, one would expect to see alterations in movement patterns (e.g., speed/quality of movement) with ratings of 6 or higher.[1]

VISUAL ANALOGUE SCALE[1,5,8]

Purpose. Similar to the numeric pain scale, the visual analogue scale (VAS) provides a quantitative "measure" of a patient's pain intensity. This instrument consists of a 10-cm line with descriptors at each end. Although the VAS has been shown to be valid and reliable, disadvantages include some patients' tendency to mark the extreme ends of the scale, psychomotor problems that preclude marking the line with a pen or pencil, and the occasional difficulty patients may have transferring their subjective experience to a straight line continuum.

Administration. Patients are instructed to make a mark through the line to represent the amount of pain they are experiencing at the present time. This scale can also be used to reflect the patient's best and worst days of pain over the past 30 days or since the onset of pain (Fig. 3-2).

Scoring. Using a centimeter scale, the distance is measured on the line from the bottom anchor upward to the patient's mark and is recorded. The greater the distance from the bottom anchor, the greater the patient's pain intensity.

Based on a 10.5-cm scale, a score of 0 to 2.9 cm is considered a low pain level; 3 to 5.9 cm, a moderate pain level; and 6 to 10.5 cm, a high pain level. In general, one would expect to see alterations in movement patterns (e.g., speed or quality of movement) with ratings of 6 or higher.[1]

McGILL PAIN QUESTIONNAIRE[12]

Purpose. This questionnaire was designed by Ronald Melzack to provide quantitative measures of clinical pain that can be treated statistically.

INSTRUCTIONS

There are many words that describe pain. Some of these are grouped below. Look at each group of words and circle any word which describes the pain you are experiencing right now. Continue until you have finished all 20 word groups. You should choose only one word from every word group but you do not have to choose a word from every word group. If none of the words in a particular word group describe your pain, go to the next word group.

1.	2.	3.	4.
Flickering	Jumping	Pricking	Sharp
Quivering	Flashing	Boring	Cutting
Pulsing	Shooting	Drilling	Lacerating
Throbbing		Stabbing	
Beating		Lancinating	
Pounding			

5.	6.	7.	8.
Pinching	Tugging	Hot	Tingling
Pressing	Pulling	Burning	Itchy
Gnawing	Wrenching	Scalding	Smarting
Cramping		Searing	Stinging
Crushing			

9.	10.	11.	12.
Dull	Tender	Tiring	Sickening
Sore	Taut	Exhausting	Suffocating
Hurting	Rasping		
Aching	Splitting		
Heavy			

13.	14.	15.	16.
Fearful	Punishing	Wretched	Annoying
Frightful	Grueling	Blinding	Troublesome
Terrifying	Cruel		Miserable
	Vicious		Intense
	Killing		Unbearable

17.	18.	19.	20.
Spreading	Tight	Cool	Nagging
Radiating	Numb	Cold	Nauseating
Penetrating	Drawing	Freezing	Agonizing
Piercing	Squeezing		Dreadful
	Tearing		Torturing

▲ **Figure 3.3** McGill Pain Questionnaire.

Administration. The questionnaire consists of 20 categories of words used to describe pain or the patient's pain experience. Patients are asked to select the words that best describe their symptoms at the time of administration. They are to choose only one word per category and only the categories that are appropriate. Patients must follow the instructions thoroughly (Fig. 3-3).

The patient must understand the meaning of the words. This may require that words be defined for the patient. The clinician must be patient and understanding to avoid hurried decisions by the patient. It takes approximately 5 to 10 minutes for the patient to complete the questionnaire.

Scoring. The word columns are divided into four categories by Melzack.[12] Columns 1 to 10 describe sensory qualities of the pain experience; columns 11 to 15 describe affective (emotional) qualities of the pain experience; column 16 consists of evaluative words that describe the subjective overall intensity of the total pain experience; the words in columns 17 to 20 are considered miscellaneous descriptors.

Four types of data can be obtained from the questionnaire:

1. Pain rating index (S). This consists of the sum total of the scale values of all the words chosen in a given category (sensory, affective, evaluative, miscellaneous).

2. Pain rating index (R). In each column, the words are numbered from top to bottom, with the first word valued at 1, the second at 2, and so forth. The values of the words chosen by the patient are added to obtain a score for each category. A total score for all categories is ob-

tained by adding together the scores for each category.

3. The number of words chosen. The number of words chosen by the patient is counted and becomes the score.
4. Present pain intensity. This is described by Melzack as the number–word combination chosen as the indicator of overall pain intensity at the time of administration of the questionnaire.[12]

In common clinical practice, the most frequently used scoring methods use steps two and three. In other words, the total score and number of words chosen represent the typical values reported by clinicians.

PAIN DRAWING[13]

Purpose. The pain drawing is an aid to document the spatial distribution of a patient's pain symptoms.

Administration. The patient is given a pain drawing (Fig. 3-4) and is asked to use the symbols (denoting separate qualities of pain) to reflect his or her current distribution of symptoms. The number of pain symbols a patient has to choose from may vary, depending on different investigators. For example, the Ransford drawing uses four symbols (numbness, pins and needles, burning, stabbing), whereas other drawings may use up to six symbols (dull, burning, numb, stabbing/cutting, tingling, cramping). We are not aware of any studies addressing the number of symbols used as an indicator of a more reliable instrument.

Scoring. Different investigators have proposed various methods of scoring, which vary in complexity. An approach consistently used in interpreting a drawing reflects the expectation that a specific musculoskeletal dysfunction will produce an anatomical symptom pattern appropriate to the structure involved, with any radicular symptoms occurring along a specific dermatomal/myotomal/sclerotomal distribution. Widespread or nonanatomical pain can be used to identify potentially chronic or inappropriate pain patients.

The reference list provides sources detailing other scoring schemes.

Low Back Pain Questionnaires

DALLAS PAIN QUESTIONNAIRE[10]

Purpose. The Dallas pain questionnaire is designed to assess the impact of chronic pain on patients' lives. Developed by Lawlis and associates, this is a 16-item visual analogue tool with the purpose of evaluating a patient's cognition about the percentage that chronic pain affects four aspects of his or her life. These aspects include daily and work-leisure activities, anxiety-depression, and social interest. Each scale is anchored at the beginning, middle, and end, with the left side indicating no interference and the right side maximal interference.

Administration. Each of the 16 items contains its own VAS. The scales are divided into five to eight small segments in which the patient is asked to mark an "X" to indicate where the pain impact falls on that continuum (Fig. 3-5).

Scoring. Scoring of the four general factors is accomplished by assigning values for each item of 0 to the left-hand segment, 1 to the next segment, 2 to the next segment, and so on to the last segment. These individual ratings are summed and multiplied by a constant for a percentage of pain impact for that general area of life events. Each of the four aspects has its own multiplier, which is indicated on the questionnaire (Table 3-1).

INSTRUCTIONS

Indicate where your pain is located and what type of pain you feel at the present time. Use the symbols to describe your pain. Do not indicate areas of pain that are not related to your present injury or condition.

Key

///	Stabbing	XXX	Burning
000	Pins and Needles	===	Numbness

▲ **Figure 3.4** Pain Drawing.

INSTRUCTIONS

Mark an "X" along the line that expresses your thoughts from 0% to 100% in each section. Read each statement carefully. There are words to help you with each statement. If you need help, please ask.

Section I: Pain Intensity
To what degree do you rely on pain medications or pain relieving substances for you to be comfortable?

None	Some	All the Time

0% (_____:_____:_____:_____:_____:_____) 100%

Section II: Personal Care
How much does pain interfere with your personal care (getting out of bed, teeth brushing, dressing, etc.)?

None (no pain)   Some   I cannot get out of bed

0% (_____:_____:_____:_____:_____:_____) 100%

Section III: Lifting
How much limitation do you notice in lifting?

None (I can lift as I did)   Some   I cannot lift anything

0% (_____:_____:_____:_____:_____:_____) 100%

Section IV: Walking
Compared to how far you could walk before your injury or back trouble, how much does pain restrict your walking now?

I can walk the same   Almost the same   Very little   I cannot walk

0% (_____:_____:_____:_____:_____:_____) 100%

Section V: Sitting
Back pain limits my sitting in a chair to:

None, pain same as before   Some   I cannot sit at all

0% (_____:_____:_____:_____:_____:_____) 100%

Section VI: Standing
How much does your pain interfere with your tolerance to stand for long periods?

None same as before   Some   I cannot stand

0% (_____:_____:_____:_____:_____:_____) 100%

Section VII: Sleeping
How much does pain interfere with your Sleeping?

None; same as before   Some   I cannot sleep at all

0% (_____:_____:_____:_____:_____:_____) 100%

_____ × 3 = _____ %

Section VIII: Social Life
How much does pain interfere with your social life (e.g., dancing, games, going out, eating with friends)?

None; same as before   Some   No activities; total loss

0% (____:____:____:____:____:____) 100%

▲ **Figure 3.5** Dallas Pain Questionnaire.

Section IX: Traveling
How much does pain interfere with traveling in a car?

None; same as before	Some	I cannot travel

0% (_____ : _____ : _____ : _____ : _____ : _____ : _____) 100%

Section X: Vocational
How much does pain interfere with your job?

None; no interference	Some	I cannot work

0% (_____ : _____ : _____ : _____ : _____ : _____ : _____) 100%

_____ × 5 = _____ %

Section XI: Anxiety/Mood
How much control do you feel that you have over demands made on you?

(No change) Total	Some	None

100% (_____ : _____ : _____ : _____ : _____ : _____ : _____) 0%

Section XII: Emotional Control
How much control do you feel you have over your emotions?

(No change) Total	Some	None

100% (_____ : _____ : _____ : _____ : _____ : _____ : _____) 0%

Section XIII: Depression
How depressed have you been since the onset of pain?

Not depressed Significantly		Overwhelmed by depression

0% (_____ : _____ : _____ : _____ : _____ : _____ : _____) 100%

_____ × 5 = _____ %

Section XIV: Interpersonal Relationships
How much do you think your pain has changed your relationship with others?

Not Changed		Drastically changed

0% (_____ : _____ : _____ : _____ : _____ : _____ : _____) 100%

Section XV: Social Support
How much support do you need from others to help you during this onset of pain
(e.g., taking over chores, fixing meals)?

None needed	Some	All the time

0% (_____ : _____ : _____ : _____ : _____ : _____ : _____) 100%

Section XVI: Punishing Response
How much do you think others express irritation, frustration or anger toward you
because of your pain?

None	Some	All the time

0% (_____ : _____ : _____ : _____ : _____ : _____ : _____) 100%

_____ × 5 = _____ %

▲ **Figure 3.5** *(Continued).*

TABLE 3.1	**Dallas Pain Questionnaire Scoring**	
FACTOR	SECTIONS	MULTIPLIER
I. Daily Activities	I–VII	3
II. Work/Leisure Activities	VIII–X	5
III. Anxiety/Depression	XI–XIII	5
IV. Social Interest	XIV–XVI	5

Regarding interpretation of the scores for each category, the 50th percentile is a "significant" interference, especially in the event that the patient attributed a major portion of variance to emotional issues. When factors I and II are greater than 50% and factors III and IV are less than 50%, medical interventions alone appear to be beneficial. When factors I and II are less than 50% and factors III and IV are greater than 50%, a behavioral approach alone has been considered most beneficial. When all factors are greater than 50%, the combination of medical and behavioral intervention is appropriate.

OSWESTRY LOW BACK PAIN DISABILITY QUESTIONNAIRE[6]

Purpose. Disability can be defined as the functional limitation of a patient's performance. This questionnaire measures a patient's perceived disability as it relates to low back pain.

Administration. The Oswestry questionnaire consists of 10 sections, with six statements contained in each section. The patient marks the one statement in each section that describes his or her limitations most accurately. The questionnaire takes approximately 3.5 to 5 minutes to complete and 1 minute to score (Fig. 3-6).

INSTRUCTIONS

Mark in each section only the <u>one box</u> which applies to you. We realize you may consider that two of the statements in any one section relate to you, but please just mark the box which most closely describes your problem.

Section 1—Pain Intensity
( ) I can tolerate the pain I have without having to use pain killers.
( ) The pain is bad but I manage without taking pain killers.
( ) Pain killers give complete relief from pain.
( ) Pain killlers give moderate relief from pain.
( ) Pain killers give very little relief from pain.
( ) Pain killers have no effect on the pain and I do not use them.

Section 2—Personal Care (Washing, Dressing, etc.)
( ) I can look after myself normally without causing extra pain.
( ) I can look after myself normally but it causes extra pain.
( ) It is painful to look after myself and I am slow and careful.
( ) I need some help but manage most of my personal care.
( ) I need help every day in most aspects of self care.
( ) I do not get dressed, wash with difficulty and stay in bed.

Section 3—Lifting
( ) I can lift heavy weights without extra pain.
( ) I can lift heavy weight but it gives extra pain.
( ) Pain prevents me from lifting heavy weights off the floor, but I can manage if they are conveniently positioned (e.g., on a table).
( ) Pain prevents me from lifting heavy weights but I can manage light to medium weights if they are conveniently positioned.
( ) I can lift only very light weights.
( ) I cannot lift or carry anything at all.

Section 4—Walking
( ) Pain does not prevent me from walking any distance.
( ) Pain prevents me walking more than one mile.
( ) Pain prevents me walking more than $1/2$ mile.
( ) Pain prevents me walking more than $1/4$ mile.
( ) I can only walk using a stick or crutches.
( ) I am In bed most of the time and have to crawl to the toilet.

Section 5—Sitting
( ) I can sit in any chair as long as I like.
( ) I can only sit in my favorite chair as long as I like.

▲ **Figure 3.6** Oswestry Low Back Pain Questionnaire.

( ) Pain prevents me from sitting more than 1 hour.
( ) Pain prevents me from sitting more than 1/2 hour.
( ) Pain prevents me from sitting more than 10 minutes.
( ) Pain prevents me from sitting at all.

Section 6—Standing
( ) I can stand as long as I want without extra pain.
( ) I can stand as long as I want but it gives me extra pain.
( ) Pain prevents me from standing for more than 1 hour.
( ) Pain prevents me from standing for more than 30 minutes.
( ) Pain prevents me from standing for more than 10 minutes.
( ) Pain prevents me from standing at all.

Section 7— Sleeping
( ) Pain does not prevent me from sleeping well.
( ) I can sleep well only by using tablets.
( ) Even when I take tablets I have less than 6 hours of sleep.
( ) Even when I take tablets I have less than 4 hours of sleep.
( ) Even when I take tablets I have less than 2 hours of sleep.
( ) Pain prevents me from sleeping at all.

Section 8—Sex Life
( ) My sex life is normal and causes no extra pain.
( ) My sex life is normal but causes some extra pain.
( ) My sex life is nearly normal but is very painful.
( ) My sex life is severely restricted by pain.
( ) My sex life is nearly absent because of pain.
( ) Pain prevents any sex life at all.

Section 9—Social Life
( ) My social life is normal and gives me no extra pain.
( ) My social life is normal but increases the degree of pain.
( ) Pain has no significant effect on my social life apart from limiting my more
    energetic interests (e.g. dancing, etc).
( ) Pain has restricted my social life and I do not go out as often.
( ) Pain has restricted my social life to my home.
( ) I have no social life because of pain.

Section 10—Travelling
( ) I can travel anywhere without extra pain.
( ) I can travel anywhere but it gives me extra pain.
( ) Pain is bad but I manage journeys over 2 hours.
( ) Pain restricts me to journeys of less than 1 hour.
( ) Pain restricts me to short necessary journeys under 30 minutes.
( ) Pain prevents me from travelling except to the doctor or hospital.

▲ **Figure 3.6** *(Continued).*

Scoring. Each section is scored on a 0-to-5 scale, with 5 representing the greatest disability. The scores for all sections are added together, giving a possible score of 50. The total is doubled and expressed as a percentage. If a patient marks two statements, the higher scoring statement is recorded as a true indication of his or her disability. If a section is not completed because it is inapplicable, the final score is adjusted to obtain a percentage (e.g., nine sections scored for a possible total of 45).

The scores have been interpreted as follows:

1. 0% to 20%: Minimal disability
2. 20% to 40%: Moderate disability
3. 40% to 60%: Severe disability
4. 60% to 80%: Crippled
5. 80% to 100%: Bed bound or displaying exaggerated or inappropriate illness behavior

For more information regarding the above classifications of disability, refer to the article by Fairbank and colleagues.[6]

INAPPROPRIATE SYMPTOMS QUESTIONNAIRE[16,17]

Purpose. This questionnaire was designed to assist in the identification of inappropriate illness behavior in patients with chronic low back pain.

Administration. The patient is asked to answer yes or no to five simple questions. Two additional re-

▲ **Figure 3.7** Inappropriate Symptoms Questionnaire.

sponses are completed by the evaluator based on information obtained from the patient's history (Fig. 3-7).

Scoring. Each affirmative response is assigned 1 point with a maximum total score of 7 points. Two or more positive responses are considered abnormal and indicative of inappropriate illness behavior. Isolated findings are of no significance.

SUMMARY

The authors' goal in this chapter is to familiarize the new and the experienced clinician in the use of pain questionnaires. "Objectifying" the pain experience provides the clinician with another tool to help initiate and modify appropriate treatment, gauge progress or lack thereof, and ultimately ascertain the efficacy of a specific treatment approach. These instruments should always be combined with other tools, such as a comprehensive musculoskeletal evaluation and assessment of function. Focused and well-directed therapy treatment should be the utmost priority for today's clinician, particularly in these times of managed care and cost containment, when we should be viewing ourselves not solely as rehabilitation experts, but also as integral case managers.

Identifying and managing inappropriate illness behavior are two of the most difficult challenges a therapist will face in clinical practice. This can be difficult for even the most experienced therapist. As seen from some of the descriptions above, pain questionnaires can be helpful aids in this identification process. However, a patient's pain profile should not be based solely on the results of one pain questionnaire. Rather, it should be based on several tools that provide a composite picture of the symptom experience. The results of these pain tools must then be correlated with the results of the musculoskeletal evaluation for these tools to have their maximum value in identifying this behavior.

REFERENCES

1. Blankenship KL: Industrial Rehabilitation—A Seminar Syllabus, 2nd printing. Macon, GA, American Therapeutics, 1990
2. Borg GAV: Psychophysical bases of perceived exertion. Med Sci Sports Exercise 14:377–381, 1982
3. Bowsher D: Acute and chronic pain and assessment. In Wells PE, et al (eds): Pain Management in Physical Therapy, pp. 11–17. East Norwalk, CT, Appleton & Lange, 1988
4. Deyo RA, Walsh NE, Schoenfeld LS, Ramamurthy S: Studies of the modified somatic perceptions questionnaire (MSPQ) in patients with back pain: Psychometric and predictive properties. Spine 14:507–510, 1989
5. Downie WW, et al: Studies with pain rating scales. Ann Rheum Dis 37:378–381, 1978
6. Fairbank JCT, et al: The Oswestry low back pain disability questionnaire. Physiotherapy 66:271–273, 1980
7. Gersh M, Echternach JL: Management of the individual with pain: Part I, physiology and evaluation. PT Magazine 62:54–63, 1996
8. Grossman SA, et al: A comparison of the Hopkins pain rating instrument with standard visual analogue scale and verbal descriptor scales in patients with cancer pain. Journal of Pain and Symptom Management 7:196–203, 1992
9. Huskisson EC: Measurement of pain. Lancet 2:1127, 1974
10. Lawlis GF, Cuencas R, Selby D, McCoy CE: The development of the Dallas pain questionnaire: An assessment of the impact of spinal pain on behavior. Spine 14:512–516, 1989
11. Mechanic D: The concept of illness behavior. J Chronic Dis 15:182–184, 1967
12. Melzak R: The McGill pain questionnaire: Major properties and scoring. Pain 1:277–299, 1975
13. Ransford AO, Cairns D, Mooney V: The pain drawing as an aid to the psychologic evaluation of patients with low back pain. Spine 1:127–134, 1976
14. Sluka KA: Pain mechanisms involved in musculoskeletal disorders. JOSPT 24:240–254, 1996
15. Uden A, Astrom M, Bergenudd H: Pain drawings in chronic back pain. Spine 13:389–939, 1988
16. Waddell G, et al: Chronic low-back pain, psychologic distress, and illness behavior. Spine 9:209–213, 1984
17. Waddell G, et al: Nonorganic physical signs in low back pain. Spine 15:117–125, 1980

4

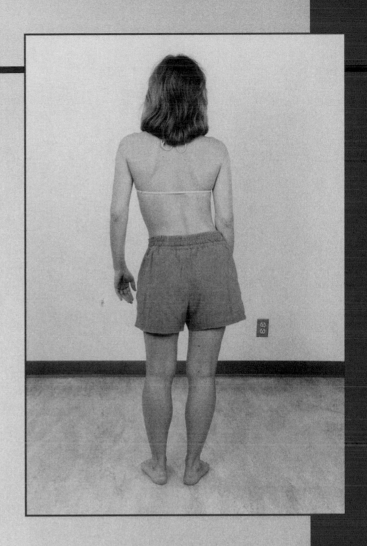

Posture

The ability to perform a postural evaluation accurately and thoroughly requires tremendous skill on the part of the examiner, because many postural abnormalities are extremely subtle in appearance. The examiner must be able to separate the parts of the body from the whole and, in turn, assess the sum of the parts in reference to their interaction in the entire anatomical structure.

Correct posture consists of alignment of the body with maximal physiological and biomechanical efficiency, which minimizes stresses and strains imparted to the supporting system by the effects of gravity. In correct posture, the gravity line passes through the axes of all joints with the body segments aligned vertically. The gravity line is represented by a vertical line drawn through the body's center of gravity, located at the second sacral vertebra (S2). It is the reference point from which gravitational effects on individual body segments are assessed.

The gravity line is an ever-changing reference line that responds to the constantly altering body position during upright posture. Although the gravity line generally does not pass through all joint axes of the human body, people with excellent posture may come close to fulfilling that criterion. Therefore, the closer a person's postural alignment lies to the center of all joint axes, the less gravitational stress is placed on the soft-tissue components of the supporting system.

ASSESSMENT

Not only is it ideal to have gravitational forces passing through the center of the joint axes, it is also advantageous for the muscles, ligaments, and other soft-tissue structures about the joints to be balanced. The strength and length of muscles involved in joint motion must be balanced. The balance is based on force couple (two or more translatory forces that in combination produce rotation) principles among muscles involved in the three cardinal planes of motion. When a force couple is out of balance, the segment moves off its axis of rotation, and there is faulty joint motion. The head, trunk, shoulders, and pelvic girdle are the most important segments to have in muscular and mechanical balance. They are the foundation from which forces are directed to the limbs.

Postural faults can be used as guidelines for identifying alterations in muscle and ligament length. For instance, round shoulders result from short or tight pectoralis major and minor muscles. Often one of the muscle groups may be tight and the antagonist elongated. For example, in lumbar lordosis, the iliopsoas muscle is tight and the abdominals are stretched. Synergistic muscles around a joint and the agonists may be unbalanced.

The primary hip flexors may be elongated, and the secondary flexors may be short. Minor alignment faults in posture limit motion and lead to tightness of muscles and other soft tissues. Muscles that are elongated often develop their maximal force in the stretched position and are weak in the normal physiological position. Kendall calls this condition stretch weakness. The body relies on the support provided by muscles and joints to minimize energy costs that further contribute to muscle imbalance and faulty posture.[1]

Alignment of body segments should be observed while the subject is standing still and during such movement as walking to detect faulty patterns of muscle activity and joint mobility. Ideally, each segment should move in the correct sequence relative to the adjoining segment, whether movement is taking place from distal to proximal segment or vice versa. During ambulation, for example, the correct timing and sequence of muscle contractions between the hip and knee joints or between the scapula and the glenohumeral joints are required for ideal movements. The better the quality of movement and the better the alignment of gravitational forces through the joint's axes, the better is the sequence of motion. When postural alignment improves, imbalances are minimized.

This chapter presents methods of evaluating standing posture using a plumb line or a posture grid. As a guide to segmental alignment, other static postures, such as sitting or getting on hands and knees, and dynamic walking postures are measured by observation and palpation. Skills necessary for accurate assessment of body alignment are acquired through an understanding of kinesiology and anatomy.

ANALYSIS

An organized, systematic approach to postural analysis involves viewing, from various perspectives, the body's anatomical alignment relative to a certain established reference line. This reference line, or gravity line, divides the body into equal front and back halves and bisects it laterally. Figures 4-1 and 4-2 demonstrate the anatomical structures that coincide with the postural reference line and the surface landmarks that coincide with established plumb lines.

In preparing to carry out postural assessment, it is important for the examiner to be aware of factors that will enhance the success and validity of the examination process:

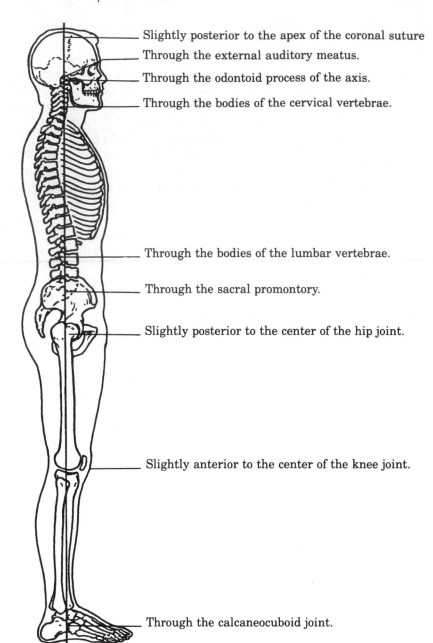

Slightly posterior to the apex of the coronal suture

Through the external auditory meatus.

Through the odontoid process of the axis.

Through the bodies of the cervical vertebrae.

Through the bodies of the lumbar vertebrae.

Through the sacral promontory.

Slightly posterior to the center of the hip joint.

Slightly anterior to the center of the knee joint.

Through the calcaneocuboid joint.

▲ **Figure 4.1** Anatomical structures related to postural reference line.

1. The postural assessment must be performed with the subject minimally clothed to ensure a clear view of the contours and anatomical landmarks used for reference. Men should be dressed only in shorts; women should wear a bra and shorts or a two-piece bathing suit. Subjects should not wear shoes or socks during the examination.

2. The examiner should instruct the subject to assume a comfortable and relaxed posture.

3. Subjects who use orthotic support or assistive devices for activities of daily living and gait should be assessed with and without them so that the examiner can determine the effectiveness of the devices in correcting posture.

4. The examiner should use whatever instruments are necessary to enhance the validity of the examination, including plumb lines, grids, rulers, tape measures, and goniometers.

5. The examiner should note relevant medical history and other information that may account for certain postural abnormalities. Also, any information regarding previous treatment relevant to planning a current program of management must be taken into consideration. Important information includes the following:

    Any history that accounts for present postural abnormalities (e.g., scoliosis, displaced fractures, congenital abnormalities)

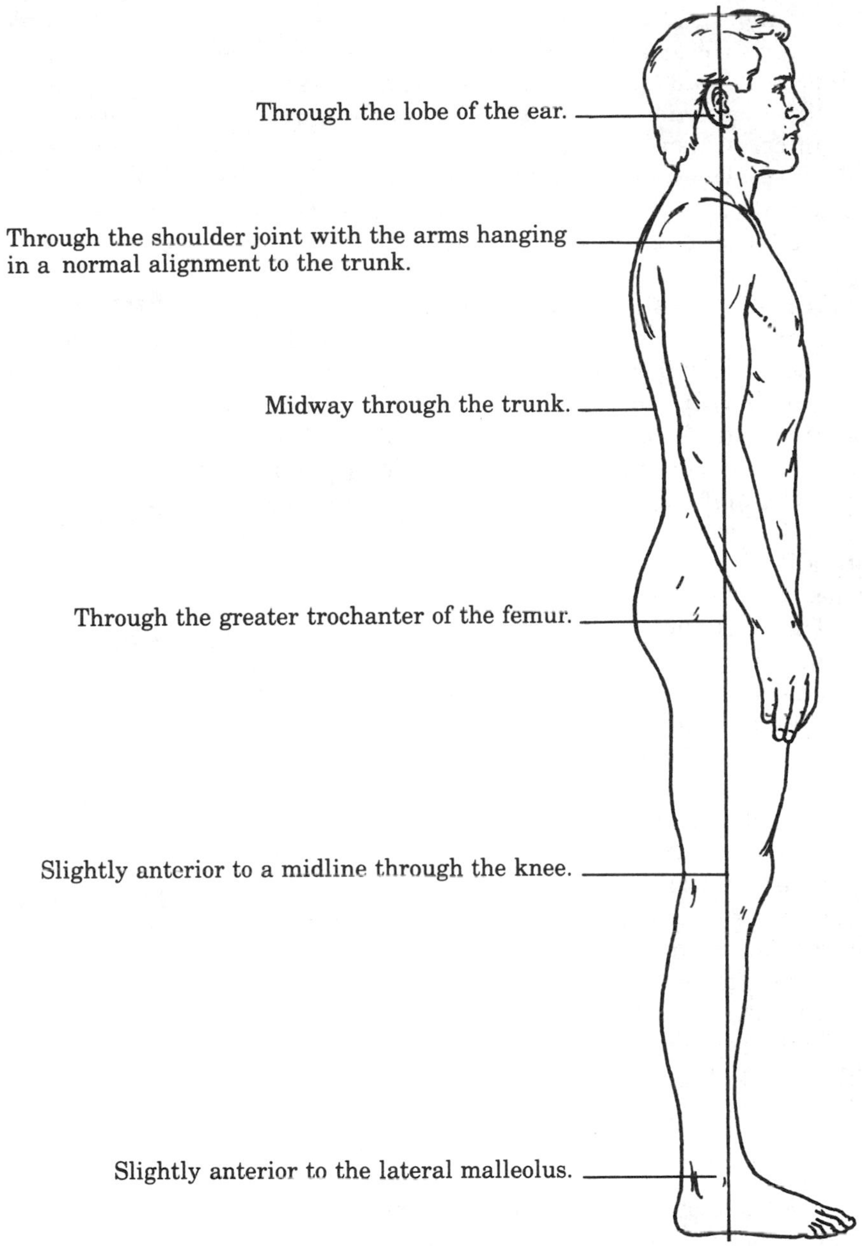

Through the lobe of the ear.

Through the shoulder joint with the arms hanging in a normal alignment to the trunk.

Midway through the trunk.

Through the greater trochanter of the femur.

Slightly anterior to a midline through the knee.

Slightly anterior to the lateral malleolus.

▲ **Figure 4.2** Surface landmarks related to dropping of plumb line.

A complete description of present symtoms

All previous treatment for the presenting postural complaints, including orthopedic and neurological therapy

The upper limb dominance of the subject, which is often responsible for asymptomatic postural deviations; for example, it is common for the shoulder and scapula on the dominant side to be lower.

Postural examination is most commonly performed by assessing the body's alignment in lateral, posterior, and anterior views. It is imperative that the examiner study the alignment of the body thoroughly from head to toe in each position. The components of the postural examination are described below.

STANDING POSTURE

Lateral View

Lateral postural assessments should be performed from both sides to detect any rotational abnormalities that might go undetected if observed from only one lateral perspective. The examiner should begin by looking at the head position relative to the previously established landmarks. Ideally, the plumb line should pass through the ear lobe and shoulder joint.

A common postural abnormality is "forward head," in which the head lies anterior to the plumb line. Forward head posture is many times associated with excessive cervical lordosis and, consequently, tight cervical extensor muscles.

The cervical spine should display normal lordosis. The examiner should note an exaggerated or a flattened lordotic curve. The examiner should next look at the shoulder area of the subject for its position relative to the plumb line reference. Shoulders that fall anterior to the plumb line are referred to as rounded shoulders—a faulty posture commonly associated with excessive thoracic kyphosis and forward head. As a result, weakness of the thoracic spine extensor musculature, the middle trapezius muscle, and the rhomboid muscles is usually present. Conversely, tightness of the intercostal, the pectoralis major and minor, and the subscapularis muscles becomes apparent.

The thoracic region should demonstrate a kyphotic thoracic curve, and the gravity, or plumb, line should approximately bisect the chest. Any abnormalities of the thoracic curve should be noted. The chest should be observed for such deformities as excessive prominence or depression. One such deformity includes pectus excavatum, or funnel chest, in which the anterior thorax and sternum are depressed. Barrel chest is represented by a large rounded rib cage and an increase of the overall anteroposterior diameter. Pigeon chest, or pectus cavinatum, gives the appearance of an anterior and downward projection of the sternum.

The abdominal region is bisected by the plumb line, and the abdomen itself should be relatively flat in the adult. A protruding abdomen is often implicated in lumbar pathologies and deserves attention.

The lumbar region should be examined for a normal lordotic appearance. Excessive lumbar lordosis is associated with an anterior pelvic tilt and consequent tightness of the hip flexor musculature. Decreased lumbar lordosis is accompanied by a posterior pelvic tilt and possible hamstring muscle tightness.

In examination of the hip, the plumb line passes posterior to the hip joint, creating an extension moment through the greater trochanter of the femur.

At the knee joint, the reference line should pass slightly anterior to the midline of the knee, thereby creating an extension moment. The subject should be observed for genu recurvatum, in which the plumb line will be found to lie far forward of the normal position. Conversely, a flexed knee posture secondary to bone or soft-tissue limitation in the kinematic chain should also be noted, in which case the plumb line falls more posteriorly than normal.

At the ankle, the plumb line lies slightly anterior to the lateral malleolus. Deviations observed may be the result of bone or soft-tissue pathology in the kinematic chain.

The feet should be examined for flat arches or supinated posture and for deformities, such as hammer toes or claw toes.

Summary of Lateral View Examination of Standing Subject and Possible Findings

HEAD AND NECK

Plumb Line. The line falls through the ear lobe to the acromion process.

Common Faults

Forward Head. The head lies anterior to the plumb line (Fig. 4-3).

Causes
- Excessive cervical lordosis
- Tight cervical extensor, upper trapezius, and levator scapulae muscles
- Elongated cervical flexor muscles

Flattened Lordotic Cervical Curve. The plumb line lies anterior to the vertebral bodies.

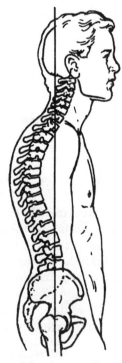

▲ **Figure 4.3** Forward head is usually accompanied by round shoulders. The external auditory meatus lies anterior to the plumb line. Cervical lordosis with accompanying forward head: The bodies of the vertebrae lie anterior to the plumb line.

Causes
- Stretched posterior cervical ligaments and extensor muscles
- Tight cervical flexor muscles

Excessive Lordotic Curve. The gravity line lies posterior to the vertebral bodies (see Fig. 4-3).

Causes
- Vertebral bodies and joints compressed posteriorly
- Anterior longitudinal ligament stretched
- Tightness of posterior ligaments and neck extensor muscles
- Elongated levator scapulae muscles

SHOULDER

Plumb Line. The line falls through the acromion process.

Common Faults

Forward Shoulders. The acromion process lies anterior to the plumb line; the scapulae are abducted (Fig. 4-4).

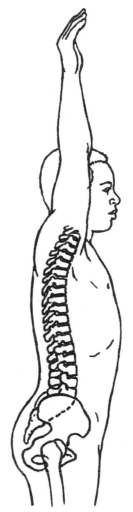

▲ **Figure 4.5** Increase in lumbar lordosis is demonstrated with the upper limbs raised above the head. Tightness of the latissimus dorsi muscle and thoracolumbar fascia prevents full shoulder joint flexion.

Causes
- Tight pectoralis major and minor, serratus anterior, and intercostal muscles
- Excessive thoracic kyphosis and forward head
- Weakness of thoracic extensor, middle trapezius, and rhomboid muscles
- Lengthened middle and lower trapezius muscles

Lumbar Lordosis. The lumbar region is flat as the subject raises arms overhead (Fig. 4-5).

Causes
- Tightness of the latissimus dorsi muscle and thoracolumbar fasciae

THORACIC VERTEBRAE

Plumb Line. The line bisects the chest symmetrically.

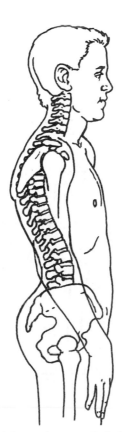

▲ **Figure 4.4** With forward, or rounded, shoulders, the acomion process of the scapula lies anterior to the plumb line.

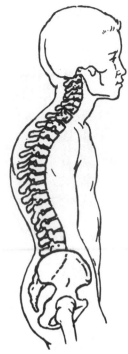

▲ **Figure 4.6** In the case of thoracic kyphosis, the thoracic vertebrae are overly flexed and the plumb line is anterior to the vertebral bodies.

Common Faults

Kyphosis. Increased posterior convexity of the vertebrae (Fig. 4-6).

Causes
- Compression of intervertebral disks anteriorly
- Stretched thoracic extensors, middle and lower trapezius muscles, and posterior ligaments
- Tightness of anterior longitudinal ligament, upper abdominal, and anterior chest muscles

Pectus Excavatum, or Funnel Chest. Depression of the anterior thorax and sternum.

Causes
- Tightness of upper abdominal, shoulder adductor, pectoralis minor, and intercostal muscles
- Bony deformities of sternum and ribs
- Stretched thoracic extensors and middle and lower trapezius muscles

Barrel Chest. Increased overall anteroposterior diameter of rib cage.

Causes
- Respiratory difficulties
- Stretched intercostal and anterior chest muscles
- Tightness of scapular adductor muscles

Pectus Cavinatum, or Pigeon Chest. The sternum projects anteriorly and downward.

Causes
- Bony deformity of the ribs and sternum
- Stretched upper abdominal muscles
- Tightness of upper intercostal muscles

LUMBAR VERTEBRAE

Plumb Line. The line falls midway between the abdomen and back and slightly anterior to the sacroiliac joint.

Common Faults

Lordosis. Hyperextension of lumbar vertebrae (Fig. 4-7).

Causes
- Anterior pelvic tilt
- Compressed vertebrae posteriorly
- Stretched anterior longitudinal ligament and lower abdominal muscles
- Tightness of posterior longitudinal ligaments and lower back extensor and hip flexor muscles

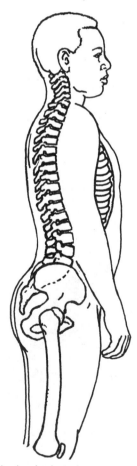

▲ **Figure 4.7** In lumbar lordosis, hyperextension of the lumbar vertebrae is associated with anterior pelvic tilt and hip flexion.

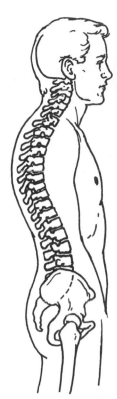

▲ **Figure 4.8** Swayback is the manifestation of lumbar flexion with associated posterior pelvic tilt, hip extension, thoracic kyphosis, and forward displacement of the pelvis.

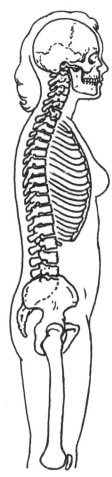

▲ **Figure 4.9** A flat back is evidence of increased lumbar flexion with associated posterior pelvic tilt and hip extension.

Sway Back. Flattening of the lumbar vertebrae (the pelvis is displaced forward) (Fig. 4-8).

Causes
- Thoracic kyphosis
- Posterior pelvic tilt
- Stretched anterior hip ligaments—hips hyper-extended
- Compression of vertebrae posteriorly
- Stretched posterior longitudinal ligaments, back extensors, and hip flexor muscles

Flat Back. Flattening of the lumbar vertebrae (Fig. 4-9).

Causes
- Posterior pelvic tilt
- Tightness of the hamstring muscles
- Weakness of the hip flexor muscles
- Stretched posterior longitudinal ligaments

PELVIS AND HIP

Plumb Line. The line falls slightly anterior to the sacroiliac joint and posterior to the hip joint through the greater trochanter, creating an extension moment.

Common Faults

Anterior Pelvic Tilt. The anterior superior iliac spines lie anterior to the symphysis pubis (Fig. 4-10).

Causes
- Increased lumbar lordosis and thoracic kyphosis
- Compression of vertebrae posteriorly
- Stretched abdominal muscles, sacrotuberous, sacroiliac, and sacrospinous ligaments
- Tightness of hip flexors

Posterior Pelvic Tilt. The symphysis pubis lies anterior to the anterior superior iliac spines (Fig. 4-11).

Causes
- Sway back with thoracic kyphosis
- Compression of vertebrae anteriorly
- Stretched hip flexor and lower abdominal muscles and joint capsule
- Tightness of hamstring muscles

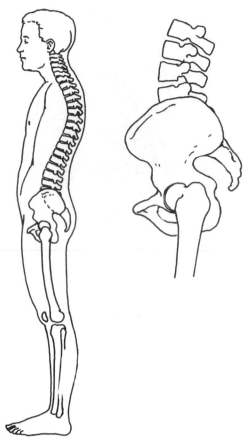

▲ **Figure 4.10** In anterior pelvic tilt, the anterior superior iliac spines project anterior to a vertical line parallel with the pubic bone. Lumbar lordosis is associated with the anterior tilt.

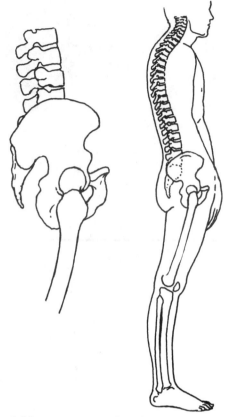

▲ **Figure 4.11** In posterior pelvic tilt, the anterior superior iliac spines are posterior to a vertical line parallel with the pubic bone.

KNEE

Plumb Line. The line passes slightly anterior to the midline of the knee, creating an extension moment.

Common Faults

Genu Recurvatum. The knee is hyperextended and the gravitational stresses lie far forward of the joint axis (Fig. 4-12).

Causes
- Tightness of quadriceps, gastrocnemius, and soleus muscles
- Stretched popliteus and hamstring muscles at the knee
- Compression forces anteriorly
- Shape of tibial plateau

Flexed Knee. The plumb line falls posterior to the joint axis (Fig. 4-13).

Causes
- Tightness of popliteus and hamstring muscles at the knee

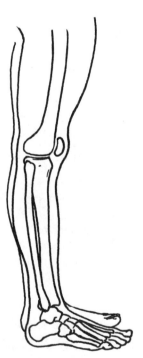

▲ **Figure 4.12** In genu recurvatum, the knees are hyperextended and the center of the joint lies posterior to the plumb line. The ankle joints are often positioned in plantar flexion.

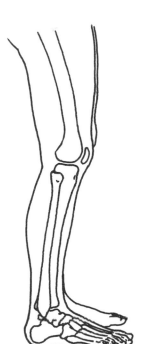

▲ **Figure 4.13** In knee flexion, the axis of the knee joint lies anterior to the plumb line. This condition is not as common as genu recurvatum.

- Stretched quadriceps and tight gastrocnemius muscles
- Posterior compression forces
- Bony and soft-tissue limitations

ANKLE

Plumb Line. The line lies slightly anterior to the lateral malleolus aligned with the tuberosity of the fifth metatarsal (Fig. 4-14).

Common Faults

Forward Posture. The plumb line is posterior to the body; body weight is carried on the metatarsal heads of the feet.

Causes
- Ankles in dorsiflexion with forward inclination of the legs; posterior musculature stretched
- Tightness of dorsal musculature
- Posterior muscles of the trunk contracted

Posterior View

In a posterior view examination, the examiner's plumb line divides the body into equal left and right halves. The following relationships are assessed.

The head should be upright, with no noticeable deviation to left or right. Lateral deviations of the head and neck may be related to torticollis or to other cervical dysfunction.

The examiner should observe the subject's shoulder height. It is considered normal to have an asymmetry in shoulder height related to hand dominance.

The scapulae are assessed for positional symmetry by observing the spines of the scapulae and the level of the inferior angles. Excessive abduction or adduction of one or both scapulae is assessed by measuring the distance from the thoracic spine to the medial scapular borders. "Winging" of the scapulae resulting from serratus anterior muscle weakness may also be evaluated from this view.

The subject's trunk is evaluated for lateral deviation to either side. Normally, the spine should lie in vertical alignment in the midline of the body.

A common cause of lateral postural deviations is scoliosis. The subject is assessed for scoliosis by marking the spinous processes from the second cervical vertebra to the lumbosacral junction. If a lateral curvature exists, the subject is instructed to bend forward from the trunk. Curvature that straightens with forward bending is termed *functional scoliosis,* whereas curvature that does not straighten is called *structural scoliosis.* Functional scoliosis is caused by muscle imbalances secondary to faulty posture or disease (such as cerebral palsy) and is not progressive. Structural scoliosis is progressive because of bony deformities. The thoracic region should also be examined for rib protrusions, which are commonly associated with scoliosis.

The pelvis and hip area are examined next for symmetry in levels of iliac crests, posterior superior

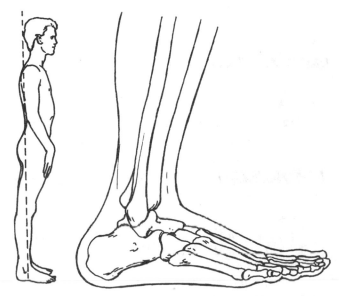

▲ **Figure 4.14** The subject with forward posture bears weight on the forefeet, and the entire body is deviated anterior to the plumb line.

iliac spines, gluteal folds, and greater trochanters. Asymmetries noted in this region may be associated with leg-length discrepancies, pelvic obliquities, scoliotic curves, hip pathology, or lumbar spine pathology. The examiner needs to be astute in understanding the pathomechanics and postural consequences of such pathologies so that he or she can make differential assessments accurately.

The region of the knee should be examined for varus or valgus postures. Valgus posture is one in which the distal segment deviates from the midline relative to the proximal segment. Varus posture is one in which the distal segment deviates toward the midline in relation to the proximal segment.

The tibias may be assessed for tibia varum as described in the section on biomechanical examination of the foot. The position of the Achilles' tendons relative to the lower third of the leg is also observed. A medially deviated Achilles' tendon is commonly found in people with pronated postures of the foot. The foot may also be assessed for pronated or supinated postures from this view.

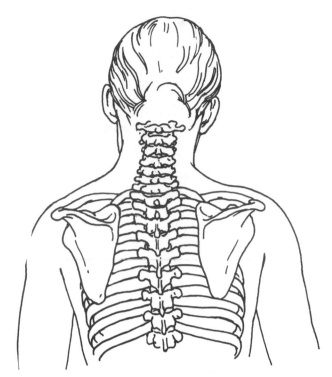

▲ **Figure 4.15** In head tilt, the head is deviated in the coronal plane to one side of the plumb line.

Summary of Posterior View Examination of Standing Subject and Possible Findings

HEAD AND NECK

Plumb Line. The midline bisects the head through the external occipital protuberance; head is usually positioned squarely over the shoulders so that the eyes remain level.

Common Faults

Head Tilt. Subject's head lies more to one side of the plumb line (Fig. 4-15).

Causes
- Tightness of lateral neck flexors on one side
- Stretched lateral neck flexors contralaterally
- Compression of vertebrae ipsilaterally

Head Rotated. The plumb line is to the right or left of the midline (Fig. 4-16).

Causes
- Tightness of the sternocleidomastoid, upper trapezius, scalene, and intrinsic rotator muscles on one side
- Elongated contralateral rotator muscles
- Compression and rotation of the vertebrae

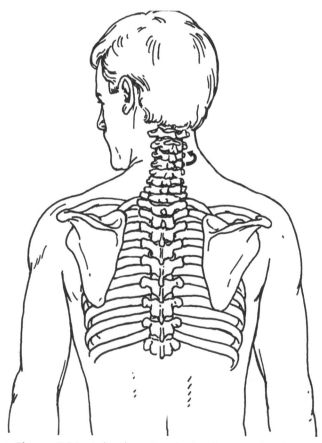

▲ **Figure 4.16** In head rotation, the head is rotated in the transverse plane to the right or left of the plumb line.

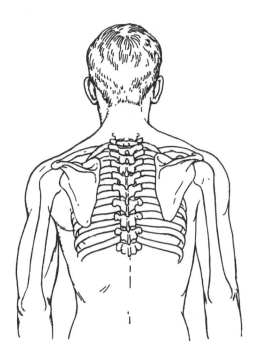

▲ **Figure 4.17** In dropped shoulder the shoulders are not level with each other in the coronal plane.

SHOULDER AND SCAPULA

Plumb Line. The line falls midway between shoulders.

Common Faults

Dropped Shoulder. One shoulder is lower than the other (Fig. 4-17).

Causes
- Hand dominance (dominant shoulder is lower)
- Short lateral trunk muscles short and high and adducted hip joint
- Tightness of the rhomboid and latissimus dorsi muscles

Shoulder Elevated. One shoulder is higher than the other.

Causes
- Tightness in the upper trapezius and levator scapulae muscles on one side; possible hypertrophy on the dominant side
- Elongated and weak lower trapezius and pectoralis minor muscles
- Scoliosis of the thoracic vertebrae

Shoulder Medial Rotation. The medial epicondyle of the humerus is directed posteriorly.

Causes
- Joint limitation in lateral rotation
- Tightness of the medial rotator muscles

Shoulder Lateral Rotation. The olecranon process faces posteriorly.

Causes
- Joint limitation in medial rotation
- Tightness of the lateral rotators

Scapulae Adducted. The scapulae are too close to the midline of the thoracic vertebrae (Fig. 4-18A).

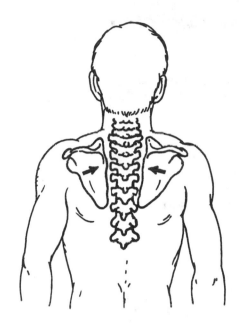

A

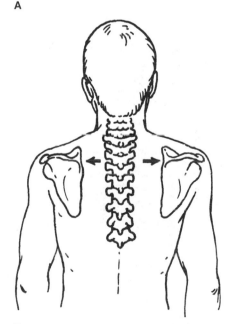

B

▲ **Figure 4.18** (**A**) In scapular adduction, the medial borders of the scapulae are adducted and elevated. (**B**) In scapular abduction, the medial borders of the scapulae lie laterally on the thorax. Scapular abduction is usually accompanied by rounded, or forward, shoulders.

Causes
- Shortened rhomboid muscles
- Stretched pectoralis major and minor muscles

Abducted Scapulae. The scapulae have moved away from the midline of the thoracic vertebrae (see Fig. 4-18*B*).

Causes
- Tightness of the serratus anterior muscle
- Lengthened rhomboid and middle trapezius muscles

Winging of the Scapulae. The medial borders of the scapulae lift off the ribs (Fig. 4-19).

Causes
- Weakness of the serratus anterior muscle

TRUNK

Plumb Line. The line bisects the spinous process of the thoracic and lumbar vertebrae.

Common Faults

Lateral Deviation (Scoliosis). The spinous processes of the vertebrae are lateral to the midline of the trunk (Fig. 4-20).

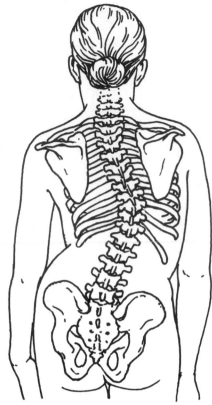

▲ **Figure 4.20** In scoliosis, the spinous processes of the vertebrae are deviated laterally from the plumb line. Uneven shoulders and pelvis are common in scoliosis.

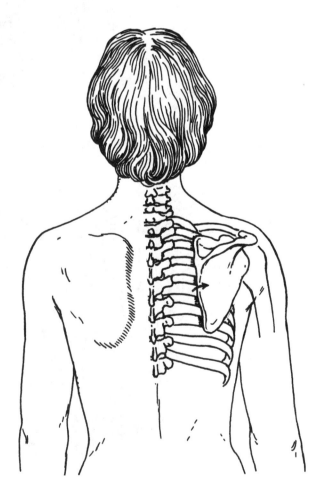

▲ **Figure 4.19** In winging of the scapula, the medial border and inferior angle of the scapula are prominent and are deviated into the transverse plane.

Causes
- Intrinsic trunk muscles shortened on one side
- Contralateral intrinsic trunk muscles lengthened
- Compression of vertebrae on the concave side
- Structural changes in ribs or vertebrae
- Leg-length discrepancy and pelvic obliquity
- Internal organ disorders

PELVIS AND HIP

Plumb Line. The line bisects the gluteal cleft, and the posterior superior iliac spines are on the same horizontal plane; the iliac crests, gluteal folds, and greater trochanters are level.

Common Faults

Lateral Pelvic Tilt. One side of the pelvis is higher than the other (Fig. 4-21).

Causes
- Scoliosis with ipsilateral lumbar convexity
- Leg-length discrepancies
- Shortening of the contralateral quadratus lumborum

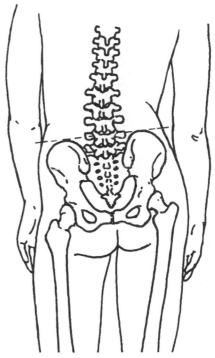

▲ **Figure 4.22** In hip abduction (coxa valga), the pelvis tilts downward on the femoral head to the same side as the abducted hip.

- Tight ipsilateral hip abductor muscles on the same side and tight contralateral hip adductor muscles
- Weakness of the contralateral abductor muscles

Pelvic Rotation. The plumb line falls to the right or left of the gluteal cleft.

Causes
- Tightness of medial rotator and hip flexor muscles on the rotated side
- Ipsilateral lumbar rotation

Hip Abducted. The greater trochanter is higher on the involved side (Fig. 4-22).

Causes
- Tightness of hip abductor muscles
- Tightness of contralateral hip adductor muscles
- Weakness of contralateral hip abductors and ipsilateral adductors

Hip Adducted. The greater trochanter is lower on the involved side (Fig. 4-23).

Causes
- Tightness of the hip adductor muscles
- Tightness of contralateral hip abductor muscles
- Weakness of contralateral adductor and ipsilateral abductor muscles

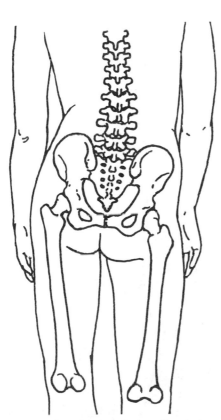

▲ **Figure 4.21** In lateral pelvic tilt, the pelvis deviates in the coronal plane to the right (left Trendelenburg's sign). Lateral tilt of the pelvis to the right is accompanied by relative left hip adduction and right hip abduction.

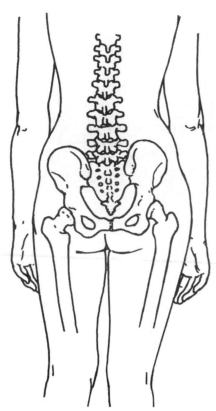

▲ **Figure 4.23** In hip adduction, the pelvis tilts on the femoral head to the side opposite the adducted hip.

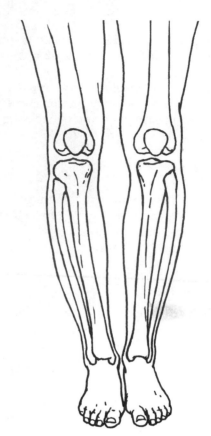

▲ **Figure 4.24** In genu varum (bowlegs), the center of the knee joint is lateral to the midline of the thigh and leg.

KNEE

Plumb Line. The plumb line lies equidistant between the knees.

Common Faults

Genu Varum. The distal segment (leg) deviates toward the midline in relation to the proximal segment (thigh); the knee joint lies lateral to the mechanical axis of the lower limb (Fig. 4-24).

Causes
- Tightness of medial rotator muscles at the hip with hyperextended knees, quadriceps, and foot everter muscles
- Compression of medial joint structures
- Femoral retroversion
- Elongated lateral hip rotator muscles, popliteus, tibialis posterior

Genu Valgum. The mechanical axis for the lower limbs is displaced laterally (Fig. 4-25).

Causes
- Tightness of the iliotibial band and the lateral knee joint structures
- Femoral anteversion

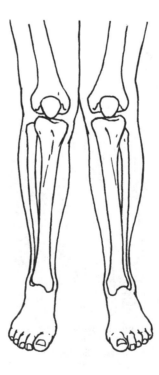

▲ **Figure 4.25** In genu valgum (knock knees), the center of the knee joint is medial to the midline of the thigh and leg.

- Lengthened medial knee joint structures
- Compression of lateral knee joint
- Foot pronation

ANKLE AND FOOT

Plumb Line. The line is equidistant from the malleoli; medially, a line (Feiss') is drawn from the medial malleolus to the head of the first metatarsal bone, and the tuberosity of the navicular bone lies on the line.

Common Faults

Pes Planus *(Pronated).* There is a decreased medial longitudinal arch, the Achilles' tendon is convex medially, and the tuberosity of the navicular bone lies below the Feiss line (Fig. 4-26).

Causes
- Shortened peroneal muscles
- Elongated posterior tibial muscle
- Stretched plantar calcaneonavicular ligament (spring)
- Structural displacement of the talus, calcaneus, and navicular bones

Pes Cavus *(Supinated).* The medial longitudinal arch is high, and the navicular bone lies above Feiss' line (Fig. 4-27).

Causes
- Shortened posterior and anterior tibial muscles
- Elongated peroneals and lateral ligaments

Anterior View

Relationships can be posturally assessed from an anterior view with the plumb line bisecting the body

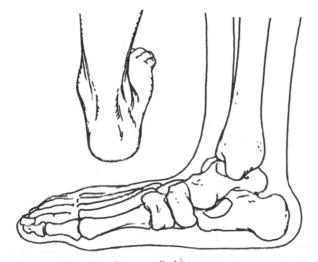

▲ **Figure 4.26** Pes planus, or flatfoot.

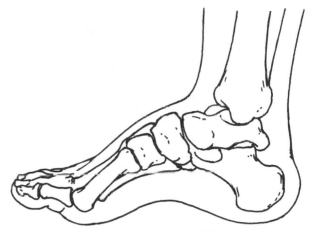

▲ **Figure 4.27** Pes cavus, or high-arched foot.

into equal left and right halves. The head and neck should lie in the midline without rotation and with no lateral deviation to either side. The mandibular region should be examined for symmetry. (See Chap. 8 for specific details.) The nose, the manubrium of the sternum, the xiphoid process of the sternum, and the umbilicus should all be vertically aligned in the midline. The margins of the upper trapezius muscles should be examined for symmetry. Noticeable unilateral hypertrophy may be indicative of upper extremity dominance, while atrophy of one upper trapezius muscle may be a result of pathology or disuse. The levels of the shoulder joint should be relatively equal, but upper limb dominance may slightly affect the symmetry. The bony components of the shoulder girdle, namely the sternoclavicular joint, the clavicle, and the acromioclavicular joint, should be examined for equality and symmetry. Prominences at either joint may be attributed to effusions secondary to joint trauma or to actual bony deformation resulting from subluxation or dislocation. Protrusions along the course of the clavicle may have occurred as a result of fractures.

The examiner assessing a subject with the upper extremities in the anatomical position should note the carrying angle of the elbow. Normally, this angle is 5 to 10 degrees in men and 10 to 15 degrees in women.

The examiner should examine the pelvic and hip region for symmetry of the iliac crest heights and notice the levels of the anterior superior iliac spines. As in the posterior assessment, asymmetries may be a result of leg-length discrepancies, pelvic obliquities, scoliosis, lumbosacral pathology, or hip pathology.

The patellae should be examined for deviations such as patella alta, "winking" patellae, or excessive lateral displacement. Most of these patellar abnormalities are related to pathomechanics within the kinematic chain of the lower extremity. The fibular heads may be palpated for symmetry, the tibia examined for torsion, and the malleoli observed for equal height.

The feet may again be examined for pronation and supination. Normally when a person stands still, there is a tendency for the feet to point outward. The angle of toeing out averages 5 to 7 degrees. The feet also may be examined in this view for such deformities as hammer toes and claw toes. The great toe should also be assessed for hallux valgus.

Summary of Anterior View Examination of Standing Subject and Possible Findings

HEAD AND NECK

Plumb Line. The line bisects the head at the midline into equal halves.

Common Faults

Lateral Tilt. See section on posterior view.

Rotation. See section on posterior view.

Mandibular Asymmetry. The upper and lower teeth are not aligned, and the mandible is deviated to one side.

Causes
- Tightness of the mastication muscles on one side
- Stretched mastication muscles on the contralateral side
- Malalignment of temporomandibular joints
- Malalignment of teeth

SHOULDERS

Plumb Line. A vertical line bisects the sternum and xiphoid process.

Common Faults

Shoulder Dropped or Elevated. See section on posterior view.

Clavicle and Joint Asymmetry

Causes
- Prominences secondary to joint trauma
- Subluxation or dislocation of sternoclavicular or acromioclavicular joints
- Clavicular fractures

ELBOWS

A line bisects the upper limbs and forms an angle of 5 to 15 degrees laterally at the elbow with the elbow extended. This angle is normal and is referred to as the carrying angle.

Common Faults

Cubitus Valgus. The forearm deviates laterally from the arm at an angle greater than 15 degrees for the woman and 10 degrees for the man.

Causes
- Elbow hyperextension
- Distal displacement of the trochlea in relation to the capitulum of the humerus
- Stretched ulnar collateral ligament

Cubitus Varus. The forearm deviates medially (adducts) from the arm at an angle of less than 15 degrees for the woman and 10 degrees for the man.

Causes
- Fracture about the elbow joint
- Inferior displacement of the humeral capitulum
- Stretched radial collateral ligament

HIP

Common Faults

Lateral Rotation. The patellae angle out (Fig. 4-28).

Causes
- Tightness of the lateral rotators and the gluteus maximus muscles
- Weakness of the medial rotator muscles
- Femoral retroversion
- Internal tibial torsion (compensated)

Medial Rotation. The patellae face inward.

Causes
- Tightness of the iliotibial band and the medial rotator muscles
- Weakness of the lateral rotator muscles
- Femoral anteversion
- External tibial torsion (compensated)

KNEE

Plumb Line. The legs are equidistant from a vertical line through the body.

Common Faults

External Tibial Torsion. Normally the distal end of the tibia is rotated laterally 25 degrees from the

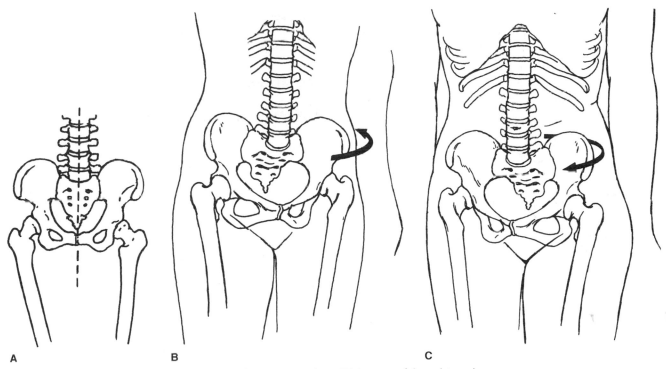

A   B   C

▲ **Figure 4.28** (**A**) Normal position for hips in the transverse plane; (**B**) Rotation of the pelvis to the right results in lateral rotation of the left hip joint. (**C**) Rotation of the pelvis to the left results in medial rotation of the left hip joint.

proximal end; excess of 25 degrees rotation is an increase in torsion and is referred to as lateral tibial torsion (toeing out) (Fig. 4-29).

Causes
- Tightness of the tensor fasciae latae muscle or iliotibial band

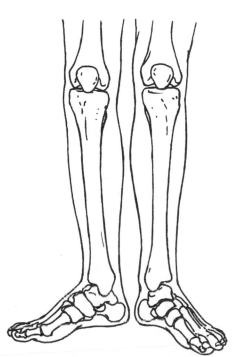

▲ **Figure 4.29** External torsion of both tibia.

- Bony malalignment (e.g., fracture)
- Cruciate ligament tear
- Femoral retroversion

Internal Tibial Torsion. The feet face directly forward or inward.

Causes
- Tightness of the medial hamstrings and gracilis muscles
- Structural deformities of the tibia (traumatic or developmental)
- Anterior cruciate ligament tear
- Femoral anteversion
- Foot pronation
- Genu valgus

ANKLE AND FOOT

Common Faults

Hallux Valgus. Lateral deviation of the first digit at the metatarsophalangeal joint (Fig. 4-30).

Causes
- Excessive medial bone growth of the first metatarsal head
- Joint dislocation
- Tight adductor hallucis muscle
- Stretched abductor hallucis muscle

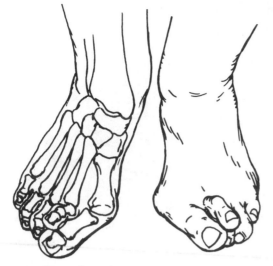

▲ **Figure 4.30** Hallux valgus.

Claw Toes. Hyperextension of the metatarsophalangeal joint and flexion of the proximal interphalangeal joints associated with pes cavus (Fig. 4-31).

Causes
- Tightness of the long toe flexors
- Shortness of the toe extensor muscles

Hammer Toes. Hyperextension of the metatarsophalangeal joints and distal interphalangeal joints and flexion of the proximal interphalangeal joints (Fig. 4-32).

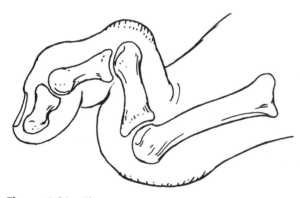

▲ **Figure 4.31** Claw toe.

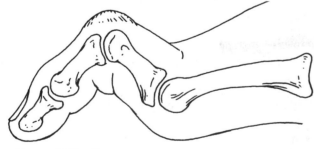

▲ **Figure 4.32** Hammer toe.

Causes
- Shortness of the toe extensors
- Lengthened lumbricals

STANDING ON ONE FOOT

Anteroposterior View

TRUNK

Common Faults

Hip Drop. Lateral tilt to the non–weight-bearing side over 5 degrees.

Cause
- Weakness of the weight-bearing gluteus medius muscle.

Lateral Trunk Shift. Toward the weight-bearing side greater than 5 degrees.

Causes
- Weakness of weight-bearing gluteus medius muscle
- Pain on weight-bearing side

Foot Pronation. See section on posterior view.

SITTING POSTURE

HIP AND PELVIS

Observation. The pelvis assumes a posterior tilt with the posterior inferior iliac spines in the same horizontal plane as the superior pubic ramus.

Common Faults

Posterior Pelvic Tilt. The superior pubic ramus is superior to the posterior inferior iliac spines.

Causes
- Lumbar vertebrae flexed excessively
- Tightness of the hamstring muscles
- Elongated low back extensors

Anterior Pelvic Tilt. The superior pubic ramus lies inferior to the posterior inferior iliac spine.

Causes
- Tightness of low back extensor muscles
- Lengthened hip extensor muscles
- Excessive lumbar lordosis

ON HANDS AND KNEES

Observation. The thoracic and lumbar vertebrae are level, the scapulae lie flat on the thorax, the hips are flexed 90 degrees and aligned over the knee joints, and ankles are in plantar flexion.

Common Faults

Winging of Scapulae. The vertebral border and inferior angle are lifted off the thorax.

Cause
- Weakness of the serratus anterior muscle.

Lumbar Lordosis. Increase in the normal curves.

Causes
- Weak or elongated abdominal muscles
- Tightness of low back extensor muscles and posterior longitudinal ligaments

Thoracic Kyphosis. Arched thoracic vertebrae.

Causes
- Tightness of anterior chest muscles and anterior longitudinal ligaments
- Weakness of upper back extensor muscles
- Vertebral deformities

Trunk Rotation or Lateral Flexion. Deviation from the midline.

Causes
- Structural or functional scoliosis
- Pelvic rotation
- Intrinsic trunk muscle weakness

Decreased Hip Flexion. Less than 90 degrees.

Causes
- Tightness of hip extensor muscles
- Increase in lumbar flexion
- Increase in posterior pelvic tilt

Increased Hip Flexion. Greater than 90 degrees.

Causes
- Weakness of hip extensor muscles
- Increase in lumbar lordosis
- Increase in anterior pelvic tilt

Hip Rotation. Not in neutral position.

Causes
- Tightness of rotator muscles
- Lumbar vertebral rotation
- Pelvic rotation left or right

External Tibial Rotation. The foot angles outward more than 25 degrees.

Causes
- Tightness of iliotibial band
- Bony deformity

Ankle Dorsiflexion. The dorsum of the foot is not resting on the floor.

Causes
- Lengthened heel cord
- Weakness of gastrocnemius and soleus muscles
- Tightness of the dorsiflexor muscles

Ankle Inversion. Subtalar and transtarsal joints are not in a neutral position, and the forefoot angles inward.

Causes
- Lengthened peroneals
- Tightness of posterior and anterior tibial muscles

Ankle Eversion. Subtalar and transtarsal joints are not in a neutral position and the forefoot angles outward.

Causes
- Lengthened anterior and posterior tibial muscles
- Tightness of peroneals

GAIT

Observation. Dynamic posture may be evaluated by watching the subject walk; observations are organized in a methodical manner (from head to toes or vice versa).

Common Faults

Stride Length and Time Inequality. Stance phase is longer on one side.

Causes
- Pain
- Lack of trunk and pelvic rotation
- Weakness of lower limb muscles
- Limitation of lower limb joints
- Uncoordinated muscle control
- Increased muscle tone

Slow Cadence. Less than average for person's age, occupation.

Causes
- Generalized weakness
- Pain or joint limitations
- Lack of voluntary motor control

Stance Phase. Less than 60% of gait cycle.

Causes
- Restricted plantar or dorsiflexion motion
- Painful or restricted knee and hip joints

Head. Erect and in the midline; for deviations, refer to discussion of standing posture.

Shoulders. Horizontal and coordinated with the arm swing; each shoulder swings reciprocally with equal motion.

Inequality

Causes
- Shoulder pathology
- Generalized muscle weakness or lack of coordination
- Emotional disturbance

Deviations. Refer to section on standing posture.

Trunk. Erect, rotates slightly with the pelvis and shoulders; for deviations, refer to discussion of standing posture.

Pelvis. Rotates slightly in the transverse plane during the swing phase of gait; drops (laterally tilts) 4 or 5 degrees on the opposite side during the stance phase; tilts anteriorly slightly during the gait cycle, except during stance, when it is level.

Excessive Pelvic Rotation. Increased rotation in the transverse plane beyond 5 degrees.

Causes
- Tight hip flexor muscles on the same side
- Limited hip joint flexion

Excessive Pelvic Drop. Lateral tilt of the pelvis beyond 5 degrees.

Causes
- Weakness of the hip abductors on the stance side
- Tightness in the quadratus lumborum on the swing side

Posterior Pelvic Tilt. Any posterior pelvic tilt in the sagittal plane.

Causes
- Sway back and flat back postures
- Tightness of the hamstring muscles
- Weakness of the hip flexor muscles

Anterior Pelvic Tilt. Occurring in the stance phase, a tilt in the sagittal plane beyond 5 degrees.

Causes
- Tightness of the hip flexor and low back extensor muscles
- Lumbar lordosis

Hip. Rotates medially during swing to midstance then rotates laterally through terminal stance.

Femur Medially Rotated. The hip remains medially rotated through terminal stance.

Causes
- Tightness of the iliotibial band
- Weakness of the lateral rotator muscles
- Femoral anteversion
- Tightness of the medial rotators

Femur Laterally Rotated. The hip remains rotated laterally during the swing phase.

Causes
- Tightness of the lateral rotators
- Femoral retroversion
- Weakness of the medial rotators

Abduction. The base of support is wide in stance, or the subject circumducts during the swing phase.

Causes
- Decrease in hip flexion or dorsiflexion motion
- Weakness in the adductor muscles
- General body weakness
- General lack of coordination or balance
- Coxa vara

Adduction. The base of support is narrowed.

Causes
- Increased tone in the adductor muscles
- Genu valgum or coxa valga deformity
- Weakness of the abductor muscles

Flexion. Exaggerated flexion during the swing phase.

Causes
- Weakness in the ankle dorsiflexor muscles
- Weakness of the hamstring muscles
- Increased hip flexor muscle tone

Knees. Extension of the knee at initial contact, followed by flexion at midstance, followed again by extension at terminal stance and flexion at preswing.

Hyperextension. Complete extension/hyperextension at midstance.

Causes
- Weakness in the quadriceps muscles
- Spasticity in the quadriceps muscles
- Weakness of the hamstring muscles
- Joint deformity

Restricted Extension. Loss of initial contact and plantar flexion.

Causes
- Joint disorders
- Meniscal derangement
- Weakness of hip extensor muscles

Exaggerated Flexion. Increase in knee flexion during the swing and midstance phases.

Causes
- Increased tone in the hamstring muscles
- Weakness of the ankle dorsiflexor muscles
- Increased tone in the hip flexor muscles

Genu Valgum. Patellae face inward.

Causes
- Femoral anteversion
- Foot pronation
- Tight iliotibial band

Genu Varum. Patellae face outward.

Causes
- Femoral retroversion
- Foot supination

Ankle. Dorsiflexion at initial contact; foot flat in midstance; dorsiflexion at terminal stance and plantar flexion at preswing.

Preswing Exaggerated. Subject walks on the toes (pes equinus) or demonstrates increase in plantar flexion.

Causes
- Pes equinus deformity
- Tightness in gastrocsoleus muscles
- Increased tone in the gastrocsoleus muscles
- Weakness in the dorsiflexor muscles
- Knee flexion increased during stance

Preswing Decreased. Subject lacks plantar flexion at terminal stance and preswing.

Causes
- Weakness of the plantar flexor muscles
- Ankle or foot pain

Foot Slap. Inability to maintain dorsiflexion at initial contact.

Causes
- Weakness of the dorsiflexor muscles
- Lack of lower limb proprioception

Foot Drop. Lack of adequate dorsiflexion during the swing phase.

Causes
- Weakness of ankle dorsiflexor muscles
- Loss of hip extension

Excessive Dorsiflexion. The subject walks on heels (pes calcaneus) or has increase in dorsiflexion during the swing phase of gait.

Causes
- Weakness of the gastrocsoleus muscle group
- Tightness of the dorsiflexor muscles
- Increased muscle tone in the dorsiflexors
- Pes calcaneus deformity

Pes Valgus. The foot turns outward, and the ankle angles medially.

Causes
- Weakness of the posterior tibial and medial ankle ligaments
- Pes planus deformity
- Femoral anteversion

Pes Varus. The ankle is angled laterally; subject walks on the lateral border of the foot.

Causes
- Weakness of the lateral compartment muscles
- Increased muscle tone in the invertors of the ankle

Foot. Weight on the lateral heel on initial contact, along the lateral border of the foot during midstance, and across the metatarsal heads during terminal stance and preswing phases.

Pronation. Decrease in the medial longitudinal arch.

Causes
- Hypermobility of foot
- Femoral anteversion
- Genu valgum
- Weakness of dorsiflexor muscles
- Tight heel cords

REFERENCES

1. Kendall HO, Kendall FP: Posture and Pain. Malabar, Robert E. Krieger, 1981.

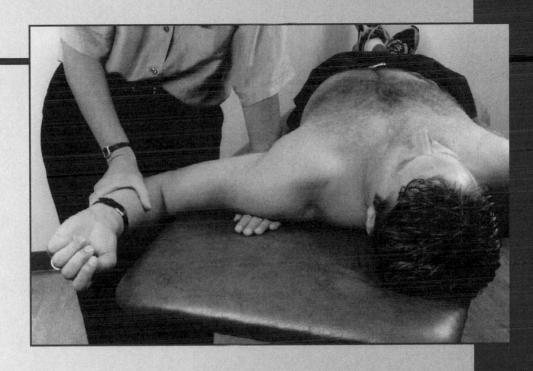

5

Shoulder

The humerus, clavicle, scapula, and sternum comprise the shoulder girdle. The bones articulate to form three joints—sternoclavicular, acromioclavicular, and glenohumeral. The scapula also forms a physiological joint by moving on the thorax, the scapulothoracic joint. These joints function in a closed-chain fashion: As the humerus moves in the glenoid fossa, the scapula rotates on the thorax and the clavicle moves on the sternum. The glenohumeral joint is a ball-and-socket synovial joint and has three degrees of freedom of movement. The sternoclavicular joint has been identified as a saddletype synovial joint with three degrees of freedom of movement. The acromioclavicular joint is a plane synovial joint having the ability to produce motion in three planes.

The shoulder complex has developed mobility at the expense of stability. The head of the humerus hangs loosely in the glenoid fossa, and the only attachment of the upper limb to the trunk is at the sternoclavicular joint. Stabilization at the shoulder is provided by the ligaments—and primarily the tendons—of the muscle that blend into the joint capsule.

GONIOMETRY

Shoulder

SHOULDER FLEXION

Motion occurs at the shoulder (glenohumeral) joint in the sagittal plane and is accompanied by motions at the sternoclavicular, acromioclavicular, and scapulothoracic joints. During glenohumeral flexion, the clavicle rises, then rotates posteriorly. To complete the range of shoulder joint flexion, the scapula rotates on the clavicle and rotates upward on the thorax approximately 60 degrees. Such accessory motions as humeral head depression, medial rotation, and posterior glide in the glenoid fossa occur simultaneously to provide smooth motion throughout the normal range. The functional range at the glenohumeral joint must include all associated motions.

Motion. Zero to 180 degrees (glenohumeral, acromioclavicular, sternoclavicular, and scapulothoracic joints).

Position. Subject lies supine, with the hips and knees flexed. The feet are flat on the table to prevent hyperextension of the lumbar vertebrae. The palm of the hand and the forearm are pronated (Fig. 5-1).

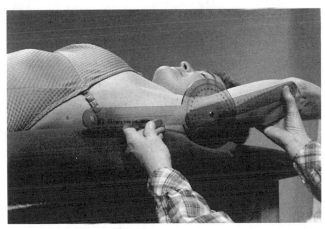

▲ **Figure 5.1** Ending position for shoulder flexion measurement.

Goniometric Alignment

Axis. At the acromion process of the scapula, through the head of the humerus.

Stationary Arm. Placed along the midaxillary line of the trunk in line with the greater trochanter of the femur.

Moving Arm. Placed along the lateral longitudinal midline of the humerus in line with the lateral epicondyle of the humerus at the beginning of the ROM and with the medial epicondyle at the end of ROM.

Stabilization. The scapula should be prevented from rising and tipping posteriorly.

Precautions

- Avoid hyperextension of the lumbar vertebrae.
- Avoid abduction at the shoulder joint and elevation of the scapula. The motion occurs strictly in the sagittal plane.
- Allow medial rotation of the shoulder joint to occur at approximately 90 degrees of shoulder flexion.
- Allow for scapular and clavicular joint motion to occur at approximately 30 degrees of shoulder flexion.
- Maintain the elbow joint in extension to prevent the long head of the triceps muscle from being stretched.

SHOULDER EXTENSION AND HYPEREXTENSION

Shoulder joint extension and hyperextension are the return from the flexion motion. In the sagittal plane, extension at the glenohumeral joint is accompanied by motions at the sternoclavicular, acromioclavicular, and scapulothoracic joints. When the shoulder joint is extending to the anatomical position, the scapula rotates downward and the clavicle depresses and rotates anteriorly. In hyperextension, the humerus rotates medially and glides anteriorly to complete the full functional range, while the humeral head remains depressed in the glenoid fossa.

Motion. 180 to 0 degrees of extension. Zero to 50 degrees of hyperextension (glenohumeral, scapulothoracic, acromioclavicular, and sternoclavicular joints).

Position

- Preferred: Subject lies prone with the head comfortably positioned without a pillow. The shoulder joint is in the anatomical position with the elbow slightly flexed, and the forearm is pronated (Fig. 5-2).
- Alternate:
    1. Subject is supine with the elbow flexed and the arm over the side of the treatment table (Fig. 5-3).

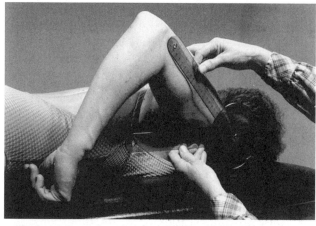

▲ **Figure 5.2** Preferred ending position for shoulder hyperextension measurement.

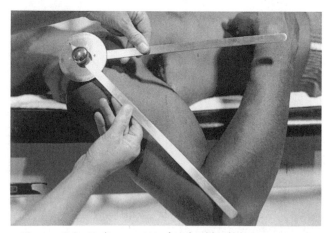

▲ **Figure 5.3** Ending position for shoulder hyperextension measurement with the subject in the supine position.

2. Subject lies on one side with the elbow slightly flexed.

Goniometric Alignment

Axis. Slightly inferior to the acromion process of the scapula in line with the humeral head.

Stationary Arm. Placed along the midaxillary line of the trunk in line with the greater trochanter of the femur.

Moving Arm. Placed along the lateral longitudinal midline of the humerus in line with the lateral epicondyle of the humerus.

Stabilization. Stabilize the scapula.

Precautions

- Avoid flexion of the thoracic vertebrae.
- Avoid abduction of the shoulder joint.
- Keep elbow slightly flexed to prevent the biceps brachii muscle from being stretched.
- Avoid scapular adduction.
- Prevent anterior tipping and elevation of the scapula.

SHOULDER ABDUCTION

Motion of shoulder joint abduction occurs in the coronal plane. Accompanying abduction of the glenohumeral joint is clavicular elevation, followed by posterior rotation. Also, the scapula rotates upward on the thorax. The combined motions of the scapula and clavicle account for approximately 60 degrees of the movement. For the complete functional range of shoulder joint abduction to occur, there is an accompanying lateral rotation of the humerus to clear the greater tubercle under the acromion process of the scapula. The head of the humerus remains depressed in the glenoid fossa and glides inferiorly during the movement.

Motion. Zero to 180 degrees (glenohumeral, sternoclavicular, acromioclavicular, and scapulothoracic joints).

Position

- Preferred: Subject is supine with the hips and knees flexed and the feet flat on the table. The upper limb being tested is placed in the anatomical position (Fig. 5-4). The elbow joint remains extended.
- Alternate: Subject sits or lies prone (Fig. 5-5).

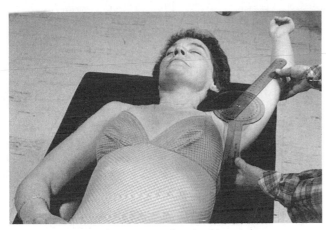

▲ **Figure 5.4** Ending position for shoulder abduction measurement.

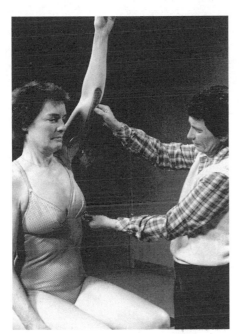

▲ **Figure 5.5** Ending position for measuring shoulder abduction from an anterior approach with the subject in a sitting position.

Goniometric Alignment

Axis. Placed on the anterior portion of the acromion process of the scapula, through the center of the head of the humerus.

Stationary Arm

- Preferred: Placed on the lateral aspect of the anterior surface of the chest, parallel to the midline of the sternum.
- Alternate: Placed on the lateral aspect of the chest, parallel to the spinous process of the vertebrae.

Moving Arm

- Preferred: Placed on the anterior aspect of the arm, parallel to the midline of the humerus, in line with the medial humeral epicondyle.
- Alternate: Placed on the posterior aspect of the arm, parallel to the midline of the humerus, in line with the lateral humeral epicondyle.

Stabilization. Stabilize the thorax.

Precautions

- Avoid spine flexion toward the contralateral side.
- Avoid elevation of the scapula.
- Permit the shoulder to rotate laterally approximately 90 degrees.
- Maintain the upper limb in the coronal plane, except for the lateral rotation.

SHOULDER ADDUCTION

Adduction at the shoulder joint is measured as the return from shoulder joint abduction. The movement occurs in the coronal plane. Accompanying motions of the clavicle and the scapula occur as they return to the anatomical position during glenohumeral adduction. The humerus rotates medially and glides superiorly in the glenoid fossa until the completion of the range of motion.

Motion. From 180 degrees to 0 degrees (glenohumeral, scapulothoracic, acromioclavicular, and sternoclavicular joints).

Position

- Preferred: Subject lies supine with the knees flexed and the feet flat on the table (Fig. 5-6).
- Alternate: Subject sits.

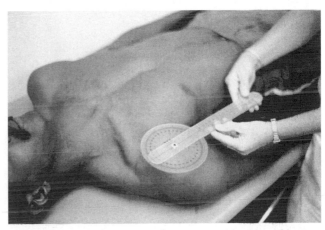

▲ **Figure 5.6** Ending position for measuring shoulder adduction.

Goniometric alignment and stabilization are the same as described for shoulder joint abduction.

Precautions

• Prevent the spine from flexing ipsilaterally.
• Avoid scapular depression.
• Permit the shoulder joint to rotate medially.

SHOULDER HORIZONTAL ADDUCTION

Horizontal adduction at the glenohumeral joint occurs in the transverse plane. The scapula abducts on the thorax, and the clavicle protracts to allow complete motion. The humeral head is depressed and glides posteriorly and laterally in the glenoid fossa.

Motion. Zero to 120 degrees of horizontal adduction from a fully horizontally abducted position (shoulder, sternoclavicular, acromioclavicular, and scapulothoracic joints). Zero to 30 degrees of horizontal adduction from the neutral position.

Position

• Preferred: Subject sits. The shoulder joint is abducted 90 degrees and the elbow flexed 90 degrees. The shoulder joint is also positioned in neutral rotation (Figs. 5-7 and 5-8).
• Alternate:
  1. Subject sits with shoulder flexed 90 degrees and internally rotated. The elbow is flexed 90 degrees.
  2. The subject lies supine, with the shoulder and elbow positioned as described above in the preferred position (Fig. 5-9).

Goniometric Alignment

Axis. Superiorly on the acromion process of the scapula through the head of the humerus.

Stationary Arm

• Preferred: Along the midline of the shoulder toward the neck (the goniometer arm must be short).
• Alternate: Along the midline of the humerus in line with the lateral epicondyle of the humerus.

Moving Arm. Along the midshaft of the humerus, in line with the lateral epicondyle of the humerus.

Stabilization. Stabilize the thorax to prevent rotation.

Precaution

• Prevent rotation of the trunk.

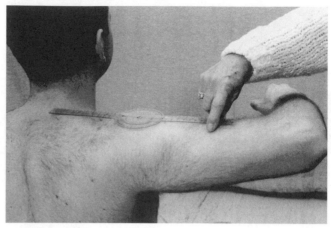

▲ **Figure 5.7** Starting position for measuring horizontal shoulder adduction with the subject in a sitting position.

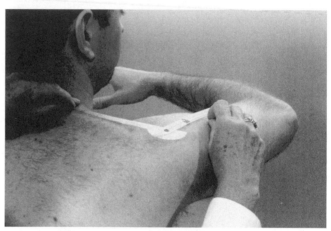

▲ **Figure 5.8** Ending position for measuring horizontal shoulder adduction with the subject in a sitting position.

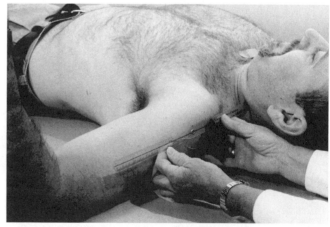

▲ **Figure 5.9** Alternate starting position for measuring horizontal shoulder adduction.

SHOULDER HORIZONTAL ABDUCTION

Horizontal abduction at the shoulder joint occurs in the transverse plane. The scapula adducts on the thorax, and the clavicle retracts to allow complete motion. The humeral head remains depressed and glides anteriorly in the glenoid fossa.

Motion. Zero to 120 degrees from a fully horizontally adducted position (sternoclavicular, acromioclavicular, and scapulothoracic). Zero to 90 degrees of horizontal abduction from the neutral position.

Position. Subject sits with the shoulder joint in neutral rotation, flexed to 90 degrees, and the elbow flexed 90 degrees.

Goniometric Alignment

Axis. Superiorly on the acromion process of the scapula through the head of the humerus.

Stationary Arm. Aligned on the midline of the shoulder toward the neck. The goniometer arm must be short.

- Alternate: Along the midline of the humerus, in line with the lateral epicondyle of the humerus.

Moving Arm. Along the midshaft of the humerus, in line with the lateral epicondyle of the humerus (see Fig. 5-7).

Stabilization. Stabilize the thorax to prevent rotation.

Precaution

- Prevent trunk rotation.

MEDIAL SHOULDER ROTATION

In the anatomical position, the motion occurs in the transverse plane. For goniometric evaluation, the shoulder joint is abducted and the elbow joint flexed 90 degrees while the subject is supine; the motion tested occurs in the sagittal plane. The evaluation position for medial rotation of the shoulder joint puts the scapula in abduction and upward rotation. During the motion of medial rotation, the scapula adducts slightly, and the humeral head glides posteriorly in the glenoid fossa.

Motion. Zero to 65 to 90 degrees.

Position

- Preferred: Subject lies supine, with the knees flexed and the feet flat on the table. The shoulder joint is abducted and the elbow flexed 90 degrees. The forearm is in midposition between supination and pronation and is perpendicular to the table top. The full length of the humerus is supported on the table. It may be necessary to place a rolled towel under the arm to keep it level (Fig. 5-10).
- Alternate: Subject is prone with the shoulder abducted 90 degrees and the elbow flexed over the edge of the table (Fig. 5-11).

Goniometric Alignment

Axis. The olecranon process of the ulna projects through the humeral shaft toward the humeral head.

Stationary Arm. Placed parallel to the tabletop or perpendicular to the floor.

Moving Arm. Along the ulnar shaft, directed toward the styloid process of the ulna.

Stabilization. Stabilize the distal end of the humerus throughout the range of motion and the scapula and thorax toward the end of the range.

Precautions

- Keep the shoulder joint abducted 90 degrees so that the olecranon process is in line with the glenoid fossa.

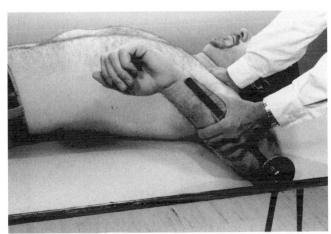

▲ **Figure 5.10** Ending position for measuring medial shoulder rotation.

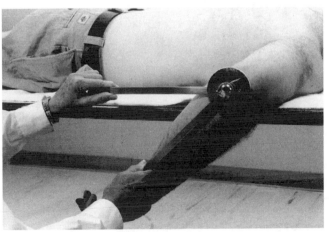

▲ **Figure 5.11** Alternate ending position for measuring medial shoulder rotation with the subject prone.

- Avoid flexion and extension at the shoulder joint.
- Avoid flexion of the vertebrae.
- Avoid elbow extension.
- Prevent elevation and anterior tipping of the scapula.

LATERAL SHOULDER ROTATION

In the anatomical position, the motion of lateral shoulder rotation occurs in the transverse plane. During goniometric evaluation, the shoulder joint is positioned in abduction, and the elbow is flexed 90 degrees; therefore, the test motion occurs in the sagittal plane. When the test is conducted with the subject in the supine position, the scapula is put in abduction and upward rotation and increases slightly in both motions during lateral rotation of the glenohumeral joint. The head of the humerus is depressed in the glenoid fossa and glides anteriorly during the motion. It may be necessary to use a rolled towel or pad to keep the humerus level.

Motion. Zero to 90 degrees.

Position

- Preferred: The position is the same as described for medial rotation of the shoulder joint (Fig. 5-12).
- Alternate: The position is the same as described for medial shoulder rotation (Fig. 5-13).

Goniometric alignment and stabilization are the same are described for shoulder joint medial rotation.

Precautions

- Keep the shoulder abducted to 90 degrees so that the olecranon process is in line with the glenoid fossa.

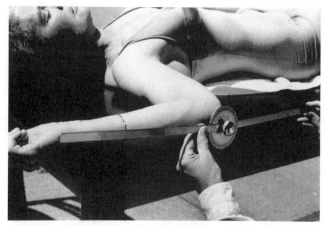

▲ **Figure 5.12** Ending position for measuring lateral shoulder rotation.

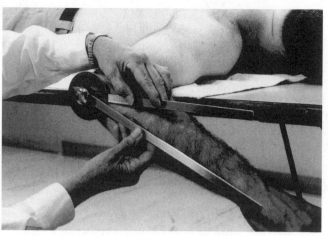

▲ **Figure 5.13** Alternate ending position for measuring lateral shoulder rotation with the subject in a prone position.

- Avoid extension of the spine.
- Avoid extension of the elbow.
- Prevent posterior tipping of the scapula.
- Avoid flexion, extension, abduction, and adduction of the shoulder joint.

Scapula

UPWARD SCAPULAR ROTATION

Upward rotation of the scapula occurs in the coronal plane around an axis in the sagittal plane. The scapulothoracic joint is not a true anatomical joint but a functional one that exists between thorax, muscle, and bony scapula. For the scapula to rotate upward, the shoulder joint must complete a motion of abduction or flexion. Motion in this joint is seldom measured, but when it is, it is usually performed with a tape measure rather than a goniometer.

Motion. The measurement is the difference in inches between the anatomical starting position and the end position. The motion of one scapula is compared to that of the other.

Position. Subject sits with the shoulder in the anatomical position. Standing and lying prone are alternate positions (Fig. 5-14).

Measuring Tape

- Starting: Place the tape parallel to and in line with a line from the inferior angle of the scapula and the spinous process of the seventh thoracic vertebra (T7).
- Ending: Following motion, measure to the inferior angle of the scapula, and calculate the difference in inches or centimeters. The difference between the two measurements is the amount of upward scapular rotation.

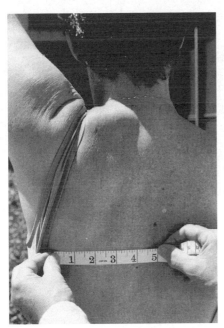

▲ **Figure 5.14** End position for measuring scapular upward rotation.

Stabilization. Stabilize the thorax.

Precautions

• Make sure the scapula does not tip.

DOWNWARD SCAPULAR ROTATION

Downward rotation occurs in the coronal plane around an axis in the sagittal plane. The scapulothoracic joint is not a true anatomical joint but a functional one necessary for complete range of motion at the shoulder joint. Downward rotation of the scapula is seldom measured.

Motion. The scapula's inferior angle moves medially when the shoulder joint is extended and adducted across the posterior trunk. The amount of motion is the difference between the starting and ending positions. It is compared with the motion in the opposite scapulothoracic joint.

Position, measuring, and stabilization are the same as scapular rotation. (Fig. 5-15).

Precaution

• Make sure the scapula is not adducted.

SCAPULAR ABDUCTION

Abduction of the scapula is a translatory motion occurring in the coronal plane at the scapulothoracic joint between the thorax, muscle, and scapula when the vertebral border of the scapula moves laterally.

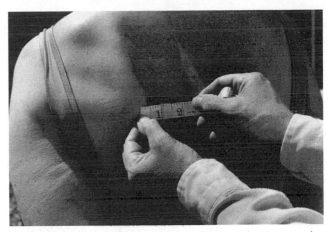

▲ **Figure 5.15** End position for measuring scapular downward rotation.

The lateral motion of the scapula is accompanied by lateral tilt as the scapula follows the curved contour of the thorax. The starting test position is 90 degrees of shoulder abduction. The scapula is rotated slightly upward. For scapular abduction to occur, the shoulder joint adducts horizontally in the transverse plane.

Motion. The scapula moves laterally on the thorax as the shoulder joint moves through a complete range of horizontal adduction. The amount of motion is determined by measuring with a tape the difference between the beginning and ending points.

Position. Subject sits with the shoulder joint abducted and the elbow flexed 90 degrees.

Measuring Tape

• Starting: Hold the tape horizontal at the level of the root of the spine of the scapula and the thoracic vertebrae.
• Ending: Measure the difference between the beginning and end points of motion following horizontal adduction of the shoulder joint. The difference between the two measurements is the total range of scapular abduction (Fig. 5-16).

Stabilization. Stabilize the trunk.

Precautions

• Avoid rotation of the shoulder joint.
• Avoid trunk rotation.

SCAPULAR ADDUCTION

The motion for scapular adduction is translatory and occurs in the coronal plane between thorax, muscle, and scapula. The motion is tested with the shoulder joint abducted 90 degrees and the scapula

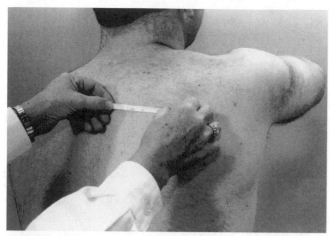

▲ **Figure 5.16** End position for measuring scapular abduction.

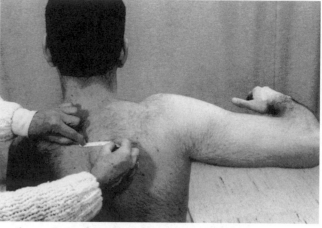

▲ **Figure 5.17** End position for measuring scapular adduction.

rotated slightly upward. The range of motion is determined when the vertebral border of the scapula moves medially toward the spinous processes of the thoracic vertebrae. Scapular adduction occurs as the shoulder joint abducts horizontally.

Motion. The scapula moves medially during horizontal abduction of the shoulder. The range of motion is the difference between the beginning and end points of the scapula's motion.

Position, measuring, stabilization, and precautions are the same as scapular abduction.

Measuring Tape

- Starting: Hold the tape horizontally between the root of the spine of the scapula and the thoracic vertebrae.
- Ending: Following horizontal abduction of the shoulder joint, measure the distance between the root of the spine of the scapula and the thoracic vertebral spinous processes. The difference between the two measurements is the range of scapular adduction (Fig. 5-17).

MUSCLE LENGTH TESTING

Shoulder Extensor Muscles

The shoulder joint is designed to provide mobility for the upper limb, unlike the hip joints, which have developed to afford stability. Usually the movements of the upper limb are performed in an open chain. The extension motion of the shoulder joint is accompanied by contraction of the scapular muscles. The muscles that extend the shoulder joint are the one-joint muscles: teres major, pec-

toralis major (sternocostal head), teres minor, and posterior deltoid. The teres major and posterior deltoid muscles seldom demonstrate limitation in length. The long head of the triceps brachii muscle is a two-joint muscle acting on the shoulder and the elbow joint. The latissimus dorsi muscle may act on the trunk, therefore crossing the vertebra, and is categorized as a multijoint muscle. Most one-joint muscles do not show a decrease in muscle length as do two-joint muscles; however, some common limitations exist. The length of the long head of the triceps muscle is described with the elbow joint.

LATISSIMUS DORSI AND TERES MAJOR

Position. The subject is standing or supine with the trunk flat against a wall or supine with the hip and knee joints flexed. The upper limbs are positioned at the side of the trunk.

Movement. The examiner flexes both upper limbs through as much range of motion as possible, keeping the limbs in the sagittal plane. The low back remains flat on the table or against the wall. If the low back arches, the motion is stopped, and the amount of shoulder joint flexion is measured.

Measurement. Inability of complete shoulder flexion should be measured with a goniometer. Landmarks used are the same as goniometry measurement for shoulder flexion. Measurement also may be recorded by indicating the amount of lumbar hyperextension when the upper limbs have completed the range of shoulder flexion in terms of minimal, moderate, or marked (Fig. 5-18).

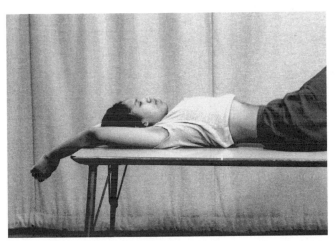

▲ **Figure 5.18** Muscle length testing for latissimus dorsi and teres major muscles.

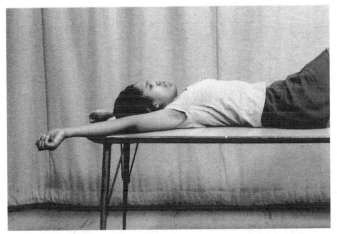

▲ **Figure 5.19** Muscle length testing for pectoralis major muscle.

Considerations

- Tightness of the pectoralis minor muscle may position the scapula in an anterior tilt, which may not allow the shoulders to flex completely.
- The anterior abdominal wall musculature may show tightness, which may depress the thorax and tend to pull the scapula anteriorly.

PECTORALIS MAJOR (STERNOCOSTAL HEAD)

The feet and low back are flat on the surface of the table.

Movement. The shoulder is laterally rotated and flexed in line with the pectoralis major muscle fibers. The range of motion is approximately 50 degrees into the sagittal plane from the frontal plane, maintaining the elbow joint in extension. A limitation in length of the muscle would exist if complete flexion at the shoulder joint did not occur.

Measurement. The lack of complete shoulder flexion should be measured with a goniometer using shoulder flexion landmarks (Fig. 5-19).

Considerations

- The anterior capsular joint structures may show limitation along with the pectoralis major muscle.
- As the muscle reaches its maximal length, the shoulder will come out of lateral rotation in an attempt to elevate completely.

Shoulder Flexor Muscles

The flexion motion at the shoulder joint is accompanied by scapular upward rotation. The muscles

that cross the shoulder joint anteriorly and produce flexion are the one-joint anterior deltoid, coracobrachialis, and clavicular head of the pectoralis major. The two-joint muscles anterior to the joint are the biceps brachii (long and short heads). The length of biceps brachii muscles is described with the elbow joint.

PECTORALIS MAJOR (CLAVICULAR HEAD)

Position. The subject is supine with the hip and knee joints flexed and the feet and low back flat on the treatment table.

Movement. The examiner horizontally abducts the shoulder joint to 90 degrees with the shoulder in lateral rotation. The elbow is slightly flexed to minimize any effect from the biceps brachii muscles. If the upper limb does not reach the surface of the table, then limitation in the pectoralis major (clavicular portion) exists (Fig. 5-20). Excessive length can

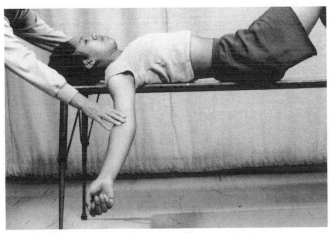

▲ **Figure 5.20** Muscle length testing with the shoulder laterally rotated for the pectoralis major muscle.

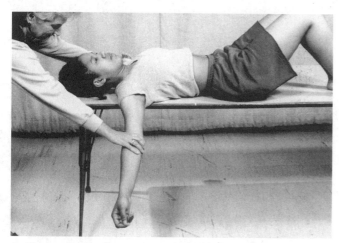

▲ **Figure 5.21** Excessive muscle length for the pectoralis major muscle.

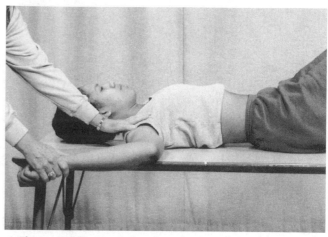

▲ **Figure 5.22** Muscle length testing for the medial rotator muscles.

be assessed by having the subject move close to the edge of the treatment table, and the upper limb will horizontally abduct beyond the edge of the table (Fig. 5-21).

Measurement. Lack of complete motion may be measured using a tape measure from the elbow to the table top.

Considerations

- The three joint biceps brachii muscles may be limited in length; therefore, slight elbow flexion should be maintained.
- Trunk rotation to the same side may occur if limitation in length exists.
- Limitations in the shoulder joint capsule or the acromioclavicular joint may accompany pectoralis major clavicular portion tightness.
- As the muscle reaches its maximal length, the shoulder will come out of lateral rotation in an attempt to elevate completely.

Shoulder Medial Rotator Muscles

The medial rotators are numerous and powerful compared to their counterpart, the lateral rotators. Also, as the shoulder joint medially rotates, the scapula abducts on the thoracic wall. Many of the muscles that were previously identified as shoulder joint extensor muscles also medially rotate the shoulder joint. The medial rotator muscles are the latissimus dorsi, pectoralis major, subscapularis, teres major and anterior deltoid.

Position. The subject is supine with the hip and knee joints flexed and the feet and low back flat on the surface of the treatment table. The shoulder

joint is abducted 90 degrees, and the elbow is flexed 90 degrees.

Movement. The shoulder joint is laterally rotated so that the dorsum of the hand is flat on the surface of the table. Excessive range would exist if lateral rotation went beyond 90 degrees.

Measurement. Lateral rotation measurement is the same as described in goniometry (Fig. 5-22).

Considerations

- If the low back remains flat on the surface of the treatment table and range of motion is compete, then the latissimus dorsi muscle is not limited in its length.
- If the latissimus dorsi length test is normal and limitation in range of motion exists, then the one-joint medial rotators are too short.
- The joint capsule and ligaments may be tight, accompanied by the limitation in length of the medial rotators.

Shoulder Lateral Rotator Muscles

The lateral rotator muscles are weak compared to the medial rotators. To allow full range of lateral shoulder joint rotation, the scapula adducts the thoracic wall. The lateral rotator muscles are teres minor, infraspinatus, and posterior deltoid. Limitation in length of the lateral rotators is much more common in an adult than a limitation in length of the medial rotator muscles.

Position. Same as above for medial rotator muscle limitation.

Movement. The examiner rotates the shoulder joint medially to allow the palm of the hand to touch

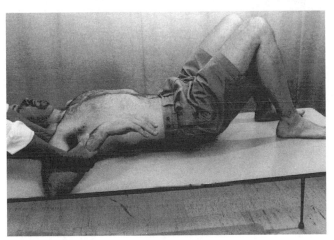

▲ **Figure 5.23** Muscle length testing for the lateral rotator muscle.

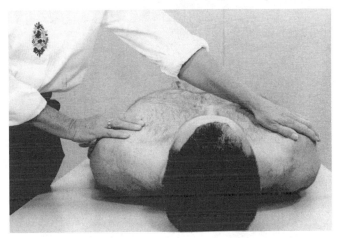

▲ **Figure 5.24** Muscle length testing for the pectoralis minor muscle.

the surface of the treatment table. The shoulder joint is firmly held by the examiner to eliminate anterior tipping of the scapula.

Measurement. The complete range of motion into medial rotation is normally 70 degrees. A goniometer is used, and the bony landmarks are the same as in goniometry (Fig. 5-23).

Considerations

- The joint capsule may also be limited in flexibility, accompanied by shortened lateral rotator muscles.
- A quick assessment for shortness of the lateral rotators is with the subject sitting and placing the hands on back. The right and left hands should touch. One could measure thumb to vertebral height.
- Anterior tipping of the scapula is not permitted for an accurate assessment of the lateral rotator muscle length.

Scapular Muscles

Of the 17 muscles attaching on the scapula, the pectoralis minor muscle tends to show limitation in length. Shortness of the pectoralis minor muscle is particularly evident in students and sedentary individuals. The levator scapulae and rhomboid muscles are discussed in the chapter on the neck.

PECTORALIS MINOR

Position. The subject assumes a supine position with the hip and knee joints flexed and the feet and low back flat on the surface of the table. The upper limbs are in the anatomical position at the side of the trunk.

Movement. The examiner observes the subject from the head of the treatment table and compares the scapulae for anterior tipping. No limitation is evident when the posterior aspect of the shoulder joint is flat on the table surface.

Measurement. The tightness of the muscle is recorded as slight, moderate, or marked. The determination is judged by the distance that exists from the surface of the table to the posterior surface of the scapula superiorly (Fig. 5-24).

Considerations

- None.

MANUAL MUSCLE TESTING

UPPER TRAPEZIUS AND LEVATOR SCAPULAE

The upper trapezius and levator scapulae muscles elevate the scapula approximately 2 in. Usually both sides are tested simultaneously, providing stabilization and resistance bilaterally. Simultaneous testing also provides an indication of symmetry. The neck and head must be observed for motion if a lesion is unilateral. To test isolated scapular elevation, the head is stabilized on the test side.

Palpation. Palpate the upper trapezius on the superior and posterior surface of the shoulders (Fig. 5-25). The levator scapula is deep to the upper trapezius in the angle formed by the upper trapezius and the sternocleidomastoid muscles. To isolate the action of the levator scapula, minimize the action of the trapezius muscle by having the subject place the hand in the small of his or her back and shrug the shoulders quickly within a limited range of motion (Fig. 5-26).

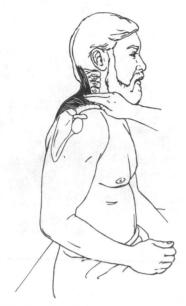

▲ **Figure 5.25** Palpating the upper trapezius muscle.

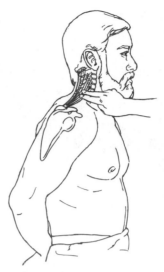

▲ **Figure 5.26** Palpating the levator scapulae muscle.

Position

Against gravity (AG): Subject sits with the arms relaxed (Fig. 5-27).

Gravity minimized (GM): Subject is supine or prone; examiner supports upper limbs and shoulders (Fig. 5-28).

Movement. Elevate the shoulders toward the ears.

Resistance. Applied superiorly on the acromion process in an inferior direction.

Stabilization. Apply resistance to both shoulders simultaneously to offer stability or unilaterally to the posterior lateral aspect of head.

Substitutions

- Serratus anterior abducts and rotates the scapula upward, appearing to elevate it.
- Pectoralis minor anteriorly tilts the scapula, as in "round shoulders."
- Anterior, middle, and posterior scalenus muscles elevate the first and second ribs.
- Major and minor rhomboid muscles elevate the scapula, with accompanying downward rotation.

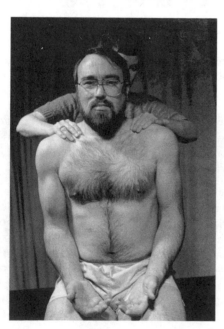

▲ **Figure 5.27** Muscle testing the upper trapezius and levator scapulae muscles in the AG sitting position.

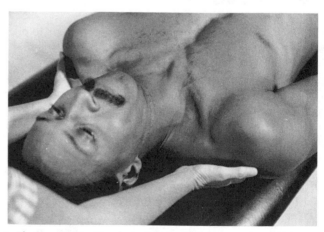

▲ **Figure 5.28** Muscle testing the upper trapezius and levator scapulae muscles in the GM supine position.

▼ Attachments of Upper Trapezius and Levator Scapulae Muscles

Muscle	Proximal	Distal	Innervation
Upper trapezius	Superior nuchal line	Lateral third of clavicle and the acromion process	Spinal accessory CN XI
	Ligamentum nuchae		
Levator scapulae	Transverse processes of upper four cervical vertebrae	Medial border of scapula at level of the scapular superior angle	Dorsal scapular C5 (C3 and C4)

MIDDLE TRAPEZIUS MUSCLE

The middle trapezius muscle adducts the scapula. The vertebral border of the scapula moves 2 in toward the spinous processes of the thoracic vertebrae. Gravitational effects on the scapula are minimal; all testing may be performed with the subject in the prone position. Results may be determined by the palpated firmness of the contraction.

Palpation. Palpate along the medial border of the scapula near the root of the spine (Fig. 5-29).

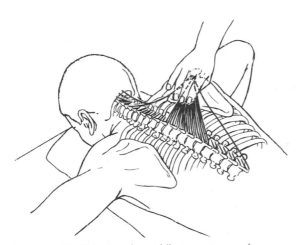

▲ **Figure 5.29** Palpating the middle trapezius muscle.

Position

AG: Subject is prone with elbow flexed over the edge of the treatment table (Fig. 5-30).
GM: Subject sits with upper limb resting on the table, shoulder joint abducted 90 degrees, and elbow flexed 90 degrees. The surface must be friction free (Fig. 5-31).

Movement. Bring scapulae together into adduction.

Resistance. Applied to the lateral border of the scapula, pushing down and out into abduction.

Stabilization. Stabilize the contralateral thorax.

Substitutions

- While sitting, the subject may rotate the trunk, giving the appearance of scapular adduction.
- The posterior deltoid muscle causes horizontal abduction of the shoulder without adducting the scapula.
- Major and minor rhomboid muscles will cause the scapula to elevate and rotate downward while adducting. Do not allow the shoulder to rotate medially.
- Lower trapezius causes the scapula to depress and rotate upward.

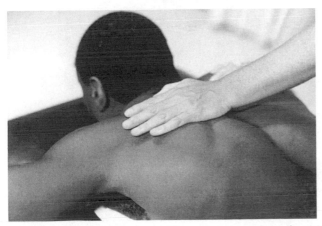

▲ **Figure 5.30** Testing the middle trapezius muscle in the AG prone position.

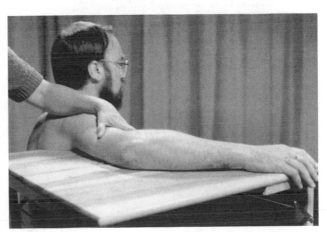

▲ **Figure 5.31** Testing the middle trapezius muscle in the GM sitting position.

▼ **Attachments of Middle Trapezius Muscle**

Muscle	Proximal	Distal	Innervation
Middle trapezius	Spinous processes of T1–T5	Superior border of scapular spine	Spinal accessory CN XI

- The rhomboids and the lower trapezius may contract synergistically to provide scapular adduction. This is monitored by palpation.
- The upper and lower fibers of the trapezius muscle contract synergistically to adduct the scapula.

LOWER TRAPEZIUS MUSCLE

The lower fibers of the trapezius muscle produce adduction and depression of the scapula. The test range of motion is 1 to 2 in. All grades are tested with the subject in the prone position. The upper limb is supported in an elevated position and aligned with the direction of the lower trapezius muscle fibers. Complete motion may be limited by a shortened pectoralis major muscle. For 0 to P or 0 to 2, the grade is determined by the firmness of muscle contraction. The subject is unable to lift the upper limb, but the scapula may depress. If the deltoid muscle is weak, the upper limb must be manually supported. Grades of 2+ to 3− are based on how far the upper limb is lifted from the table; for grade F to N or 3 to 5, resistance is applied.

Palpation. Palpate medial to the root of the spine and the medial border of the scapula; this portion of the muscle forms a triangle (Fig. 5-32).

Position

AG and GM: Subject lies prone, with the shoulder abducted 130 degrees. If shoulder range of motion is limited, the upper limb may be placed over the side of the table and manually supported (Figs. 5-33 and 5-34).

Movement. Subject lifts the upper limb off the table.

Resistance. Applied to the lateral angle of the scapula in a forward and outward direction.

Stabilization. Stabilize the thorax on the opposite side.

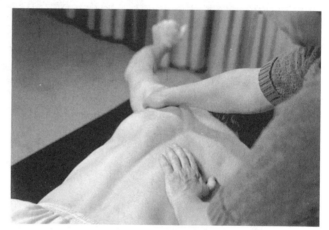

▲ **Figure 5.33** Testing the lower trapezius muscle in the AG prone position.

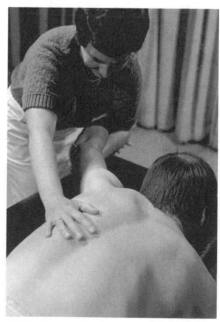

▲ **Figure 5.34** Testing the lower trapezius muscle in the GM prone position.

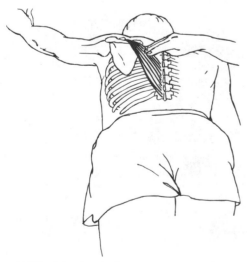

▲ **Figure 5.32** Palpating the lower trapezius muscle.

▼ Attachments of Lower Trapezius Muscle

Muscle	Proximal	Distal	Innervation
Lower trapezius	Spinous processes of T6–T12	Apex or root and inferiorly on the scapular spine	Spinal accessory CN XI

Substitutions

- Posterior deltoid will raise the upper limb without depressing or adducting the scapula.
- Latissimus dorsi is indirectly an accessory muscle in depression of the scapula through its attachment on the humerus.
- Pectoralis major (sternal head) is indirectly (through its attachment on the humerus) an accessory muscle for depression of the scapula.

MAJOR AND MINOR RHOMBOID MUSCLES

The major and minor rhomboid muscles produce the motions of scapular adduction and downward rotation. The test range consists of the inferior angle of the scapula moving approximately 1 in toward the spinous processes of the vertebrae. The effect of gravity on scapular motion is minimal; therefore, palpation and strength measurement may be performed with the subject in the prone position.

Palpation. Place the subject's hand in the lumbar area of the back to relax the overlying trapezius muscle, and palpate beneath and along the medial border of the scapula (Fig. 5-35).

Position

AG: Subject lies prone with the hand resting on the lumbar spine (Fig. 5-36).

GM: Subject sits, with the hand resting on the lumbar spine (Fig. 5-37).

Movement. Lift the hand off the back.

Resistance. Applied to the vertebral border of the scapula, pushing into abduction and upward rotation.

Stabilization. Stabilize the thorax on the opposite side.

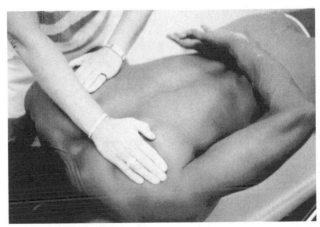

▲ **Figure 5.36** Testing the major and minor rhomboid muscles in the AG prone position.

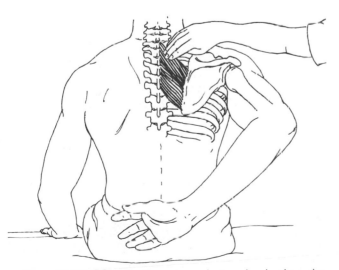

▲ **Figure 5.35** Palpating the major and minor rhomboid muscles.

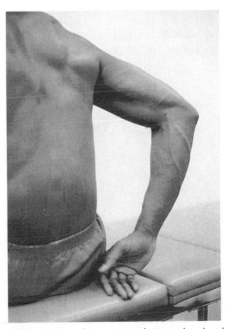

▲ **Figure 5.37** Testing the major and minor rhomboid muscles in the GM sitting position.

▼ Attachments of Major and Minor Rhomboid Muscles

Muscle	Proximal	Distal	Innervation
Major rhomboid	Spinous processes of T2–5	Medial border between the root and inferior angle of the scapula	Dorsal scapular C4 and C5
Minor rhomboid	Ligamentum nuchae Spinous process of C7–T1	Medial border at root of scapula	Dorsal scapular C4 and C5

Substitutions

- Wrist extensors: By pressing the hand against the lumbar area of the back, the subject lifts the upper limb without moving the scapula.
- Middle trapezius adducts the scapula with no rotation.
- Posterior deltoid causes the shoulder to abduct horizontally and may give the appearance of scapular adduction.
- Latissimus dorsi and teres major adduct and extend the shoulder with no effect on scapular rotation.
- Levator scapulae is an accessory muscle to downward scapular rotation and adduction, but it does not participate in the action unless the scapula is positioned in upward rotation.

SERRATUS ANTERIOR MUSCLE

The serratus anterior muscle produces the motion of abduction of the scapula with accompanying upward rotation. The test range is 2 to 3 in of the scapula sliding on the thorax. The serratus anterior muscle is a major fixator of the scapula to the thorax. Minimal weakness is difficult to detect. Standing, pushing against a wall, or performing a prone push-up may reveal "winging" of the scapula.

Palpation. Palpate along the midaxillary line adjacent to the inferior angle of the scapula (Fig. 5-38).

Position

AG: Subject lies supine with the shoulder flexed 90 degrees and the elbow joint completely flexed (Fig. 5-39).

GM: Subject sits with the upper limb resting on the table, the shoulder in 90 degrees of flexion, and the elbow extended (Fig. 5-40).

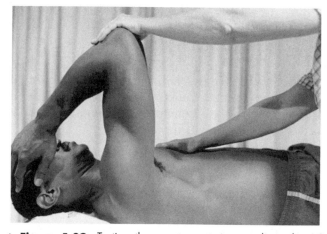

▲ **Figure 5.39** Testing the serratus anterior muscle in the AG supine position.

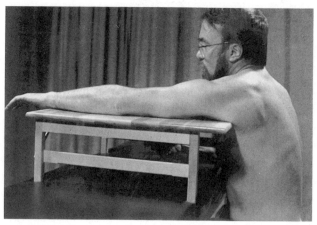

▲ **Figure 5.40** Testing the serratus anterior muscle in the GM sitting position.

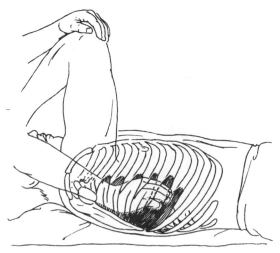

▲ **Figure 5.38** Palpating the serratus anterior muscle.

▼ Attachments of Serratus Anterior Muscle

Muscle	Proximal	Distal	Innervation
Serratus anterior	Anterior surface of the upper eight or nine pairs of ribs	Costal surface and vertebral border of the scapula	Long thoracic C6 and 7 (C5)

Movement. Reach forward or protract the shoulder joint so the scapula slides forward on the thorax.

Resistance. Applied to the elbow, pushing the scapula down into adduction.

Stabilization. Stabilize the contralateral thorax. With the subject in the sitting position, stabilize the thorax to prevent anterior displacement of the trunk.

Substitutions

- In the sitting position, the subject may move the upper limb forward by flexing the vertebrae.
- Rotation of the trunk may occur while sitting.
- Pectoralis minor is an accessory muscle for scapular downward rotation and abduction.

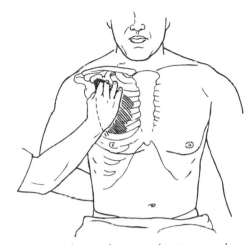

▲ **Figure 5.41** Palpating the pectoralis minor muscle.

PECTORALIS MINOR MUSCLE

The pectoralis minor muscle is tested during anterior tipping of the scapula. It is a muscle that rotates the scapula downward and assists the serratus anterior muscle during scapular abduction. The test range is approximately 10 degrees.

Palpation. Palpate inferior to the coracoid process of the scapula toward the lateral end of the clavicle. The subject is positioned with the hand resting on the lumbar region of the back to relax the pectoralis major muscle. The subject is asked to raise the hand from the lumbar region (Fig. 5-41).

Position

AG: The subject lies supine with the hand on the lumbar region of the trunk (Fig. 5-42).
GM: The subject sits with the hand resting on the small of the back (Fig. 5-43).

Movement. Tip the scapula forward, as in rounding the shoulders.

Resistance. Applied to the acromion process, pushing into the posterior tip of the scapula.

Stabilization. Stabilize the ipsilateral thorax.

Substitutions

- In the sitting position, the subject may flex the trunk forward.

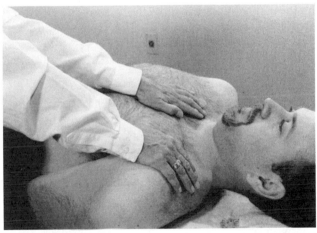

▲ **Figure 5.42** Testing the pectoralis minor muscle in the AG supine position.

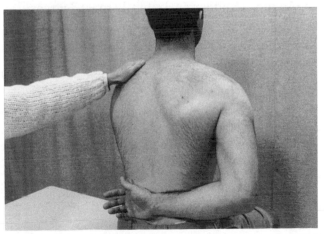

▲ **Figure 5.43** Testing the pectoralis minor muscle in the GM sitting position.

Muscle	Proximal	Distal	Innervation
Pectoralis minor	Coracoid process	Second through fifth ribs	Medial and lateral pectoral C7 (C6 and C7)

- In the supine position, the subject may flex the wrist or fingers, giving the appearance of anterior tipping of the scapula.
- In the sitting position the subject may hyperextend the shoulder joint.

ANTERIOR DELTOID MUSCLE

The anterior deltoid muscle flexes the humerus in the sagittal plane to 180 degrees; however, the test range of motion is to 90 degrees of shoulder flexion. Another test movement for the anterior deltoid muscle is horizontal adduction at the shoulder joint. Shoulder flexion motion is accompanied by medial rotation of the humerus and upward rotation of the scapula.

Palpation. Palpate the anterior deltoid inferior to the lateral third of the clavicle. It contracts strongly during the motion of resisted horizontal adduction (Fig. 5-44).

Position

AG: Subject sits with the shoulder in neutral or internal rotation and the elbow flexed (Fig. 5-45).

GM: Subject is in sidelying position with the upper limb supported and the shoulder in the neutral position, elbow flexed (Fig. 5-46).

Movement

- Flex the shoulder to 90 degrees.
- Adduct shoulder horizontally to 90 degrees.

Resistance. Applied immediately proximal to the elbow, pushing down into shoulder extension or horizontal abduction.

Stabilization. Stabilize the opposite shoulder.

Substitutions

- Biceps brachii may substitute. Prevent this by not letting the subject rotate the shoulder laterally.
- Subject may elevate the shoulder and lean forward to give the appearance of shoulder flexion.
- Subject may quickly extend the shoulder, then relax, giving the appearance of shoulder flexion.

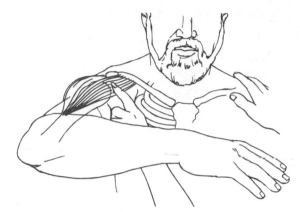

▲ **Figure 5.44** Palpating the anterior deltoid muscle.

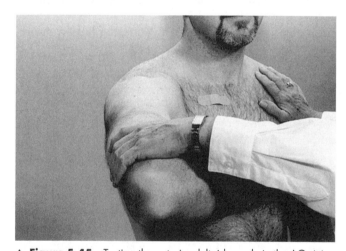

▲ **Figure 5.45** Testing the anterior deltoid muscle in the AG sitting position.

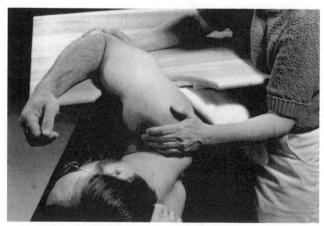

▲ **Figure 5.46** Testing the anterior deltoid muscle in the GM sidelying position.

▼ **Attachments of Anterior Deltoid Muscle**			
Muscle	Proximal	Distal	Innervation
Anterior deltoid	Anterior and superior surfaces of lateral third of clavicle	Deltoid tuberosity of the humerus	Axillary C5 (C6)

- Subject may attempt to compensate for the lack of shoulder motion by moving the scapula.
- Coracobrachialis is an accessory muscle for both shoulder flexion and horizontal adduction.
- Pectoralis major (clavicular head) is an accessory muscle for shoulder joint flexion and horizontal adduction.

CORACOBRACHIALIS MUSCLE

The coracobrachialis muscle is tested as a shoulder flexor if the joint is in less than 90 degrees of flexion or as a shoulder joint extensor if the upper limb is greater than 90 degrees of flexion from the horizontal plane. The test range is usually 90 degrees of shoulder flexion with the joint in lateral rotation. The scapula rotates upward during shoulder joint motion.

Palpation. The coracobrachialis is palpated by initially identifying the short head of the biceps brachii, following the tendon proximally into the axilla to the inferior border of the pectoralis major muscle. With the shoulder flexed overhead the subject resists extension and adduction (Fig. 5-47).

Position

AG: Subject sits with the shoulder joint in lateral rotation; the elbow is flexed with the forearm pronated (Fig. 5-48).

GM: Subject is in a sidelying position with the shoulder joint rotated laterally, the elbow flexed 90 degrees, and the forearm pronated (Fig. 5-49).

Movement. Flex the shoulder joint 90 degrees.

Resistance. Applied to the anterior and medial arm immediately proximal to the elbow joint, pushing into extension and abduction.

Stabilization. Stabilize the opposite shoulder.

Substitutions

- Minimize the action of the biceps brachii as a shoulder joint flexor.
- Anterior deltoid also flexes at the shoulder joint.
- Subject may extend the trunk.

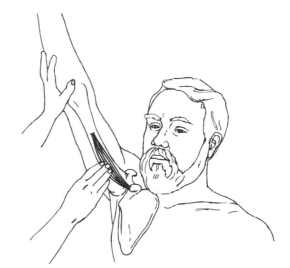

▲ **Figure 5.47** Palpating the coracobrachialis muscle.

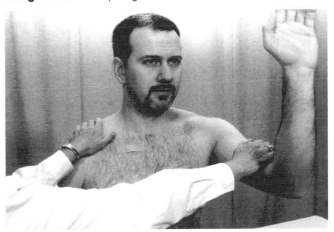

▲ **Figure 5.48** Testing the coracobrachialis muscle in the AG sitting position.

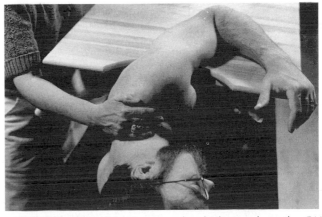

▲ **Figure 5.49** Testing the coracobrachialis muscle in the GM sidelying position.

▼ Attachments of Coracobrachialis Muscle

Muscle	Proximal	Distal	Innervation
Coracobrachialis	Coracoid process of scapula	Medial surface of midshaft of humerus	Musculocutaneous C6 (C5 and C7)

- Subject may quickly extend the shoulder joint, then relax, giving the appearance of shoulder joint flexion.
- Subject may attempt to compensate for the lack of shoulder motion by abducting and rotating the scapula upward.

LATISSIMUS DORSI MUSCLE

The latissimus dorsi, a versatile muscle of the shoulder joint, functions in medial rotation, adduction, and extension. The test motion is extension of the shoulder joint from 90 degrees of flexion to 0 degrees of extension. The shoulder is positioned in medial rotation and adduction. The scapula is allowed to rotate downward.

Palpation. Palpate along the midaxillary line on the trunk; the fiber direction is longitudinal (Fig. 5-50).

Position

AG: Subject lies prone, with the shoulder flexed and medially rotated over the edge of the table (Fig. 5-51).
GM: Subject is in a sidelying position, with upper limb supported, in 90 degrees of shoulder flexion and medial rotation and with elbow flexed (Fig. 5-52).

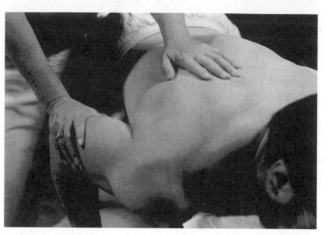

▲ **Figure 5.51** Testing the latissimus dorsi muscle in the AG prone position.

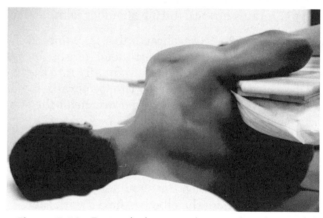

▲ **Figure 5.52** Testing the latissimus dorsi muscle in the GM sidelying position.

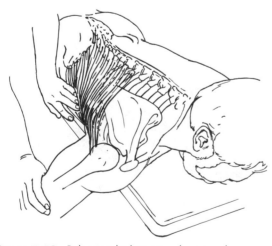

▲ **Figure 5.50** Palpating the latissimus dorsi muscle.

Movement. Extend the shoulder, allowing the elbow to flex.

Resistance. Applied to the posterior arm just proximal to the elbow.

Stabilization. Stabilize the thorax.

Substitutions

- The scapula adducts with no shoulder motion.
- The scapula tips anteriorly and abducts.
- Teres major is an accessory muscle to shoulder joint extension and contracts against resistance.
- Posterior deltoid, triceps (long head), and pectoralis major (sternal head) are also accessory muscles for shoulder joint extension.

▼ Attachments of Latissimus Dorsi Muscle

Muscle	Proximal	Distal	Innervation
Latissimus dorsi	Spinous processes of T6–12 Lumbar and sacral vertebrae Ribs 8 through 12 Thoracolumbar fascia Posterior lip of iliac crest (Occasionally) inferior angle of scapula	Medial lip of intertubercular groove of humerus	Thoracodorsal C6 and C7 (C8)

TERES MAJOR MUSCLE

The teres major muscle is evaluated as a shoulder joint adductor or extensor. It is also a prime mover for shoulder joint medial rotation. The test motion is 90 degrees of adduction, with the shoulder joint extended and medially rotated.

Palpation. Palpate lateral to the inferior angle of the scapula; the fiber direction is horizontal (Fig. 5-53).

Position

AG: Subject lies prone with the shoulder medially rotated and the hand resting on the lower back (Fig. 5-54).
GM: The teres major muscle is not tested in a GM position, because it will contract only against resistance.

Movement. Adduct and extend the shoulder joint.

Resistance. Applied proximal to the elbow joint, pushing shoulder into abduction.

Stabilization. Stabilize upper trunk.

Substitutions

- The scapula adducts without shoulder motion.
- The shoulder joint rotates laterally.
- Latissimus dorsi, pectoralis major, and teres minor also adduct the shoulder joint.

SUPRASPINATUS MUSCLE

The supraspinatus muscle is tested during elevation of the humerus in the frontal plane to 90 degrees.

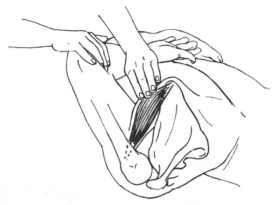

▲ **Figure 5.53** Palpating the teres major muscle.

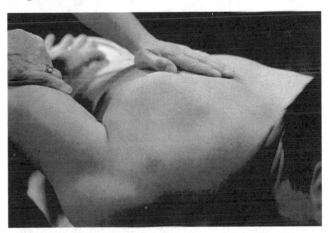

▲ **Figure 5.54** Testing the teres major muscle in the AG prone position.

The motion is normally accompanied by upward rotation of the scapula.

Palpation. Place fingers above the spine of the scapula, with shoulder in the plane of the scapula, which is approximately 30 degrees into the sagittal plane from the frontal plane (Fig. 5-55).

▼ Attachments of Teres Major Muscle

Muscle	Proximal	Distal	Innervation
Teres major	Posterior surface of scapular inferior angle	Crest of lesser tubercle of humerus	Lower subscapular C6 (C7)

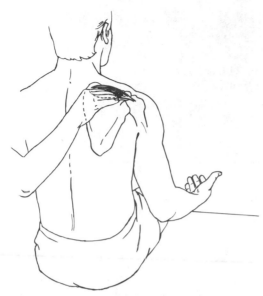

▲ **Figure 5.55** Palpating the supraspinatus muscle.

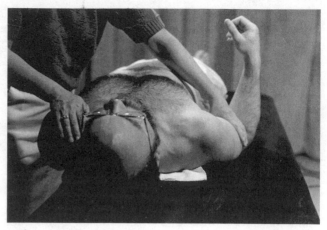

▲ **Figure 5.57** Testing the supraspinatus muscle in the GM supine position.

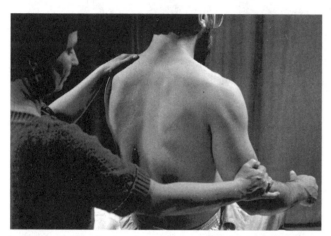

▲ **Figure 5.56** Testing the supraspinatus muscle in the AG sitting position.

Position

AG: Subject sits with the shoulder in neutral rotation and the elbow flexed (Fig. 5-56).

GM: Subject is supine with upper limb supported, shoulder in neutral rotation, and elbow flexed (Fig. 5-57).

Movement. Ask the subject to abduct the shoulder joint within a 30-degree range.

Resistance. Applied to the lateral arm immediately proximal to the elbow.

Stabilization. Stabilize the opposite shoulder.

Substitutions

- Prevent substitution by biceps brachii by not letting the shoulder rotate laterally.
- Serratus anterior may elevate the acromion process, giving the appearance of shoulder abduction.
- Scapular elevation and lateral flexion of the trunk to the opposite side may give the appearance of shoulder abduction.
- Trunk flexes to the same side.
- Deltoid abducts the shoulder joint.

MIDDLE DELTOID MUSCLE

The three portions of the deltoid muscle are tested during shoulder joint abduction in the coronal plane. The anterior and posterior portions are also tested as horizontal adductors and horizontal abductors, respectively. The test range of motion for the middle deltoid muscle is 90 degrees. The motion is accompanied by upward scapular rotation.

Palpation. Palpate laterally and inferior to the acromion process (Fig. 5-58).

Position

AG: Subject sits with the shoulder joint in neutral and the elbow flexed 90 degrees (Fig. 5-59).

▼ Attachments of Supraspinatus Muscle			
Muscle	**Proximal**	**Distal**	**Innervation**
Supraspinatus	Supraspinatus fossa	Superior surface of greater tubercle of humerus	Suprascapular C5 (C4 and C6)

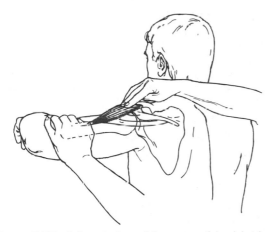

▲ **Figure 5.58** Palpating the middle portion of the deltoid muscle.

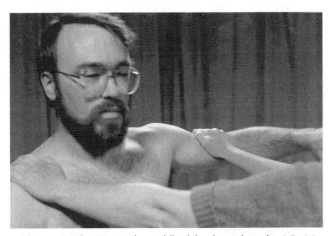

▲ **Figure 5.59** Testing the middle deltoid muscle in the AG sitting position.

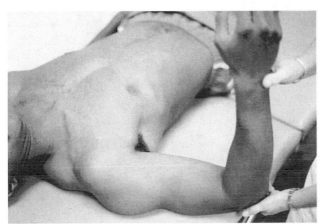

▲ **Figure 5.60** Testing the middle deltoid muscle in the GM supine position.

GM: Subject is supine with the upper limb supported and the elbow flexed 90 degrees (Fig. 5-60).

Movement. Abduct shoulder to 90 degrees in the coronal plane.

Resistance. Applied to the lateral arm immediately proximal to the elbow.

Stabilization. Stabilize the opposite shoulder.

Substitutions

- Prevent substitution by biceps brachii by keeping the shoulder joint in neutral rotation.
- Supraspinatus is also a shoulder joint abductor.
- Serratus anterior may abduct the scapula, giving the appearance of shoulder abduction.
- Trunk flexion to the same side may occur.

POSTERIOR DELTOID MUSCLE

The posterior portion of the deltoid muscle produces the test motion of shoulder horizontal abduction in the transverse plane from a flexed position. The starting position is 90 degrees of shoulder flexion. The shoulder moves into 120 degrees of abduction in the transverse plane.

Palpation. Palpate below and lateral to the spine of the scapula, crossing the shoulder joint posteriorly (Fig. 5-61).

Position

AG: Subject is prone with the shoulder flexed over the edge of the table and the elbow relaxed (Fig. 5-62).

GM: Subject sits with the upper limb supported on a table, the shoulder and elbow flexed 90 degrees (Fig. 5-63).

Movement. Horizontal abduction from 90 degrees of shoulder flexion to 120 degrees of abduction in the transverse plane.

Resistance. Applied to the posterior arm immediately proximal to the elbow.

Stabilization. Stabilize the scapula on the same side.

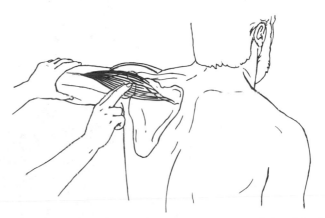

▲ **Figure 5.61** Palpating the posterior portion of the deltoid muscle.

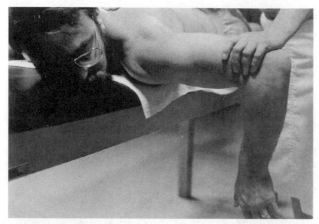

▲ **Figure 5.62** Testing the posterior deltoid muscle in the AG prone position.

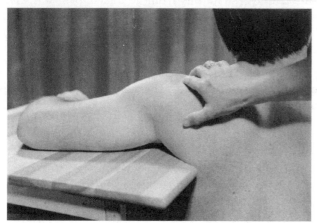

▲ **Figure 5.63** Testing the posterior deltoid muscle in the GM sitting position.

Substitutions

- Adduction of the scapula without horizontally abducting the shoulder can occur.
- In the GM position, the trunk may rotate, and the subject may throw the upper limb posteriorly, giving the appearance of horizontal adduction. Prevent this motion by stabilizing the trunk.
- Long head of the triceps is an accessory muscle; movement may be attempted by extending the elbow.

PECTORALIS MAJOR MUSCLE

The pectoralis major muscle is tested during horizontal adduction of the shoulder joint, in which the shoulder is positioned in 90 degrees of abduction. Motion occurs in the transverse plane toward 90 degrees of shoulder joint flexion.

Palpation. Palpate the pectoralis major (clavicular) muscle immediately inferior to the medial end of the clavicle. Sternal portion of the pectoralis major is palpated in the anterior axillary fold, against a resistance into extension and adduction (Fig. 5-64).

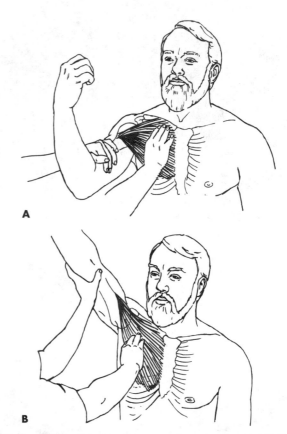

▲ **Figure 5.64** Palpating the pectoralis major muscle: (**A**) Clavicular portion; (**B**) sternal portion.

▼ Attachments of Middle Deltoid and Posterior Deltoid Muscles			
Muscle	**Proximal**	**Distal**	**Innervation**
Middle deltoid	Superior lateral surface of the acromion process of the scapula	Deltoid tuberosity of the humerus	Axillary C5 (C6)
Posterior deltoid	Inferior lip of spine of scapula	Deltoid tuberosity of the humerus	Axillary C5 (C6)

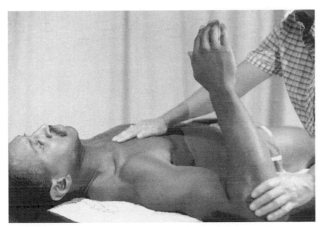

▲ **Figure 5.65** Testing the clavicular head of the pectoralis major muscle in the AG supine position.

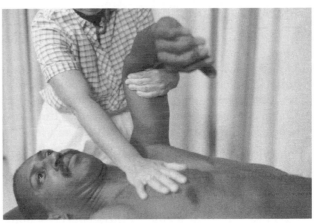

▲ **Figure 5.66** Testing the sternal head of the pectoralis major muscle in the AG supine position.

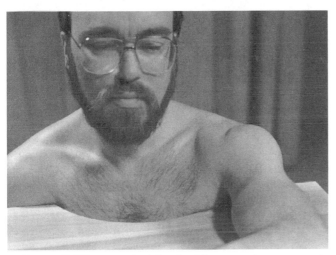

▲ **Figure 5.67** Testing both heads of the pectoralis major muscle in the GM sitting position.

Movement

- Sternal head: Horizontal adduction and extension from 90 degrees of abduction, moving toward the opposite shoulder in a diagonal direction.
- Clavicular head: Horizontal adduction with flexion from 90 degrees of abduction, moving toward the opposite shoulder in a diagonal direction.

Resistance. Applied to the anteromedial arm immediately proximal to the elbow.

Stabilization. Stabilize the contralateral shoulder or the ipsilateral trunk.

Substitutions

- Prevent the subject from twisting the trunk and throwing the upper limb using momentum by stabilizing the trunk.
- Anterior deltoid is an accessory muscle to the motion of horizontal adduction.
- Coracobrachialis and biceps brachii are accessory muscles to the motion of horizontal adduction.

Position

AG: Subject is supine with shoulder in neutral rotation and 90 degrees of abduction with elbow flexed (Figs. 5-65 and 5-66).

GM: Subject sits with shoulder in neutral rotation and 90 degrees of abduction, elbow flexed 90 degrees, and upper limb supported (Fig. 5-67).

▼ Attachments of Pectoralis Major Muscle (Clavicular and Sternal)			
Muscle	**Proximal**	**Distal**	**Innervation**
Pectoralis major (clavicular)	Anterior surface of medial half of clavicle	Inferior crest of greater tubercle of humerus	Lateral and medial pectoral C6 (C5)
Pectoralis major (sternal)	Anterior surface of sternum, costal cartilages of upper six pairs of ribs	Superior crest of greater tubercle of humerus	Lateral and medial pectoral C7 and C8 (T1)

SUBSCAPULARIS MUSCLE

The subscapularis muscle is tested during the movement of medial rotation of 60 degrees, with the shoulder joint positioned in 90 degrees of abduction and the elbow flexed over the edge of the table. A towel roll or the examiner's hand may be placed under the test elbow for comfort. Motion may be limited by tightness of the lateral rotators of the shoulder.

Palpation. Palpate with subject inclined forward so that the scapula abducts (slides forward) on the thorax by the weight of the arm. Place fingers on the costal surface of the scapula, beyond the latissimus dorsi muscle. Ask for medial rotation of the shoulder (Fig. 5-68).

Position

AG: Subject is prone with the shoulder abducted and the elbow flexed over the edge of the table (Fig. 5-69).

GM: Subject is prone with the shoulder flexed over the edge of the table (Fig. 5-70).

Movement. Medial rotation of the shoulder joint to 60 degrees.

Resistance. Applied immediately proximal to the wrist on the anterior surface of the forearm.

Stabilization. Stabilize the humerus and thorax with your hand and forearm.

Substitutions

• Prevent abduction of the scapula by stabilizing it.

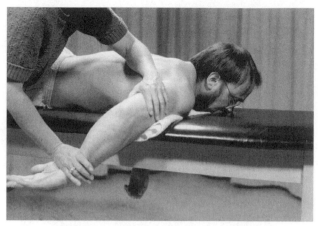

▲ **Figure 5.69** Testing the subscapularis muscle in the AG prone position.

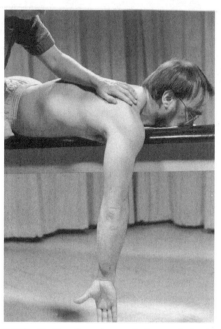

▲ **Figure 5.70** Testing the subscapularis muscle in the GM prone position.

• The subject may use momentum by laterally rotating the shoulder joint followed by relaxation, giving the appearance of medial rotation.
• Pronation of the forearm may give the appearance of medial rotation.
• Pectoralis major, teres major, and latissimus dorsi muscles are also medial rotators of the shoulder joint.

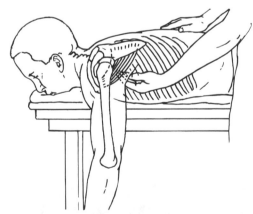

▲ **Figure 5.68** Palpating the subscapularis muscle.

▼ Attachments of Subscapularis Muscle			
Muscle	**Proximal**	**Distal**	**Innervation**
Subscapularis	Subscapular fossa of the scapula	Lesser tubercle of humerus	Upper and lower subscapular C6 (C5 and C7)

INFRASPINATUS AND TERES MINOR MUSCLES

The infraspinatus and the teres minor muscles produce the motion of lateral rotation of the shoulder joint through the test range of 90 degrees. For grades AG, the shoulder is abducted 90 degrees with the arm resting on the table and the elbow flexed 90 degrees. For grades GM, the shoulder is flexed over the edge of the table. A rolled towel or the examiner's hand is placed under the elbow joint for comfort.

Palpation. With subject in a prone position with the shoulder abducted and the elbow flexed over the edge of the table, palpate inferior to the spine of the scapula for the infraspinatus and along the lateral border of the scapula superior to the inferior angle of the scapula for the teres minor muscle. The two are often indistinguishable (Fig. 5-71).

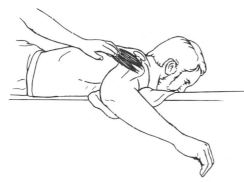

▲ **Figure 5.71** Palpating the infraspinatus and teres minor muscles.

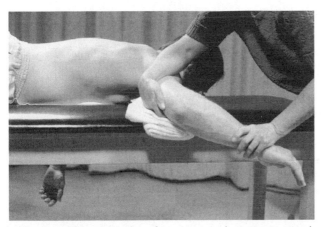

▲ **Figure 5.72** Testing the infraspinatus and teres minor muscles in the AG prone position.

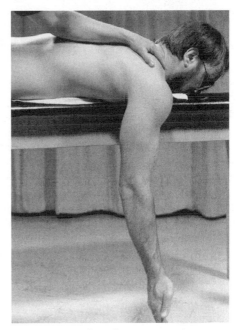

▲ **Figure 5.73** Testing the infraspinatus and teres minor muscles in the GM prone position.

Position

AG: Subject lies prone with the elbow flexed over the edge of the table (Fig. 5-72).
GM: Subject lies prone with the shoulder flexed over the edge of the table (Fig. 5-73).

Movement. Rotate the shoulder laterally 90 degrees.

Resistance. Applied immediately proximal to the wrist on the extensor surface of the forearm.

Stabilization. Stabilize the humerus and the thorax.

Substitutions

- Posterior deltoid can cause shoulder hyperextension.
- Supination of the forearm may give the appearance of lateral rotation.
- Subject may use momentum of medial rotation, giving the appearance of lateral rotation.
- Posterior deltoid is an accessory muscle to the motion of lateral rotation.

▼ Attachments of Infraspinatus and Teres Minor Muscles

Muscle	Proximal	Distal	Innervation
Infraspinatus	Infraspinatus fossa of scapula	Posterior on greater tubercle	Suprascapular C5 (C6)
Teres minor	Upper portion of lateral border of scapula	Inferior on posterior aspect of greater tubercle of humerus	Axillary C5 (C6)

CLINICAL ASSESSMENT

Observation and Screening

The shoulder complex should be examined from both a posterior and anterior view.

A posterior view of the subject allows visualization of bony landmarks, including the thoracic spine, scapula, acromioclavicular (AC) joint, and soft-tissue structures, including the upper trapezius, supraspinatus, infraspinatus, teres major and minor, and posterior and middle portions of the deltoid muscle. Particular attention should be given to areas of muscular atrophy, which could indicate disuse or peripheral nerve injury or pathology.

The scapula should be examined for evidence of "winging" due to serratus anterior weakness or long thoracic nerve injury. Winging occurs when the vertebral border of the scapula projects posteriorly away from the thoracic wall (see Chap. 4). Sprengel's deformity, a congenitally elevated or undescended scapula, results from poorly developed scapular muscles or from a fibrous band replacing scapular muscles.[5]

An anterior view of the shoulder complex allows for observation of bony landmarks, including the sternoclavicular (SC) joint, clavicle, AC joint, and coracoid process. The anterior and middle portions of the deltoid are also visible from this view. The SC and AC joints should be observed for any joint asymmetry, indicating joint disruption. Separation of the AC joint often results in a visible "step off" deformity in which the clavicle sits superiorly relative to the acromion. The clavicle should be examined for any asymmetry of its bony contour, which could indicate current or past fracture. Flattening of the normally rounded contour of the deltoid is often evident in cases of glenohumeral dislocation. Atrophy of the deltoid may also represent disuse or an axillary nerve injury or pathology.

Palpation and Surface Anatomy

Palpation of the following structures and skeletal landmarks is essential to provide the examiner with complete, accurate information relative to assessment of pathology in the shoulder complex:

1. The scapula may be examined from behind the subject and from the side. Landmarks to be included in palpation are the inferior angle, spine of the scapula, vertebral border, acromion process, and coracoid process (Fig. 5-74).
2. The clavicle is examined from the front by palpating the lateral end where it articulates with the acromion, following the course of the bone to its medial end where it articulates with the manubrium of the sternum (Fig. 5-75).

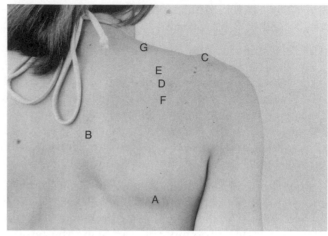

A - Inferior Angle of Scapula   E - Supraspinatus Muscle
B - Vertebral Border of Scapula   F - Infraspinatus Muscle
C - Acromion   G - Upper Trapezius Muscle
D - Spine of Scapula

▲ **Figure 5.74** Surface anatomy of the posterior shoulder.

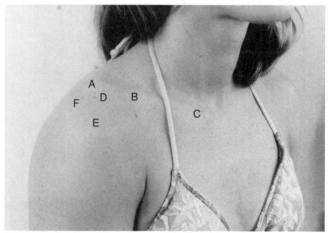

A = Acromioclavicular Joint   D = Coracoid Process
B = Clavicle   E = Bicipital Groove
C = Sternoclavicular Joint   F = Humeral Head

▲ **Figure 5.75** Surface anatomy of the anterior shoulder.

3. The proximal humerus should be assessed by palpating the greater tuberosity, lesser tuberosity, and the bicipital groove, which transmits the tendon of the long head of the biceps brachii muscle.
4. The SC, AC, and glenohumeral joints should be palpated for symmetry.

In assessing musculoskeletal pathology involving the shoulder, the examiner must be able to palpate the tendons of the rotator cuff musculature in addition to the tendon of the long head of the biceps brachii muscle.

1. The supraspinatus tendon is palpated approximately 2 cm inferior to the anterolateral acromion. The subject should be supine or half-sitting with the shoulder internally ro-

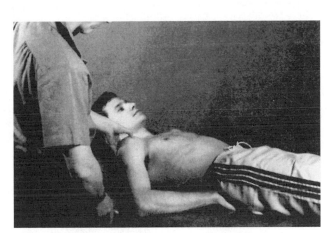

▲ **Figure 5.76** Palpating the supraspinatus tendon.

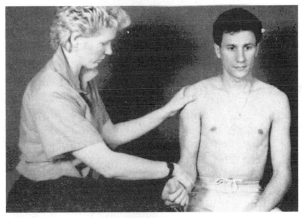

▲ **Figure 5.78** Palpating the tendon of the long head of the biceps.

tated and the hand placed behind the back. This position exposes the tenoperiosteal junction and tendon, allowing for greater ease of palpation (Fig. 5-76). The musculotendinous portion of the supraspinatus can be palpated just posterior to the distal clavicle and anterior to the suprascapular spine.

2. The infraspinatus tendon is palpated with the subject prone on elbows and the weight shifted over the shoulder being examined, placing the shoulder in a position of horizontal adduction and external rotation. This positioning displaces the tendinous insertion posteriorly and inferiorly to the acromion. The examiner palpates the spine of the scapula, follows it laterally to the posterolateral acromion, and then drops 1 cm inferiorly to locate the infraspinatus tendon (Fig. 5-77).

3. The tendon of the long head of the biceps brachii can be located between the greater and lesser tuberosities, where it lies within the bicipital (intertubercular) groove (Fig. 5-78). Placing the shoulder in 10 degrees of internal rotation situates the bicipital groove anteriorly. Additionally, internal and external rotation of the shoulder may assist the examiner in locating the

greater and lesser tuberosities. It is questionable as to whether direct palpation of the biceps tendon is possible because this area is somewhat covered by the anterior deltoid muscle.

Active and Passive Movements

The motions to be assessed both actively and passively at the shoulder complex include the following:

1. Sternoclavicular joint:
   a. Elevation
   b. Depression
   c. Protraction
   d. Retraction
2. Scapulothoracic joint:
   a. Elevation
   b. Depression
   c. Abduction
   d. Adduction
   e. Upward rotation
   f. Downward rotation
3. Glenohumeral joint:
   a. Flexion
   b. Extension
   c. Abduction
   d. Adduction
   e. Internal rotation
   f. External rotation
   g. Horizontal abduction
   h. Horizontal adduction

Contractile Testing

The contractile testing that should be performed at the shoulder includes the following:

1. Flexion
2. Extension
3. Abduction
4. Adduction

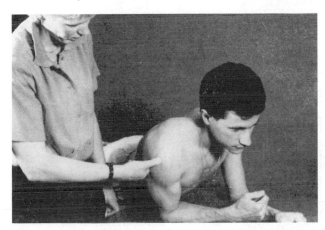

▲ **Figure 5.77** Palpating the infraspinatus tendon.

5. Internal rotation
6. External rotation
7. Horizontal abduction
8. Horizontal adduction

SPECIAL CLINICAL TESTS

APLEY'S SCRATCH TESTS

Indication. Apley's tests are designed to provide the examiner with a quick, nonspecific active functional assessment of shoulder girdle mobility.

Method

Abduction and External Rotation. The subject is instructed to reach behind the head and touch the superior medial border of the scapula on the contralateral side (Fig. 5-79).

Adduction and Internal Rotation. The subject is asked to bring the tested arm behind the back and touch the inferior angle of the opposite scapula with the hand (Fig. 5-80).

Results. The ability to perform these tests demonstrates good functional ability of the glenohumeral complex. These tests are highly correlated to a person's ability to do basic activities of daily living, including combing hair and reaching a wallet in the back pocket. Difficulty in assuming these positions indicates limitations of movement somewhere in the shoulder complex.

PAINFUL ARC SYNDROME

Indication. Painful arc should be detected during the course of a peripheral joint assessment. The arc

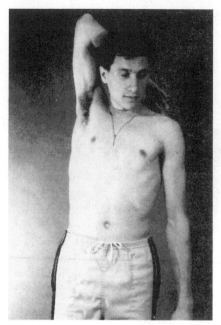

▲ **Figure 5.79** Apley's scratch test (abduction and external rotation).

is primarily found in the motion of shoulder joint abduction, although flexion may also demonstrate this defect. The pain associated with this syndrome is mechanical, resulting from pinching of structures between the acromial arch and the coracoacromial ligament.

Method. Usually no pain is associated with abduction of the shoulder until approximately 70 to 90 degrees, at which point the greater tuberosity must pass beneath the coracoacromial arch to complete full, painless abduction (Fig. 5-81). Inflamed struc-

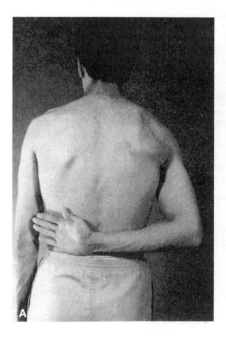

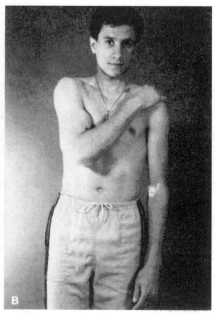

▲ **Figure 5.80** (**A** and **B**) Adduction and internal rotation in Apley's scratch test.

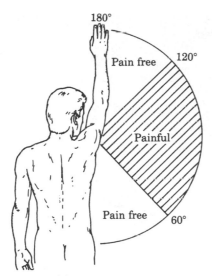

▲ **Figure 5.81** Painful arc.

tures in the suprahumeral space or faulty biomechanics compromise an already restricted area allowed for smooth motion. As a result, structures are pinched, creating pain that may continue through the range until approximately 120 degrees. At this point, the pinched structures have passed under the coracoacromial arch, thereby allowing pain-free movement through the completion of shoulder abduction.

Results. The subject experiences no pain-pain-no pain in the range of motion of the shoulder. A painful arc may be evident during passive or active motion.

TESTS FOR THE BICEPS BRACHII MUSCLE

Speed's Test

Indication. Speed's test is indicated for assessing the presence of bicipital tendinitis.

Method. The subject sits or stands while flexing the shoulder approximately 60 degrees with the elbow extended and the forearm supinated. The examiner isometrically resists shoulder flexion with resistance applied to the distal ventral forearm of the subject (Fig. 5-82).

Results. Pain localized to the area of the bicipital groove indicates a positive test for bicipital tendon pathology, usually inflammation.

Yergason's Test

Indication. Yergason's test[19] evaluates for bicipital tendinitis in the bicipital groove.

Method. The subject may be examined while sitting or standing (Fig. 5-83). The elbow is stabilized against the trunk as it is held in 90 degrees of flex-

ion. The examiner resists forearm supination from a fully pronated position while simultaneously resisting external rotation.

Results. Pain experienced by the subject during the resisted muscle contraction in the area of the bicipital groove represents a positive test. During the test, the bicipital tendon may displace out of the groove, possibly indicating a tear of the transverse humeral ligament. A more definitive means of assessing the transverse humeral ligament is described below.

Transverse Humeral Ligament Test (Booth and Marvel Test)

Indication. The transverse humeral ligament test[4] may be beneficial in assessing the integrity of the transverse humeral ligament, which is responsible

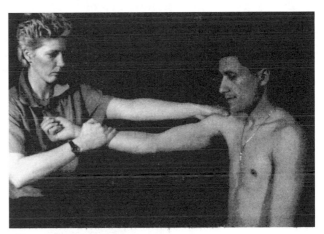

▲ **Figure 5.82** Speed's test.

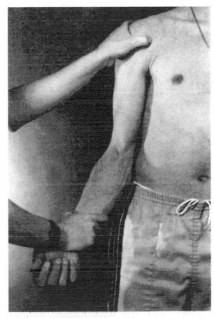

▲ **Figure 5.83** Yergason's test.

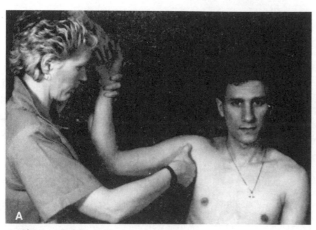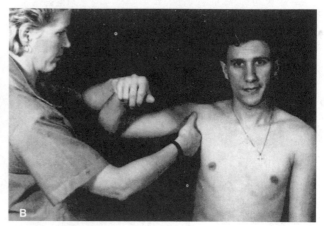

▲ **Figure 5.84** Transverse humeral ligament test. (**A**) Starting position; (**B**) end position.

for stabilizing the long head of the biceps tendon in the bicipital groove.

Method. The subject's shoulder is placed in abduction and external rotation (Fig. 5-84). In this position, the examiner palpates over the tendon in the bicipital groove while internally and externally rotating the subject's shoulder. In individuals who do not possess sufficient shoulder range of motion to achieve the standard position, an alternative is to place the shoulder in adduction with the arm stabilized against the trunk.

Results. The biceps tendon palpated popping in and out of the groove during the motions of rotation indicates a positive result for a rupture of the transverse humeral ligament.

Lippman's Test

Indication. Lippman's Test[11] is designed to assess bicipital tendinitis.

Method. The subject either sits or stands with the elbow flexed 90 degrees. The examiner displaces the biceps tendon from side to side in the bicipital groove (Fig 5-85). DeAnquin described a variation of this test in which the examiner palpates the biceps tendon in the groove while simultaneously creating movement stresses by internally and externally rotating the humerus (Fig. 5-86).

Results. A positive test is indicated by the subject experiencing sharp pain of the long head of the biceps tendon in the area of the bicipital groove.

Ludington's Test

Indication. Ludington's test[12] is performed in suspected cases of rupture of the long head of the biceps brachii.

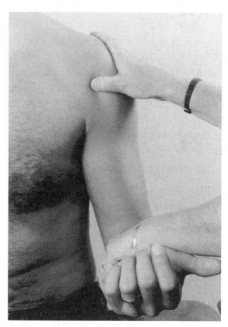

▲ **Figure 5.85** Lippman's test.

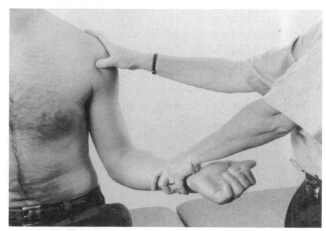

▲ **Figure 5.86** DeAnquin's test.

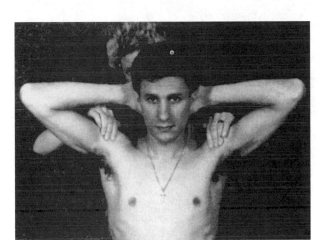

▲ **Figure 5.87** Ludington's test.

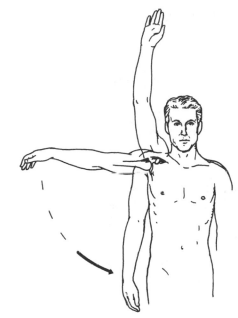

▲ **Figure 5.88** Drop arm test.

Method. The subject clasps the hands behind the head, allowing the interlocked grip to support the weight of the upper extremities (Fig. 5-87). The subject is then directed to contract and relax the biceps brachii muscle alternately, while the examiner palpates the biceps tendon proximally in the bicipital groove.

Results. Palpation of the unaffected biceps tendon during contraction is possible, while no palpable contraction is evident on the involved side. This finding is typical of a rupture of the long head of the biceps brachii.

TESTS FOR THE SUPRASPINATUS MUSCLE

Drop Arm Test

Indication. The drop arm test is used as an adjunctive technique in the assessment of a rotator cuff tear, specifically of the supraspinatus contractile unit.

Method. The subject either stands or sits with the shoulder placed in the fully abducted position. The subject is asked to slowly lower the limb from the fully abducted position back down to the side (Fig. 5-88).

Results. The ability to control the lowering of the upper limb back to an adducted position represents a negative test for involvement of the supraspinatus tendon. A positive result is confirmed when lowering the limb creates pain or the limb drops uncontrollably to the side from the abducted position of approximately 90 degrees.

Supraspinatus Test

Indication. A suspected tear within the supraspinatus contractile unit is the indication for the supraspinatus test.[14]

Method. The subject sits with the shoulder in 90 degrees of abduction and the glenohumeral joint in neutral rotation. The examiner provides isometric resistance to shoulder abduction in this position. Next, the subject's shoulder is rotated internally (so that the thumbs point toward the floor) and horizontally adducted 30 degrees into the scapular plane (Fig. 5-89). The examiner again resists shoulder abduction, looking for pain or weakness. This test should be repeated at 45 degrees of scapular plane abduction to eliminate the possibility of a painful response secondary to impingement.

Results. A positive test is represented by pain or weakness during resisted abduction of the shoulder, indicating a lesion to the supraspinatus or suprascapular nerve dysfunction. Additionally, if the level of pain decreases or ceases when the test is per-

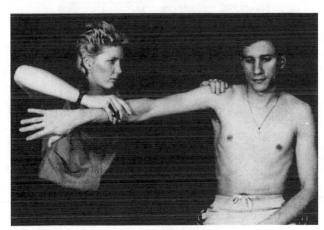

▲ **Figure 5.89** Supraspinatus test.

formed in 45 degrees of scapular plane abduction, the examiner should suspect impingement of the subdeltoid bursa.

TESTS FOR IMPINGEMENT

Neer Test

Indication. The Neer test[15] is indicated in suspected cases of shoulder impingement involving the long head of the biceps tendon.

Method. The examiner passively and forcibly flexes the subject's shoulder forward, thereby jamming the greater tuberosity against the antero-inferior surface of the acromion process (Fig. 5-90).

Results. A positive test result is indicated by the subject's painful response, indicating impingement of the long head of the biceps tendon.

Kennedy-Hawkins Test

Indication. Kennedy-Hawkins test[10] is used in assessing impingement pathology of the shoulder, involving the supraspinatus tendon.

Method. The subject's shoulder and elbow joints are flexed to 90 degrees. The examiner then forcibly internally rotates the shoulder, jamming the supraspinatus against the anterior portion of the coracacromial ligament (Fig. 5-91).

Results. Pain represents a positive test for supraspinatus impingement.

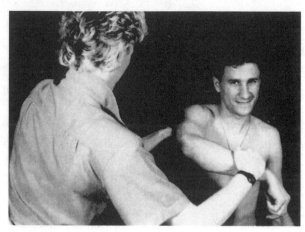

▲ **Figure 5.91** Hawkins' test.

Impingement Sign

Indication. The impingement sign test is useful in assessing impingement of the shoulder, involving either the supraspinatus or long head of the biceps.

Method. The subject sits while the examiner passively and forcibly horizontally adducts the shoulder from a starting position of 90 degrees of flexion (Fig. 5-92).

Results. Pain at the extreme of horizontal adduction represents a positive test for impingement of either or both the supraspinatus or long head of the biceps.

Impingement Relief Test

Indication. This test is useful in confirming impingement syndromes.

Method. The subject performs a movement or function involving the shoulder that produces the impingement symptoms. The examiner then de-

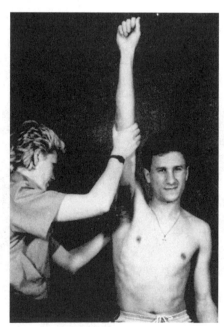

▲ **Figure 5.90** Neer's test.

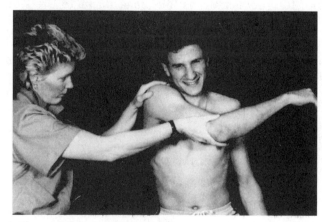

▲ **Figure 5.92** Impingement sign.

presses the humeral head as the subject repeats the same active or functional movement.

Results. Comparison of symptoms is made between the two testing situations. A noted decrease in pain intensity in the range of shoulder impingement with the humeral head depressed indicates a positive test for impingement syndrome.

TESTS FOR SHOULDER STABILITY

Anterior Apprehension Test

Indication. The apprehension test[6] is indicated in suspected cases of anterior shoulder subluxation or dislocation.

Method. The subject lies supine on the examining table. The examiner passively abducts the shoulder to approximately 90 degrees and then superimposes shoulder external rotation (Fig. 5-93A). The examiner should be careful to support the joint anteriorly in subjects who, by virtue of medical history or previous dislocations, are predisposed to shoulder instability.

Results. The combination of excessive shoulder abduction and external rotation is a common mechanism of injury in shoulder dislocation. As the combined motions of abduction and external rotation are initiated, the subject reacts by sensing that dislocation is about to occur and demonstrates a facial expression of apprehension (see Fig. 5-93B), accompanied by resistance to further motion of the shoulder. Following performance of this test, the examiner can apply a posterior pressure to the humeral head while repeating the mechanics of the anterior apprehension test. This posterior force applied to the humeral head reduces the anterior displacement of the humeral head relative to the glenoid. A decrease in the level of pain or apprehension indicates a positive relocation test.

Fulcrum Test

Indication. The fulcrum test[13] is designed to assess anterior glenohumeral instability.

Method. The subject is positioned supine with the shoulder abducted to 90 degrees and externally ro-

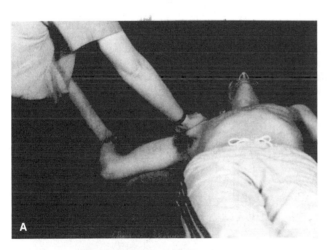

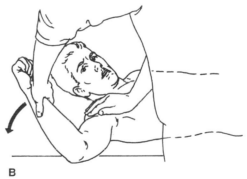

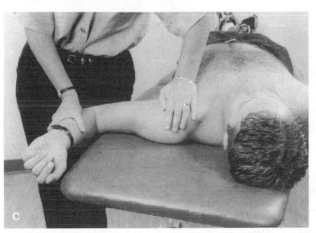

▲ **Figure 5.93** **(A)** Shoulder apprehension test. **(B)** A look of apprehension on patient's face is a positive finding. **(C)** Relocation test.

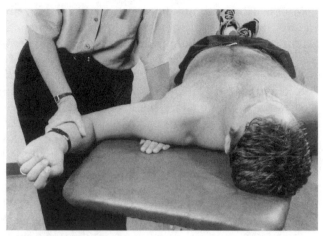

▲ **Figure 5.94** Fulcrum test.

tated. The examiner places one hand posterior to the humeral head while externally rotating and extending the arm over the fulcrum, which further stresses the capsuloligamentous complex (Fig. 5-94).

Results. Pain, apprehension, or excessive humeral head displacement is representative of a positive test.

Anterior Drawer Test

Indication. The anterior drawer test[9] is useful in the assessment of increased or decreased translation of the humeral head relative to the glenoid.

Method. The subject is seated with forearms resting on the thighs. The examiner grips the humeral head anteriorly with the fingers and posteriorly with the thumb. The other hand stabilizes the scapula (Fig. 5-95). The humeral head is then passively moved anteromedially and posterolaterally in line with the glenoid.

Results. A positive test occurs with pain, clicking, or an increase or decrease in humeral head translation.

Clunk Test (Labral Test)

Indication. The clunk test[3] is useful in the assessment of a glenoid labral tear.

Method. The subject is positioned supine with the shoulder fully abducted. The examiner grasps the distal humerus with one hand while the other hand is placed proximally over the posterior shoulder. Simultaneously, the examiner moves the humeral head anteriorly with the proximal hand while externally rotating the humerus with the distal hand (Fig 5-96).

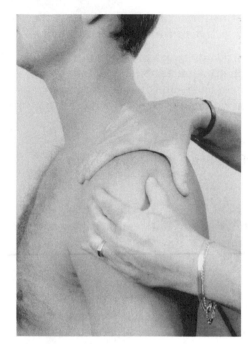

▲ **Figure 5.95** Anterior drawer test.

Results. The presence of a "clunk" or grinding sensation at the glenohumeral joint indicates a positive test for a labral tear. This test is important because a torn glenoid labrum can contribute to anterior instability of the shoulder.

Rockwood Test for Anterior Instability

Indication. The Rockwood test[15] is indicated in suspected cases of anterior instability.

Method. The subject is seated with the examiner standing behind. The subject's arm is positioned by the side as the examiner passively externally rotates

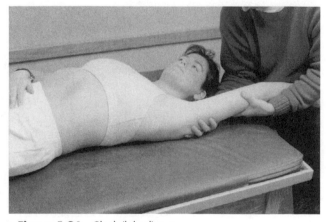

▲ **Figure 5.96** Clunk (labral) test.

the shoulder. The shoulder is then repositioned at angles of 45, 90, and 120 degrees of abduction and again passively externally rotated (Fig. 5-97).

Results. At 0 degrees of abduction, the subject should not experience apprehension. At 45 and 120 degrees of abduction, the subject exhibits some apprehension and pain. However, at 90 degrees of abduction, the subject must demonstrate significant apprehension and posterior pain.

Posterior Drawer Test

Indication. The posterior drawer test[9] is useful in the evaluation of posterior humeral head translation relative to the glenoid.

Method. Subject and examiner positioning is the same as for the anterior drawer test. The examiner passively displaces the humeral head in a posterior direction. Care must be taken to avoid excessive pressure over the bicipital groove, which could cause pain.

Results. Pain, clicking, or an increase or decrease in humeral head translation indicates a positive test. Posterior humeral head translation is normally greater than anterior translation, in that half of the humeral head can normally be displaced posteriorly.

Posterior Apprehension Test

Indication. The posterior apprehension test[6] is used in the assessment of posterior instability of the shoulder.

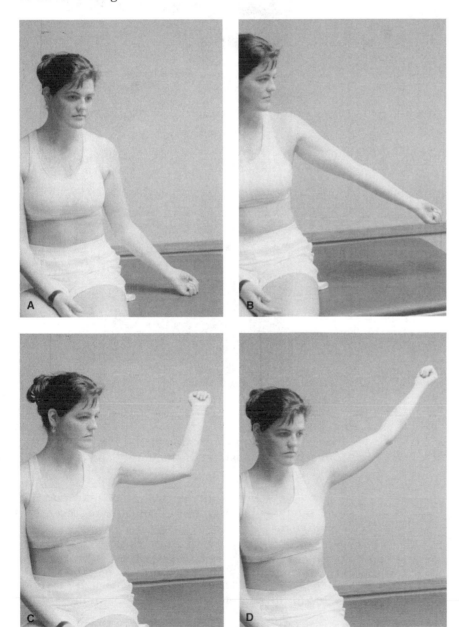

▲ **Figure 5.97** Rockwood test. **(A)** 0 degrees abduction. **(B)** 45 degrees abduction. **(C)** 90 degrees abduction. **(D)** 120 degrees abduction.

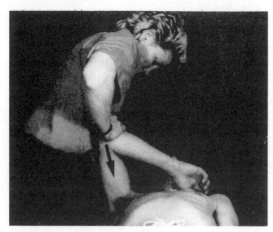

▲ **Figure 5.98** Posterior apprehension test.

Method. The subject lies supine, with the shoulder flexed and internally rotated and with the elbow flexed and resting on the trunk (Fig. 5-98). A posterior force is transmitted by the examiner through the subject's elbow.

Results. A look of apprehension and resistance to further movement constitutes a positive result indicative of posterior dislocation.

Jerk Test

Indication. The jerk test[13] is indicated in cases of suspected posterior shoulder instability.

Method. The subject is seated with the shoulder flexed 90 degrees and internally rotated with the elbow in approximately 90 degrees of flexion. The examiner applies one hand to the elbow and produces an axial load through the humerus to the glenohumeral joint. The examiner then moves the shoulder into horizontal adduction while maintaining the axial load (Fig. 5-99).

Results. A positive test occurs when the shoulder suddenly jerks during the movement of horizontal adduction, representing the humeral head slipping off the glenoid. On return of the shoulder to the start position of 90 degrees of flexion, a second jerk may be experienced, representing a reduction of the humeral head.

Push-Pull Test

The Push-Pull Test[13] is performed in subjects with suspected posterior glenohumeral joint instability.

Method. The subject is positioned supine with the shoulder placed at 90 degrees of scapular plane abduction. The examiner grasps the subject's wrist with one hand while the other hand is placed anteriorly near the humeral head. The examiner simulta-

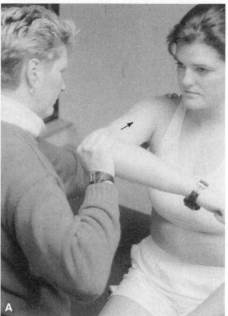

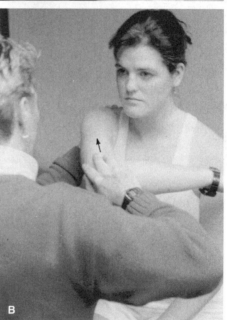

▲ **Figure 5.99** (**A** and **B**) Jerk test.

neously pulls upward through the long axis of the forearm while pushing the humeral head posteriorly (Fig. 5-100).

Results. Subject apprehension or displacement of the humeral head greater than 50% represents a positive test.

Sulcus Sign

Indication. Assessment of the sulcus sign[13] is indicated in the assessment of inferior instability

Method. The subject is seated with the upper limb relaxed by the side. The examiner grasps the fore-

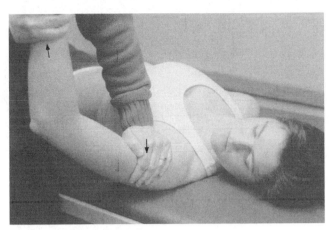

▲ **Figure 5.100** Push-pull test.

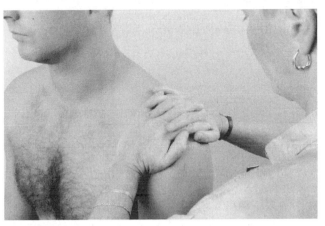

▲ **Figure 5.102** AC shear test.

arm and exerts an inferior distraction force through the limb (Fig. 5-101).

Results. A visible sulcus appearing at the glenohumeral joint space indicates a positive test for inferior instability.

Feagin Test

Indication. Feagin's test[15] is indicated in suspected cases of anteroinferior instability.

Method. The subject can be standing or seated with the shoulder abducted 90 degrees and the distal forearm resting on the examiner's shoulder. The examiner cups or clasps the hands together on the top of the subject's proximal humerus and exerts an anteroinferior force to the humerus.

Results. A response of apprehension indicates a positive test.

AC Shear Test

Indication. The AC shear test[6] is designed to assess pathology of the AC joint.

Method. The subject is seated or standing while the examiner's hands are cupped with the base of one hand over the spine of the scapula and the other anteriorly over the clavicle (Fig. 5-102). The examiner then squeezes the heels of the hands together.

Results. A positive test is indicated by pain or abnormal movement in the AC joint.

TESTS FOR THORACIC OUTLET SYNDROME

Adson's Maneuver

Indication. Adson's maneuver,[1] a thoracic outlet test, is used to rule out compression of the neurovascular bundle secondary to a cervical rib or abnormalities of scalene musculature.

Method. The subject's head is extended and rotated toward the side being tested. The examiner palpates the radial pulse while extending and externally rotating the shoulder (Fig. 5-103). The subject

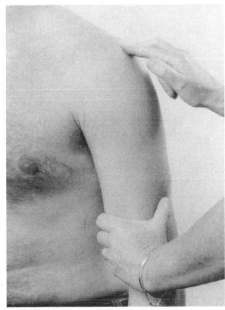

▲ **Figure 5.101** Sulcus sign.

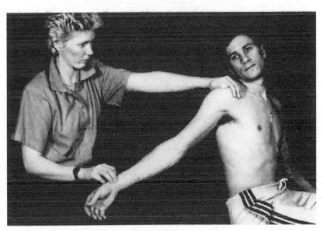

▲ **Figure 5.103** Adson's maneuver.

is instructed to take a deep breath and hold it while the examiner continues to palpate the pulse.

Results. A diminution or disappearance of the radial pulse is a positive result for thoracic outlet syndrome.

Costoclavicular Syndrome Test

Indication. The costoclavicular syndrome test[8] is used when compromise of the thoracic outlet might be attributed to entrapment of the subclavian artery and brachial plexus as they pass between the clavicle and the first rib.

Method. The examiner palpates the radial pulse and continues to do so while depressing and retracting the subject's shoulder complex (Fig. 5-104).

Results. A positive result is the same as that for Adson's maneuver, above.

Shoulder Girdle Relief Position

Indication. This test is indicated in conjunction with the costoclavicular test in assessment of thoracic outlet syndrome.

Method. The subject is either seated or standing with the arms crossed. The examiner grasps the subject's arms and passively moves the shoulder girdle superiorly and anteriorly, thereby enlarging the costoclavicular interval. This position is maintained for 30 seconds.

Results. Reproduction of paresthesias or numbness to the affected upper limb indicates a positive test.

Hyperabduction Syndrome Test (Wright Maneuver)

Indication. The hyperabduction syndrome test[18] is performed in cases of suspected thoracic outlet syn-

drome due to entrapment of subclavian vessels and the brachial plexus beneath the tendon of the pectoralis minor and the coracoid process.

Method. The upper limb being tested is placed and maintained in a position of shoulder hyperabduction as the examiner palpates the radial pulse (Fig. 5-105).

Results. Positive results are the same as those for Adson's maneuver.

Halstead's Maneuver

Indication. Halstead's maneuver is used to assess for thoracic outlet syndrome.

Method. The subject hyperextends the head and rotates it away from the side being tested (Fig. 5-106). The subject's radial pulse is palpated as the examiner exerts a downward traction force on the upper limb being assessed.

Results. Diminution or absence of the radial pulse represents a positive result.

Allen's Test

Indication. Allen's test[2] is performed to confirm or rule out thoracic outlet syndrome.

Method. The subject's shoulder is abducted 90 degrees with the elbow flexed 90 degrees (Fig. 5-107). The examiner palpates the radial pulse as the subject is instructed to rotate the head away from the tested side.

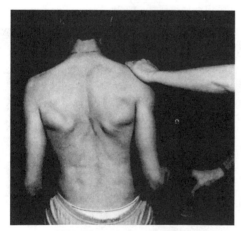

▲ **Figure 5.104** Costoclavicular syndrome test.

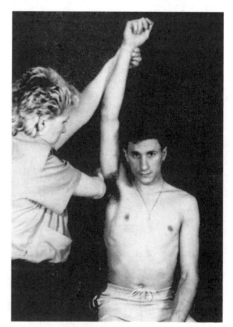

▲ **Figure 5.105** Hyperabduction syndrome test.

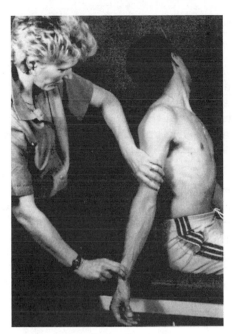

▲ **Figure 5.106** Halstead's maneuver.

Results. A positive result is noted if the radial pulse weakens or disappears when the subject rotates the head.

Roos Test (Elevated Arm Stress Test)

Indication. Roos test[16,17] is used in the assessment of thoracic outlet syndrome.

Method. The subject stands with both shoulders abducted to 90 degrees and externally rotated with the elbows flexed to 90 degrees. The subject slowly opens and closes the hands for a 3-minute period (Fig. 5-108).

Results. A positive test for thoracic outlet syndrome is indicated by the inability to maintain the upper limb position, ischemic pain, numbness or paresthesia of the limb, or heaviness of the arm.

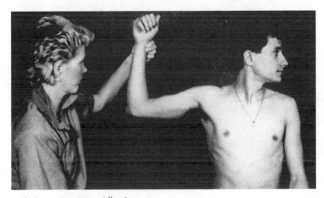

▲ **Figure 5.107** Allen's test.

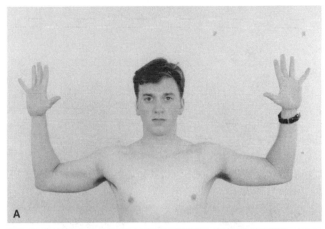
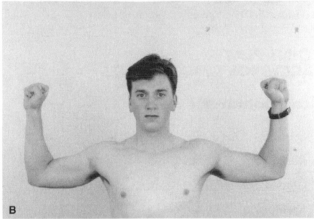

▲ **Figure 5.108** (**A** and **B**) Roos test.

Upper Limb Tension Test

Indication. The upper limb tension test[7] is designed to stress the brachial plexus and dura of the cervical spine.

Method. The subject lies supine while the examiner applies movements to the upper limb and neck that progressively stretch the brachial plexus and dura. Initially, the examiner abducts and externally rotates the shoulder posterior to the frontal plane, which stabilizes the should girdle in depression. Next, the elbow is passively extended, the forearm supinated, the wrist extended, and the fingers are placed into extension (Fig. 5-109). Finally, if tolerated, the subject can side bend the head to the contralateral side.

Results. As the progressive stretch is performed, the subject may experience reproduction of symptoms, including pain, paresthesias, or numbness in the upper limb. An indication as to the severity of the problem is evident in the amount of elbow extension tolerated by the subject as compared to the uninvolved side.

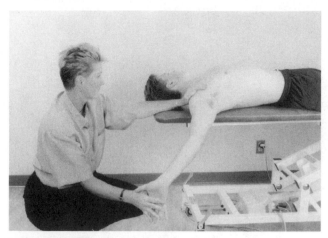

▲ **Figure 5.109** Upper limb tension test.

JOINT PLAY (ACCESSORY MOVEMENTS)

Scapulothoracic Joint

Superior Glide (Fig. 5-110A)

Restriction. Elevation.

Open-Packed Position. Anatomical position.

Positioning. The subject is in the sidelying position with the test scapula uppermost. The examiner stands at the side of the table facing the subject and stabilizes the upper limb with the distal forearm and the body. Intrinsic stabilization is also provided by the position of the subject and location of the scapula.

Movement. The therapist uses one hand to mobilize the scapula by holding the inferior angle at the web space. The other hand grasps the superior aspect of the scapula by cupping the acromion process. The scapula moves in a superior direction.

Inferior Glide (see Fig. 5-110B)

Restriction. Depression.

Positioning. The subject is in a sidelying position with the scapula being treated uppermost. The examiner stands at the side of the table facing the subject and stabilizes the upper limb being tested with the distal forearm and the body. Intrinsic stabilization is also provided by the subject's position and the location of the scapula.

Movement. One of the therapist's hands mobilizes the scapula by holding the inferior angle with the web space. The other hand grasps the superior aspect of the scapula by cupping over the acromion. The scapula is moved in an inferior direction.

Lateral Glide (Fig. 5-111A)

Restriction. Abduction.

Positioning. As for inferior glide.

Movement. The therapist's one hand grips around the inferior angle of the scapula. The index and middle finger of the other hand grip the superior medial aspect of the scapula, while the thumb holds the scapula superolaterally. The scapula is moved in a lateral direction.

Medial Glide (see Fig. 5-111B).

Restriction. Adduction.

Positioning. As for inferior glide.

Movement. As for lateral glide, except that the scapula is moved in a medial direction.

Lateral and Superior Glide (Fig. 5-112A)

Restriction. Abduction and upward rotation.

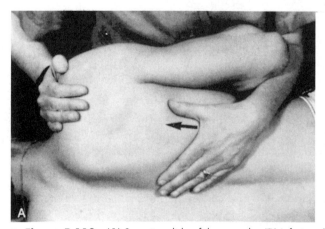
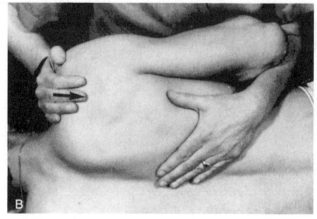

▲ **Figure 5.110** (**A**) Superior glide of the scapula. (**B**) Inferior glide of the scapula.

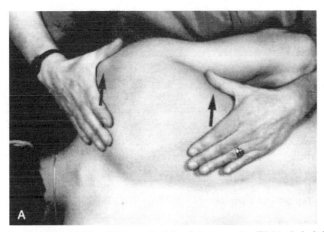

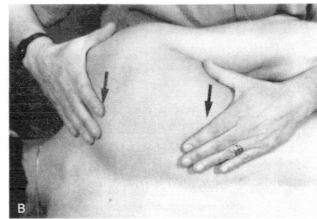

▲ **Figure 5.111** (**A**) Lateral glide of the scapula. (**B**) Medial glide of the scapula.

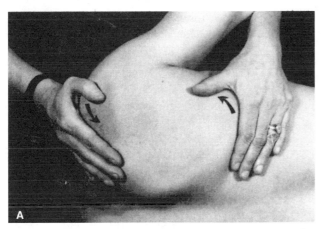

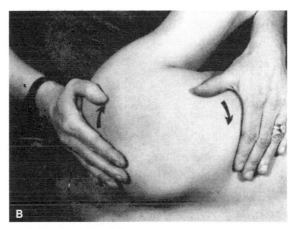

▲ **Figure 5.112** (**A**) Lateral and superior glide of the scapula. (**B**) Medial and inferior glide.

Positioning. As for inferior glide.

Movement. As for lateral glide, except that the scapula is moved laterally and superiorly; the therapist primarily controls the motion at the inferior angle.

Medial and Inferior Glide (see Fig. 5-112B)

Restriction. Adduction and downward rotation.

Positioning. As for inferior glide.

Movement. As for inferior glide, except that the scapula is moved medially and inferiorly with the therapist primarily controlling the motion at the inferior angle.

Glenohumeral Joint

Distraction (Lateral) (Fig. 5-113)

Restriction. General hypomobility.

Open-Packed Position. Fifty-five to 70 degrees abduction; 30 degrees horizontal adduction.

Positioning. The subject lies supine; a strap is applied to stabilize the scapula. The web space of the mobilizing hand is placed high in the axilla with the

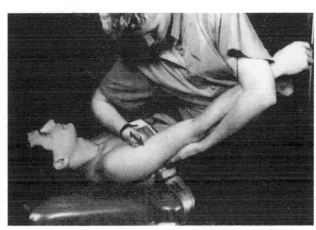

▲ **Figure 5.113** Distraction of the glenohumeral joint.

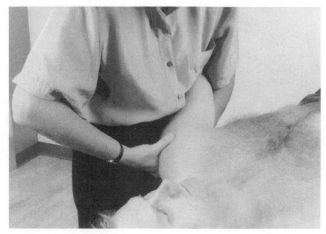

▲ **Figure 5.114** Inferior glide.

forearm placed across the body. The other limb is used only to support the subject's upper limb and maintain the resting position.

Movement. The mobilizing hand in the axilla imposes a lateral distracting force to the humeral head, thereby moving it away from the glenoid fossa.

Inferior Glide (Fig. 5-114)

Restriction. Abduction.

Positioning. The subject lies supine; a strap is applied to stabilize the scapula. The therapist places the web space of the mobilizing hand superiorly around the humeral head. The other limb is used only to support the subject's upper limb and maintain the resting position.

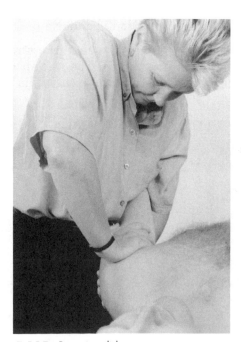

▲ **Figure 5.115** Posterior glide.

Movement. The mobilizing hand applies an inferiorly directed force to the subject's humeral head.

Posterior Glide (Fig. 5-115)

Restriction. Internal rotation.

Positioning. The subject lies supine; a stabilizing wedge is placed along the spine of the scapula extending to the acromion process. The mobilizing hand is cupped anteriorly over the humeral head with the ulnar border as close to the joint space as possible. The other hand is placed posterior on the humeral head. The subject's arm is stabilized against the examiner's trunk at the wrist.

Movement. The mobilizing hand applies a posterior force to the subject's humeral head.

Anterior Glide (Fig. 5-116)

Restriction. External rotation.

Positioning. The subject lies prone; a stabilizing wedge is placed beneath the coracoid process. The mobilizing hand is placed posteriorly over the humeral head, with the ulnar border of the hand as close to the joint space as possible. The other hand is used to support the subject's upper limb and to maintain the resting position.

Movement. The mobilizing hand applies an anterior force to the subject's humeral head.

Posterior Inferior Glide (see Fig. 5-115)

Restriction. Flexion.

Positioning. The subject lies supine; a stabilizing wedge is placed along the spine of the scapula extending to the acromion process. A strap is also applied to stabilize the scapula and trunk. The mobi-

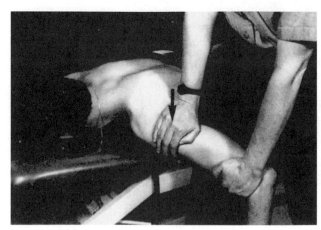

▲ **Figure 5.116** Anterior glide of the humerus.

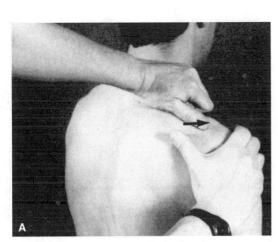
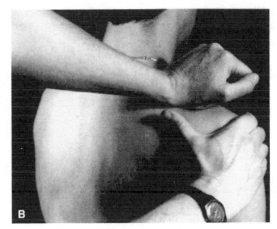

▲ **Figure 5.117** Two methods of performing ventrolateral glide of the clavicle.

lizing hand is placed over the superior anterior humeral head with the ulnar border of the hand as close to the joint space as possible.

Movement. The mobilizing hand applies a posterior inferior force to the subject's humeral head. This movement is best described as a scooping of the joint so that the motion describes a C shape.

Acromioclavicular Joint

Ventrolateral Glide (Fig. 5-117A)

Restriction. General hypomobility.

Open-Packed Position. Anatomical.

Positioning. The subject may be seated or prone for this test. The stabilizing hand of the therapist is placed around the acromion process, humeral head, and coracoid process. The thumb of the mobilizing hand is placed on the posterior aspect of the lateral clavicle. An alternate position is to place the heel of the mobilizing hand posteriorly on the lateral aspect of the clavicle (see Fig. 5-117*B*).

Movement. A ventrolateral force is applied to the posterior aspect of the lateral clavicle.

Sternoclavicular Joint

Superior Glide (Fig. 5-118)

Restriction. Depression.

Open-Packed Position. Anatomical.

Positioning. The subject lies supine. The therapist places the palmar surface of one thumb on the inferior aspect of the medial clavicle. The other thumb is placed on top, providing reinforcement to the mobilizing thumb.

Movement. A superior force is applied to the inferior surface of the medial clavicle.

Inferior Glide (Fig. 5-119)

Restriction. Elevation.

Positioning. The subject lies supine. The therapist places the palmar surface of one thumb on the supe-

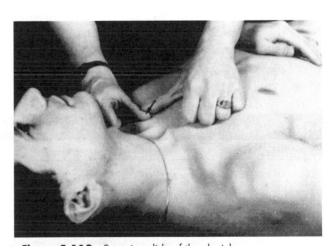

▲ **Figure 5.118** Superior glide of the clavicle.

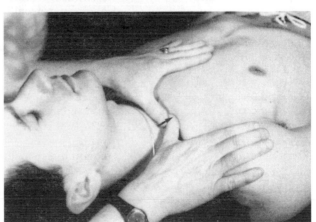

▲ **Figure 5.119** Inferior glide of the clavicle.

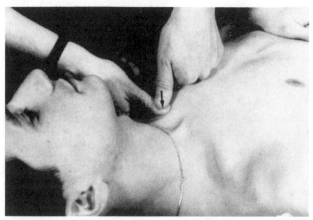

▲ **Figure 5.120** Posterior glide of the clavicle.

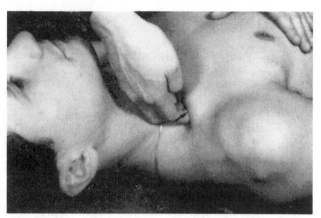

▲ **Figure 5.121** Anterior glide of the clavicle.

rior aspect of the medial clavicle. The other thumb is placed on top, providing reinforcement to the mobilizing thumb.

Movement. An inferior force is applied to the superior surface of the medial clavicle.

Posterior Glide (Fig. 5-120)

Restriction. Retraction.

Positioning. The subject lies supine. The therapist places the palmar surface of one thumb on the anterior aspect of the medial clavicle. The other thumb is placed on top, providing reinforcement to the mobilizing thumb.

Movement. A posterior force is applied to the anterior surface of the medial clavicle.

Anterior Glide (Fig. 5-121)

Restriction. Protraction.

Positioning. The subject lies supine. The therapist hooks the palmar surface of the distal phalanges of digits two and three around the superior clavicle, reaching as far onto the posterior surface of the lateral end as possible.

Movement. An anterior force is applied to the posterior surface of the medial clavicle.

Table 5-1 provides a summary of joint play of the shoulder complex.

TABLE 5.1	**Summary of Joint Play of the Shoulder Complex**		
GLIDE	RESTRICTION	FIXED BONE	MOVING BONE
Scapulothoracic Joint			
Superior	Elevation	Thorax	Scapula
Inferior	Depression	Thorax	Scapula
Lateral	Abduction or protraction	Thorax	Scapula
Medial	Adduction or retraction	Thorax	Scapula
Upward rotation	Upward rotation	Thorax	Scapula
Downward rotation	Downward rotation	Thorax	Scapula
Distraction	General hypomobility	Thorax	Scapula
Glenohumeral Joint			
Distraction	General hypomobility	Glenoid	Humerus
Anterior	External rotation	Glenoid	Humerus
Posterior	Internal rotation	Glenoid	Humerus
Inferior	Abduction	Glenoid	Humerus
Posteroinferior	Flexion	Glenoid	Humerus
Anteroinferior	Extension	Glenoid	Humerus
Dorsolateral	Horizontal adduction	Glenoid	Humerus
Acromioclavicular Joint			
Ventrolateral	General hypomobility	Acromion process	Clavicle
Sternoclavicular Joint			
Superior	Depression	Manubrium	Clavicle
Inferior	Elevation	Manubrium	Clavicle
Ventral	Protraction	Manubrium	Clavicle/disc
Dorsal	Retraction	Manubrium	Clavicle/disc

REFERENCES

1. Adson AW, Coffey JR: Cervical rehabilitation. Ann Surg 85:839, 1927
2. Allen EV: Thromboangitis obliterans: Methods of diagnosis of chronic occlusive arterial lesions distal to the wrist with illustrative cases. Am J Med Sci 178:237–244, 1929
3. Andrews JR, Gillogly S: Physical examination of the shoulder in throwing athletes. In Zarins B, Andrews JR, Carson WG (eds): Injuries to the Throwing Arm. Philadelphia, W.B. Saunders, 1985.
4. Booth RE, Marvel JP: Differential diagnosis in shoulder pain. Orthop Clin North Am 6:353, 1975
5. Cavendish ME: Congenital elevation of the scapula. J Bone Joint Surg 54B:395, 1972
6. Davies GJ, Gould A, Larson RL: Functional examination of the shoulder girdle. Phys Sports Med 9:82–104, 1981
7. Elvey RL: The investigation of arm pain. In Grieve GP (ed): Modern Manual Therapy of the Vertebral Column. Edinburgh, Churchill Livingstone, 1986
8. Falconer MA, Weddell G: Costoclavicular compression of the subclavian artery and vein. Lancet 2:539, 1943
9. Gerber C, Ganz R: Clinical assessment of instability of the shoulder. J Bone Joint Surg 66B:551–556, 1984
10. Hawkins RJ, Kennedy JC: Impingement syndrome in athletes. Am J Sports Med 8:151–158, 1980
11. Lippman RK: Frozen shoulder: Periarthritis, bicipital tenosynovitis. Arch Surg 47:283, 1943
12. Ludington NA: Rupture of the long head of the biceps tendon cubiti muscle. Ann Surg 77:358, 1923
13. Matsen FA, Thomas SC, Rockwood CA: Glenohumeral instability. In Rockwood CA, Masen FA (eds): The Shoulder. Philadelphia, W.B. Saunders, 1990
14. Neer CSM, Welsh RP: The shoulder in sports. Orthop Clin North Am 8:583–591, 1977
15. Rockwood CA: Subluxations and dislocations about the shoulder. In Rockwood CA, Green DP (eds): Fractures in Adults—1. Philadelphia, J.B. Lippincott, 1984
16. Roos DB: Congenital anomalies associated with thoracic outlet syndrome. Am J Surg 132:771–778, 1976
17. Roos DB: The place for scalenectomy and first rib resection in thoracic outlet syndrome. Surgery 92:1077, 1982
18. Wright IS: The neurovascular syndrome produced by hyperabduction of the arms. Am Heart J 29:1–19, 1945
19. Yergason RM: Supination sign. J Bone Joint Surg 13:160, 1931

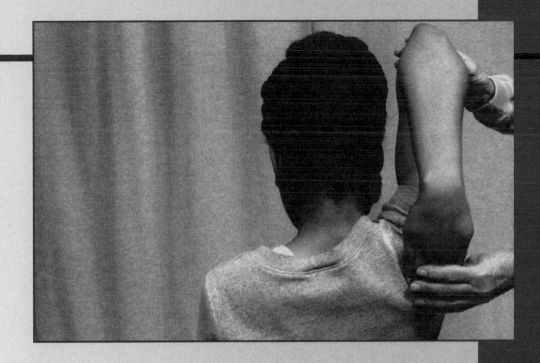

6

Elbow and Forearm

The elbow joint, an intermediate joint between the shoulder and the hand, permits lengthening and shortening of the upper limb. It is a structurally stable joint and, with its musculature, is designed primarily to position the hand. It allows the hand to be brought close to the face for eating or placed at a distance for reaching. Many of the muscles that act on the wrist and shoulder cross the elbow joint, aid in providing stability, and enhance the function of the hand.

The elbow joint moves in one plane of motion around a single axis. The motions produced at the elbow joint are flexion and extension. The head of the radius articulates with the capitulum of the humerus. The ulna articulates with the trochlea of the humerus. The axis of motion is transverse in a plane through the trochlea and the capitulum. The trochlea extends more distally than the capitulum; therefore when the elbow is extended and the forearm supinated, the forearm deviates laterally in relation to the humerus. This deviation accounts for what is termed the carrying angle. The axis lies immediately distal to the lateral and medial epicondyle of the humerus.

The radius and ulna are connected both proximally and distally. The two joints act together and form a uniaxial joint, producing the motion of supination and pronation. Most of the motion occurs because the radius rotates on the ulna. When the two bones are parallel, the forearm is supinated. When the radius crosses over the ulna, the forearm is pronated. The hand follows the movement of the radius. The axis of motion of the radioulnar joints is vertical through the head of the radius (proximally) and through the head of the ulna (distally), permitting one degree of freedom of motion.

GONIOMETRY

ELBOW FLEXION

The elbow is a double-hinge joint. The test motion occurs in the sagittal plane, between the radius moving on the humeral capitulum and the trochlear notch of the ulna on the olecranon fossa. As motion occurs, the head of the radius glides anteriorly on the capitulum. A roll is placed under the humerus to keep it level with the glenoid fossa.

Motion. From 0 to 145 degrees into flexion.

Position. Subject lies supine, with the upper limb parallel to the lateral midline of the trunk and the forearm in the anatomical position. The arm is positioned as close to the trunk as feasible.

Goniometric Alignment (Fig. 6-1)

Axis. Over the lateral epicondyle of the humerus.

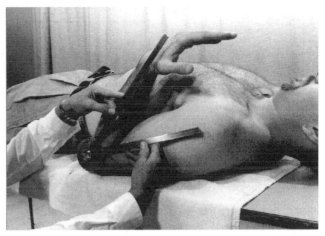

▲ **Figure 6.1** Goniometric alignment. End position for elbow flexion.

Stationary Arm. Placed along the lateral midline of the humerus in line with the acromion process of the scapula.

Moving Arm. Placed along the lateral midline of the radius in line with the styloid process of the radius.

Stabilization. The distal end of the humerus is stabilized.

Precautions

- Prevent shoulder joint flexion.
- Note position of the forearm if not in the anatomical position.

ELBOW EXTENSION AND HYPEREXTENSION

Elbow extension, the return from elbow joint flexion, occurs in the sagittal plane between radius and humerus and ulna and humerus. As the motion occurs, the head of the radius glides in a posterior direction. Hyperextension of the elbow joint is often accompanied by an increase in the carrying angle, particularly in women. The amount of motion available is determined by the articulation between the ulnar olecranon process and the fossa of the humerus.

Motion. From 145 to 0 degrees (note any hyperextension).

Position. Subject lies supine with the arm parallel to the lateral midline of the trunk and the forearm supinated.

Goniometric alignment, stabilization, and precautions are the same as described for elbow joint flexion (Fig. 6-2).

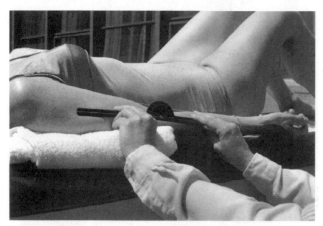

▲ **Figure 6.2** End position for elbow joint extension.

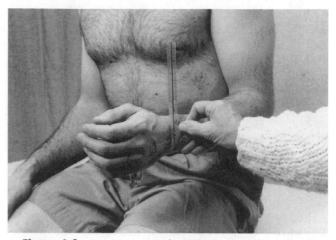

▲ **Figure 6.3** Starting position for radioulnar pronation.

RADIOULNAR PRONATION

In the anatomical position, the pronation motion occurs in the transverse plane. The forearm is positioned midway between supination and pronation with the elbow flexed to 90 degrees. Motion occurs between the head of the radius spinning on the capitulum of the humerus and on the radial notch of the ulna. The distal end of the radius glides over the head of the ulna at the inferior radioulnar joint. In this position, the radius is crossed over the ulna. Minimal motion of abduction of the ulna accompanies pronation at the proximal joint, and none occurs at the inferior radioulnar joint.

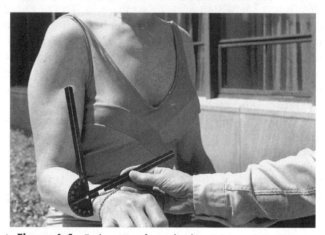

▲ **Figure 6.4** End position for radioulnar joint pronation.

Motion. From 0 to 90 degrees from midforearm position into full pronation.

Position

- Preferred: Subject sits or lies supine with the elbow flexed to approximately 90 degrees and the arm held close to the side of the trunk. The forearm is positioned midway between supination and pronation.
- Alternate: The subject is in the preferred position holding a pencil vertically in the hand.

Goniometric Alignment (Figs. 6-3 to 6-6)

Axis

- Preferred: Lateral to the ulnar styloid process.
- Alternate: Third metacarpal head, citing the third metacarpal and between the radioulnar joints.

Stationary Arm

- Preferred: Placed at the level of the dorsal aspect of the wrist and parallel to the long axis of

the humerus, with the protractor directed away from the trunk at the level of the wrist.
- Alternate: Placed perpendicular to the table top.

Moving Arm

- Preferred: Placed across the dorsum of the wrist on a line between and proximal to the styloid processes of the radius and the ulna.
- Alternate: Placed parallel to the long axis of the pencil. The subject must have good to normal grip.

Stabilization. Stabilize the distal end of the humerus.

Precautions

- Keep the elbow close to the side of the trunk.
- Avoid shoulder abduction and medial rotation.
- Avoid lateral flexion of the trunk toward the opposite side.
- Avoid wrist and finger motion when using the alternate method of measuring.

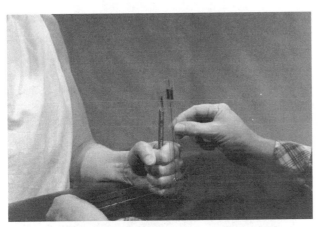

▲ **Figure 6.5** Alternate starting position for radioulnar joint pronation.

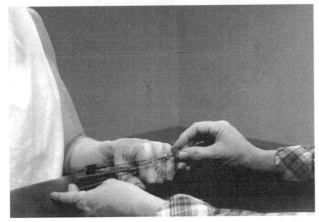

▲ **Figure 6.6** Alternate end position for radioulnar joint pronation.

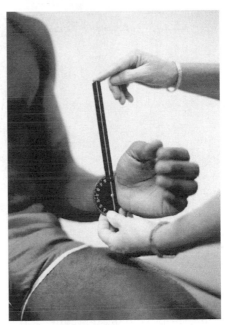

▲ **Figure 6.7** Starting position for radioulnar joint supination.

RADIOULNAR SUPINATION

The test motion of supination at the radioulnar joints occurs in the transverse plane. The pivoting motions exist between the head of the radius on the capitulum of the humerus and the proximal ulna. Distally, the radius glides over the head of the ulna until the two bones lie parallel. The shoulder and elbow joints are positioned as for pronation.

Motion. From 0 to 90 degrees into supination.

Position

- Preferred: Subject sits or lies supine, with the elbow flexed to 90 degrees and the arm held close to the side. The forearm is positioned midway between supination and pronation.
- Alternate: Same as preferred position, except that the subject holds a pencil in the vertical position. Good grip is essential.

Goniometric alignment and stabilization are the same as described for pronation (Figs. 6-7 to 6-10).

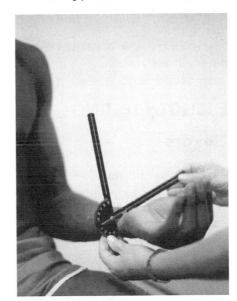

▲ **Figure 6.8** End position for radioulnar joint supination.

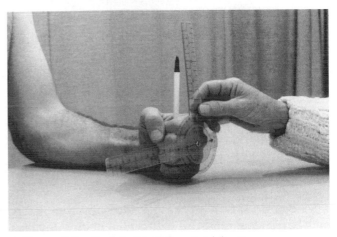

▲ **Figure 6.9** Goniometric alignment stabilization.

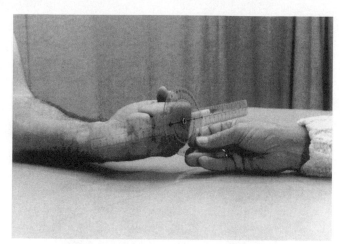

▲ **Figure 6.10** Goniometric alignment stabilization.

Precautions

- Avoid lateral flexion of the trunk to the same side as the measurement.
- Avoid adduction and lateral rotation of the shoulder joint.
- Avoid wrist and finger motions when using the alternate test method.

MUSCLE LENGTH TESTING

Elbow Flexors

The elbow joint links the shoulder and the forearm. It allows the forearm to assume any position by shortening or lengthening the upper limb. This ability allows the hand to be brought close to the face. The three-joint biceps brachii muscles cross anterior to the shoulder joint proximally and anterior to the elbow joint inferiorly; it also crosses the radioulnar joint. The one-joint elbow flexor muscles are the brachialis and brachioradialis.

BICEPS BRACHII MUSCLES (LONG AND SHORT HEADS)

Position. The subject is sitting in a straight-back chair or supine with the shoulder off the edge of the treatment table.

Movement. The examiner positions the shoulder joint in hyperextension, forearm pronated, and allows the elbow joint to extend. If the elbow joint does not completely extend, the biceps brachii muscle is limited in its length.

Measurement. With the shoulder joint completely hyperextended, measure with a goniometer any lack of elbow joint extension (Fig. 6-11).

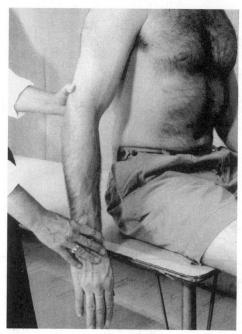

▲ **Figure 6.11** Muscle length testing for the biceps brachii muscle.

Considerations

- If the forearm is supinated, then the full length of the biceps brachii muscle is not maintained.
- The one-joint elbow flexors (brachialis and brachioradialis) may demonstrate limitation in length, but they are not influenced by the position of the shoulder joint.
- Capsular joint structures anterior to the joint will limit elbow extension regardless of shoulder joint position if they are shortened.
- The multijoint wrist extensor muscles also may influence range of motion at the elbow joint; therefore, the wrist joint is in a relaxed position and not flexed.

Elbow Extensor Muscles

The elbow joint extensor muscles are the triceps brachii, in which the long head crosses the shoulder joint posteriorly. The anconeus and the lateral and medial heads of the triceps brachii only cross the elbow joint. The triceps brachii muscle is much more powerful when the shoulder and elbow joints are flexed.

TRICEPS BRACHII AND ANCONEUS MUSCLES

Position. The subject is in a supine or in a sitting position with the shoulder completely flexed. The subject must be close to the head of the treatment table to allow the forearm and hand to clear the table.

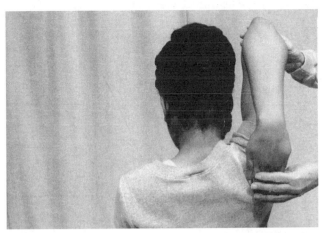

▲ **Figure 6.12** Muscle length testing for triceps brachii and anconeus muscle.

Movement. The examiner flexes the elbow joint, completely stabilizing the shoulder joint in flexion.

Measurement. A limitation in elbow flexion is measured using a goniometer (Fig. 6-12).

Considerations. If elbow flexion limitation exists without the shoulder completely flexed, then the one-joint extensor muscles or posterior capsular structures are limiting the motion.

MANUAL MUSCLE TESTING

BICEPS BRACHII, BRACHIALIS, AND BRACHIORADIALIS MUSCLES

The biceps brachii muscle is tested during the motion of elbow flexion to 90 degrees from complete extension. Against-gravity (AG) grades are determined with the subject sitting, and gravity-minimized (GM) evaluation may be done with the subject in a side-lying, supine, or sitting position. The forearm is positioned in supination. The biceps brachii also flexes the shoulder joint, and if the shoulder joint were allowed to rotate laterally, the biceps brachii would assist in shoulder joint abduction. The brachioradialis muscle participates in the motion of elbow flexion only if resistance is applied or if the motion is performed rapidly.

Palpation

Biceps Brachii. With the forearm in a supinated position, palpate the arm anteriorly for the muscle belly or the cubital fossa for the tendon of insertion; each head may be palpated proximally on the arm. The long head is on the anterior surface of the humerus, lateral to the lesser tuberosity; the short head is medial on the arm, directed toward the coracoid process (Fig. 6-13).

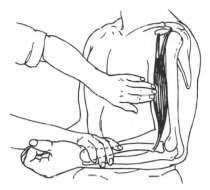

▲ **Figure 6.13** Palpation for the biceps brachii muscle.

Brachialis. With the forearm pronated to minimize the action of the biceps, place fingers either lateral or medial to the common biceps tendon immediately proximal to the cubital fossa and push the relaxed biceps to one side. Flex the elbow with as little effort as possible, and feel the contraction of the brachialis deep to the biceps tendon (Fig. 6-14).

Brachioradialis. With the forearm in midposition between supination and pronation and the elbow in 90 degrees of flexion, apply resistance. The muscle is superficial and can be palpated along its course. It forms the lateral border of the cubital fossa. It is best felt just lateral to the biceps tendon at the level of or proximal to the elbow (Fig. 6-15).

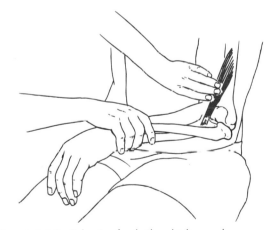

▲ **Figure 6.14** Palpation for the brachialis muscle.

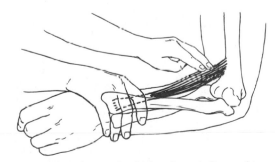

▲ **Figure 6.15** Palpation for the brachioradialis muscle.

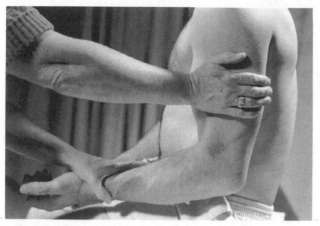

▲ **Figure 6.16** AG sitting position, testing the three anterior arm muscles simultaneously.

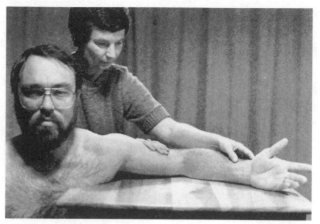

▲ **Figure 6.17** GM sitting position, testing the three anterior arm muscles simultaneously.

Position

AG: Subject is sitting, with the upper limb in the anatomical position (Fig. 6-16). To isolate each elbow flexor, the subject is positioned with (1) the forearm supinated for the biceps brachii, (2) the forearm pronated for the brachialis, and (3) the forearm in midposition for the brachioradialis muscle.

GM: Subject is sitting, with the arm supported in 90 degrees of abduction, shoulder in neutral rotation, elbow extended, and the forearm supinated (Fig. 6-17).

Movement. Flex elbow to 90 degrees with the forearm in supination.

Resistance. Applied immediately proximal to the wrist on the anterior forearm.

Stabilization. The arm is stabilized.

Substitutions

- The subject may extend the shoulder, causing passive flexion of the elbow.
- The subject may quickly extend the elbow and relax it, giving the appearance of flexion.

- Pronator teres causes the forearm to pronate as flexion occurs.
- Wrist and finger extensors and flexors originating from both the medial and lateral epicondyles can cause substitue motions.

TRICEPS BRACHII (LONG, LATERAL, AND MEDIAL HEADS), ANCONEUS MUSCLES

The triceps and anconeus muscles produce the movement of elbow extension from complete elbow flexion. The test range is 145 degrees of elbow extension. Resistance must be applied to palpate for contraction of the long and lateral heads of the triceps muscle. The medial head contracts any time during elbow extension.

Palpation

Triceps Brachii. The proximal portion of the long head is felt as it emerges beneath the posterior deltoid muscle. The lateral head, the strongest, is felt distal to the posterior deltoid muscle. The medial head is covered by the other two heads but is felt distal on the posterior arm on either side of the common triceps tendon (Figs. 6-18 to 6-20).

▼ Attachments of Biceps Brachii, Brachialis, and Brachioradialis Muscles			
Muscle	**Proximal**	**Distal**	**Innervation**
Biceps brachii			
Long head	Supraglenoid tubercle of scapula	Tuberosity of radius and bicipital aponeurosis	Musculocutaneous C6 (C5)
Short head	Coracoid process apex	Same as above	Same as above
Brachialis	Distal half of anterior surface of humerus	Tuberosity and coronoid process of ulna	Musculocutaneous small branch of radial C6 (C5)
Brachioradialis	Proximal two thirds of lateral supracondylar ridge of humerus	Base of styloid process of radius	Radial C6 (C6 and 7)

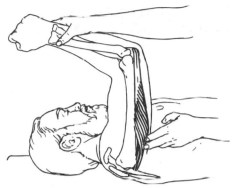

▲ **Figure 6.18** Palpation for the long head of the triceps brachii muscle.

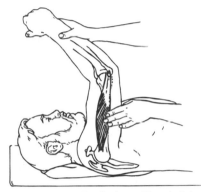

▲ **Figure 6.19** Palpation for the lateral head of the triceps brachii muscle.

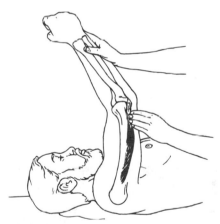

▲ **Figure 6.20** Palpation for the medial head of the triceps brachii muscle.

Anconeus. Between the lateral epicondyle and the olecranon process of the ulna, it is deep to the tendinous sheath of the triceps.

Position

AG: Subject lies supine with the shoulder flexed 90 degrees and the elbow fully flexed (Fig. 6-21).

GM: Subject sits with the shoulder supported in 90 degrees of flexion and medial rotation

with the elbow flexed and the forearm neutral (Fig. 6-22).

Movement. Extend elbow from 145 degrees of flexion.

Resistance. Applied immediately proximal to the wrist on the posterior forearm.

Stabilization. The arm is stabilized.

Substitutions

- Subject may further flex the shoulder, causing passive extension of the elbow.
- Subject may quickly increase flexion of the elbow, giving the appearance of extension.
- In the GM position, subject may abduct the shoulder joint.

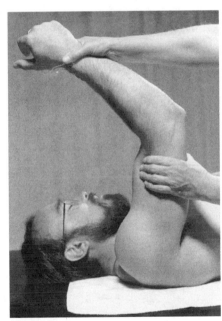

▲ **Figure 6.21** AG supine position; testing the three heads of the triceps brachii muscle simultaneously.

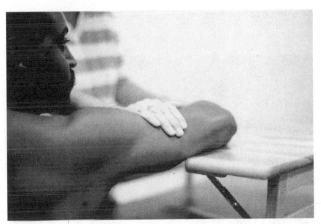

▲ **Figure 6.22** GM sitting position; testing the three heads of the triceps brachii muscle.

▼ Attachments of Triceps Brachii and Anconeus Muscles

Muscle	Proximal	Distal	Innervation
Triceps brachii			
Long head	Infraglenoid tubercle of scapula	Olecranon process of ulna	Radial C7 and 8 (C6)
Lateral head	Lateral and proximal surface of upper one half of humeral shaft above radial groove	Olecranon process of ulna	Radial C7 and 8 (C6)
Medial head	Distal two thirds of medial and posterior aspects of humerus below radial groove	Olecranon process of ulna	Radial C7 and 8 (C6)
Anconeus	Lateral humeral epicondyle	Lateral surface of ulnar olecranon process and upper posterior shaft of ulna	Radial C7 and 8 (C6)

SUPINATOR MUSCLE

The supinator muscle produces the movement of supination at the radioulnar joints. With a starting position in full pronation, the full range is 180 degrees.

Palpation. The supinator is a deep muscle, extending under the common extensor muscles from the lateral epicondyle. Relax the wrist and finger extensors and push them laterally. Place fingers under extensor muscles as much as possible (Fig. 6-23).

Position

AG: Subject sits with the arm at the side of the trunk and the elbow flexed 90 degrees (Fig. 6-24).

GM: Subject is prone with the shoulder supported in 90 degrees of abduction, the elbow flexed 90 degrees, and the forearm perpendicular to the table (Figs. 6-25 and 6-26).

• Alternate: Subject sits with the shoulder supported in 90 degrees flexion.

Movement. From full pronation to full supination in the GM position and from full pronation to neutral forearm position for AG position.

Resistance. Applied immediately proximal to the wrist into pronation.

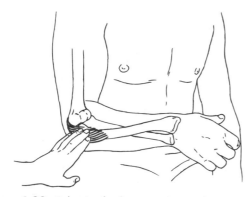

▲ **Figure 6.23** Palpation for the supinator muscle.

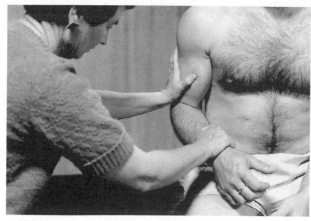

▲ **Figure 6.24** AG sitting position; testing the supinator muscle.

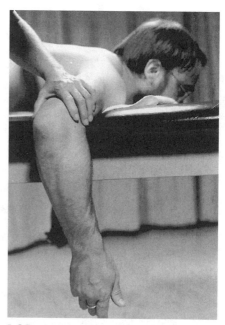

▲ **Figure 6.25** GM prone position; testing the supinator muscle.

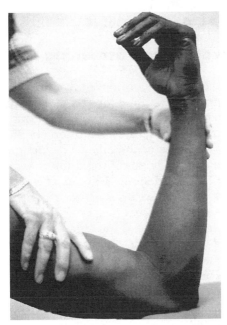

▲ **Figure 6.26** Alternate GM sitting position; testing the supinator muscle.

Stabilization. The arm is stabilized with the elbow close to the trunk.

Substitutions

- Subject may flex trunk laterally toward the same side and adduct the shoulder.
- Brachioradialis supinates from a completely pronated position to neutral.
- Subject may laterally rotate the shoulder joint and move elbow across chest.

PRONATOR TERES, PRONATOR QUADRATUS MUSCLES

The pronator teres and pronator quadratus muscles produce the motion of pronation at the radioulnar joints from the starting position of supination. The complete range of motion for pronation is 180 degrees.

Palpation

- Palpate the pronator teres on the medial surface of the cubital fossa; the fibers run laterally to the radius (Fig. 6-27).
- The pronator quadratus muscle is too deep to be palpated.

Position

AG: Subject sits, with the arm against the trunk and the elbow flexed to 90 degrees (Fig. 6-28).
GM: Subject sits, with the shoulder and elbow flexed to 90 degrees and the forearm perpendicular to the table (Figs. 6-29 and 6-30).
- Alternate: Subject is prone with the shoulder abducted 90 degrees.

Movement. In the GM position, the motion is from full supination to full pronation. In AG, it is from full supination to neutral, midway between supination and pronation.

Resistance. Applied immediately proximal to the wrist into supination.

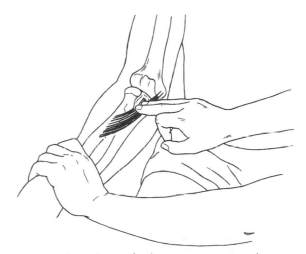

▲ **Figure 6.27** Palpation for the pronator teres muscle.

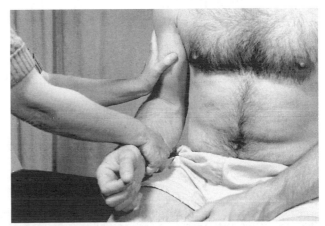

▲ **Figure 6.28** AG sitting position; testing the pronator teres muscle.

▼ **Attachments of Supinator Muscle**			
Muscle	Proximal	Distal	Innervation
Supinator	Lateral epicondyle of humerus, radial collateral and annular ligaments, and supinator crest of ulna	Lateral surface of upper third of radial shaft	Radial C6 (C5)

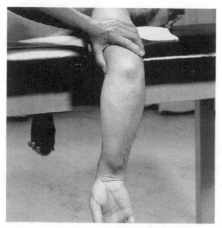

▲ **Figure 6.29** GM prone position; testing the pronator teres muscle.

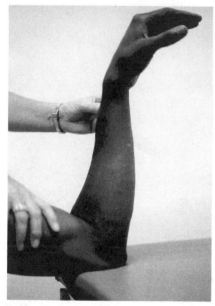

▲ **Figure 6.30** Alternate GM sitting position; testing the pronator teres muscle.

Stabilization. Stabilize the arm, keeping the elbow next to the trunk.

Substitutions

• Subject may flex trunk to contralateral side, abduct and medially rotate the shoulder.
• The end range may be completed by wrist flexors.

CLINICAL ASSESSMENT

Observation and Screening

All clothing should be removed from the upper limb being examined to allow for complete visualization of the elbow area. With the subject standing in the anatomical position, the examiner should observe the carrying angle of the elbow. This angle, formed by the longitudinal axes of the humerus and ulna, is normally 5 to 10 degrees in men and 10 to 15 degrees in women.[2] An excessive carrying angle, referred to as cubitus valgus, is present when these normal carrying angle values are exceeded. Cubitus varus, a decrease in the carrying angle, is identified when the angulation is less than the normal values. A cubitus varus at the angle is commonly referred to as a gunstock deformity.

Another focus in the observation of the elbow is the relationship of the olecranon, medial epicondyle, and lateral epicondyle. These three landmarks should normally line up in a horizontal fashion when the elbow is fully extended. In a position of 90 degrees of elbow flexion, these same three bony landmarks normally form an isosceles triangle.[1]

Palpation and Surface Anatomy

In examining the elbow and forearm complex, the examiner needs to be familiar with the location of various bony and soft-tissue landmarks (Fig. 6-31). The structures that should be examined in the subject evaluation follow:

1. Medial epicondyle of the humerus
2. Lateral epicondyle of the humerus
3. Groove that transmits the ulnar nerve
4. Lateral supracondylar ridge of the humerus
5. Olecranon process of the ulna
6. Radial head
7. Cubital fossa
8. Common flexor origin on the medial epicondyle
9. Proximal attachments of the wrist extensor musculature
10. Radial styloid

▼ Attachments of Pronator Teres and Pronator Quadratus Muscles			
Muscle	**Proximal**	**Distal**	**Innervation**
Pronator teres	Proximal portion of medial epicondyle of humerus and medial side of coronoid process of ulna	Midradial shaft on lateral side	Median C7 (C6)
Pronator quadratus	Anterior surface and distal quarter of ulna	Anterior surface and distal quarter of radius	Median C8 (T1)

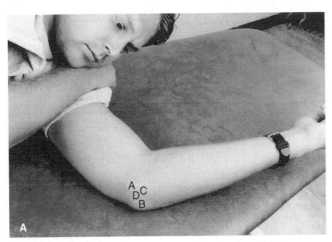

A = Medial Epicondyle
B – Olecranon Process
C = Common Flexor Tendon
D = Ulnar Groove

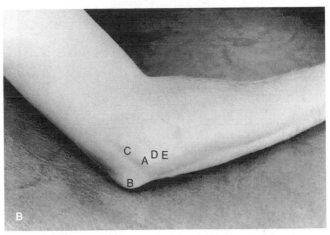

A = Lateral Epicondyle
B = Olecranon Process
C = Origin of Extensor Carpi Radialis Longus Muscle
D = Origin of Extensor Carpi Radialis Brevis Muscle
E = Radial Head

▲ **Figure 6.31** **(A)** Medial epicondyle. **(B)** Radial head.

11. Ulnar styloid
12. Ulnar head
13. Lister's tubercle on the dorsal radius, which transmits the extensor pollicis longus tendon

Active and Passive Movements and Contractile Testing

The motions to be assessed during active and passive movement of the elbow and forearm joints include the following:

1. Elbow flexion
2. Elbow extension
3. Forearm supination
4. Forearm pronation

Contractile testing includes the following:

1. Elbow flexion
2. Elbow extension
3. Forearm supination
4. Forearm pronation

SPECIAL CLINICAL TESTS

REFLEX TESTING

Biceps Brachii Reflex

Indication. The biceps brachii reflex test is used to assess the integrity of the reflex innervated by the C5 nerve root.

Method. The subject's forearm is placed over the examiner's opposite forearm, so that the weight of the subject's arm and forearm is borne by the examiner. The elbow being assessed is positioned in some degree of flexion. The examiner supports the sub-

ject's arm along the medial elbow, places the thumb distally on the biceps brachii tendon, and depresses the tendon (Fig. 6-32). With the triangular end of the reflex hammer, the examiner strikes the thumbnail, depressing the tendon. For all reflex tests, it is imperative that the subject be relaxed.

Results. A normal response is one in which there is a flexion response of the elbow comparable to that on the uninvolved side. Unsuccessful attempts to elicit the reflex are an indication that there may be pathological involvement of the C5 nerve root. An excessive response may be an indication of an upper motor neuron lesion, whereas a diminished response may reflect lower motor neuron involvement.

Brachioradialis Reflex

Indication. The brachioradialis reflex test is used to assess the integrity of the C6 nerve root.

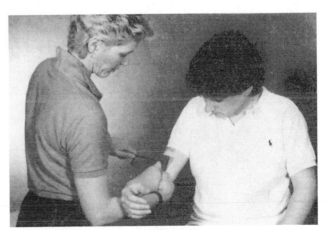

▲ **Figure 6.32** Testing the biceps tendon reflex.

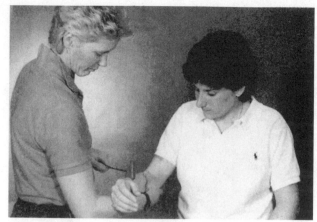

▲ **Figure 6.33** Testing the brachioradialis tendon reflex.

Method. The subject's upper limb is positioned as described for the biceps brachii reflex. Using the broad side of the hammer, the examiner strikes the radial side of the forearm just above the styloid process over the brachioradialis tendon (Fig. 6-33).

Results. A normal reflex will elicit a response of elbow flexion. Absent, depressed, or exaggerated movement indicates involvement of the C6 nerve root.

Triceps Reflex

Indication. The triceps reflex is associated with function of the C7 nerve root.

Method. The subject's position is the same as described previously. Using the triangular end of the hammer, the examiner taps the triceps tendon just proximal to the olecranon process (Fig. 6-34).

Results. The normal reflex response is elbow extension. Abnormalities of this reflex indicate the possibility of a lesion of the C7 nerve root.

TESTS FOR LIGAMENT INSTABILITY

Valgus Stress Test

Indication. The valgus stress test is used to assess the stability of the medial (ulnar) collateral ligament.

Method. The subject's elbow is positioned in slight flexion with the forearm supinated. The examiner places one hand on the lateral aspect of the elbow joint and the other medially on the midportion or distal forearm (Fig. 6-35). It is helpful to internally rotate the soft-tissue mass of the arm and to maintain that position during testing. This tends to allow for greater ease in the application of a valgus force by not allowing for any shoulder rotation. The examiner then imparts a valgus force to the elbow by pulling the forearm away from the body, using the elbow as a fulcrum.

Results. The test is positive if either the subject experiences pain or gapping is felt or seen by the examiner along the medial aspect of the elbow. The uninvolved side is tested as a base for comparison.

Varus Stress Test

Indication. The varus stress test assesses the stability of the lateral (radial) collateral ligament.

Method. The subject's elbow is slightly flexed and the forearm supinated. One of the examiner's hands is positioned on the medial aspect of the elbow joint, while the other is placed along the radial forearm, either at midshaft or distally (Fig. 6-36). It is helpful to rotate externally the soft-tissue mass of the arm and to maintain that position during testing. This tends to allow for greater ease in the application of a varus force by not allowing for any shoulder rotation. A varus force is applied by adducting the forearm relative to the arm, using the elbow as a fulcrum.

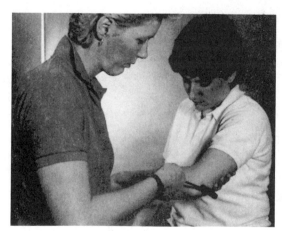

▲ **Figure 6.34** Testing the triceps tendon reflex.

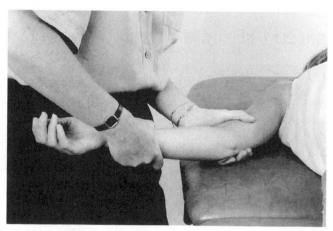

▲ **Figure 6.35** Valgus stress test.

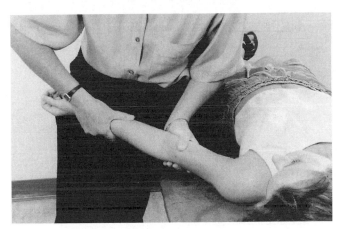

▲ **Figure 6.36** Varus stress test.

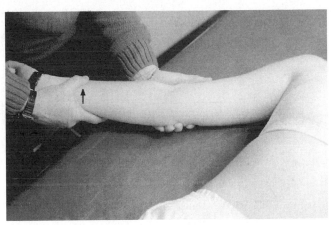

▲ **Figure 6.37** Valgus extension overload test.

Results. Pain or excessive gapping of the lateral aspect of the joint is a positive sign.

Valgus Extension Overload Test

Indication. This clinical test can aid in the determination of an osteophyte or loose body being the source of posteromedial elbow pain.

Method. The subject may be positioned supine or sitting. The examiner places the elbow in full extension while exerting a valgus stress (Fig. 6-37). This combination of movements and forces simulates those that occur during the acceleration phase of the pitching motion. As the force is applied, the examiner should palpate the posteromedial aspect of the olecranon for tenderness or crepitus.

Results. Pain over the posterior or posteromedial aspects of the olecranon represents a positive test.

NEUROLOGICAL TESTS

Tinel's Sign

Indication. Tinel's sign at the elbow is designed to assess the integrity of the ulnar nerve where it lies in the ulnar groove between the olecranon process and the medial epicondyle.

Method. The examiner taps the ulnar nerve where it lies in the ulnar groove (Fig. 6-38).

Results. A tingling sensation within the distribution of the ulnar nerve in the forearm and hand constitutes a positive result, indicating ulnar nerve involvement in the form of a neuroma or neuritis.

Pinch Grip Test

Indication. The pinch grip test assesses the possibility of a lesion in the anterior interosseous nerve (branch of the median nerve), which may be the result of entrapment of the nerve where it passes between the two heads of the pronator teres.

Method. The subject is asked to pinch the tip of the thumb to the tip of the index finger (Fig. 6-39A).

Results. If the subject is unable to pinch tip to tip, but instead pinches by approximating the pads of the distal phalanges, the test result is considered positive (see Fig. 6-39B).

Elbow Flexion Test

Indication. The elbow flexion test is performed to determine the presence of cubital tunnel syndrome, in which the ulnar nerve becomes entrapped between the two heads of the flexor carpi ulnaris muscle.

Method. The subject may be positioned sitting, supine, or standing for this test. The elbow being examined is maximally flexed and held in that position for 5 minutes. The position of maximal flexion results in an increase in the stretch of the ulnar nerve within the cubital tunnel.

Results. Provocation of tingling or paresthesias within the ulnar nerve distribution in the forearm and hand indicates a positive test.

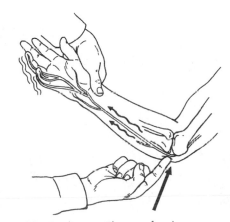

▲ **Figure 6.38** Tinel's sign. This tests for ulnar nerve entrapment.

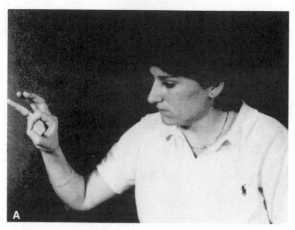

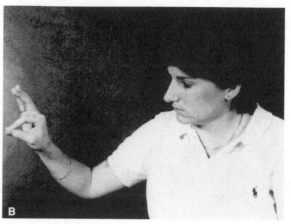

▲ **Figure 6.39** (**A**) Pinch grip test. Normal response is the ability to pinch the tip of the thumb to the tip of the index finger. (**B**) Lesion of the anterior interosseous nerve results in pinching of the pads of the distal phalanges of the thumb and index finger rather than the tips.

Test for Pronator Teres Syndrome

Indication. This test is designed to assess entrapment of the median nerve by the pronator teres muscle, which passes over it.[3]

Method. The subject is seated with the elbow flexed to 90 degrees. The examiner vigorously resists forearm pronation while the elbow is extended (Fig. 6-40).

Results. A positive test occurs with production of tingling or paresthesias within the median nerve distribution of the forearm and hand.

TESTS FOR LATERAL EPICONDYLITIS (TENNIS ELBOW)

Method 1

Indication. Method 1 test is designed to detect inflammation in the musculature originating on and around the lateral epicondyle by imposing stress through contraction.

Method. The forearm is pronated and the elbow slightly flexed. The examiner resists wrist extension and finger extension in various ways (Fig. 6-41A–C). The following testing positions are used:

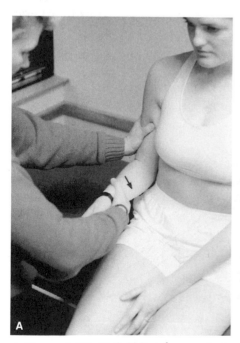

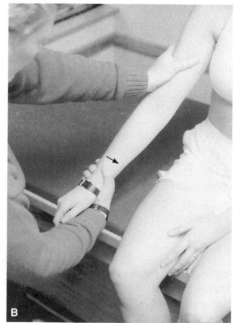

▲ **Figure 6.40** (**A & B**) Tests for pronator teres syndrome.

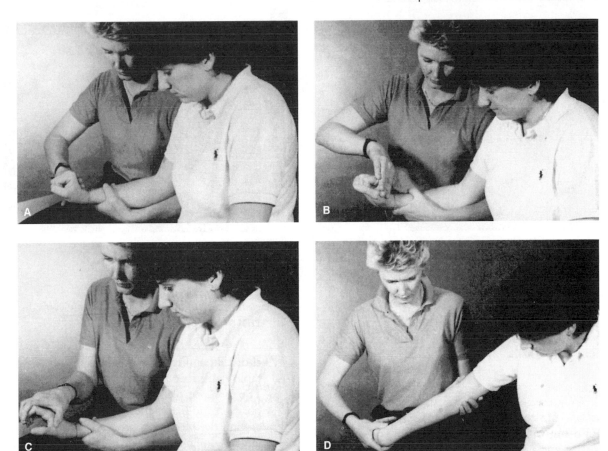

▲ **Figure 6.41** (**A–C**) Contractile testing of the wrist extensor musculature. (**D**) Flexibility testing of the wrist extensor musculature.

1. Wrist extension and radial deviation to assess the extensor carpi radialis longus and brevis
2. Wrist extension and ulnar deviation to assess the extensor carpi ulnaris
3. Finger extension to assess the extensor digitorum

Results. A positive result is sudden pain in the origin of the muscles being contracted. Because the extensor carpi radialis brevis is often involved in pathology, it is important to differentiate this structure from the extensor carpi radialis longus by palpating and recognizing the specific site of pain. In involvement of the extensor carpi radialis longus, pain is felt above the lateral epicondyle, where it originates on the supracondylar ridge. Conversely, the extensor carpi radialis brevis responds with localization of pain at its origin on the lateral epicondyle.

Method 2

Indication. Method 2 identifies inflammation in the extensor musculature of the wrist and hand originating on and about the lateral epicondyle. It requires stressing the musculature by elongation or stretching.

Method. The examiner extends the elbow and causes the subject's forearm to pronate while simultaneously flexing and deviating the wrist toward the ulna (see Fig. 6-41D). It is important that these motions be performed to the end ranges of motion to ensure complete stretching of the extensor musculature.

Results. A positive result is pain elicited at or near the lateral epicondyle. The specific tendon can be found in the manner described in the previous test. The position of the subject for this test may also be used in treatment as flexibility conditioning.

TEST FOR MEDIAL EPICONDYLITIS (GOLFER'S ELBOW)

Method 1

Indication. Method 1 is used to assess inflammation of the common flexor tendons of the wrist by stressing the musculature with contraction.

Method. The subject is positioned with the elbow in slight flexion and the forearm supinated (Fig. 6-42A). The examiner then resists flexion of the wrist.

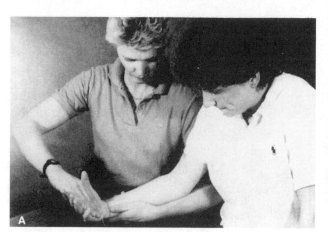

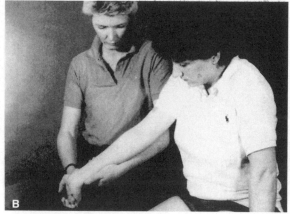

▲ **Figure 6.42** (**A**) Contractile testing of the wrist flexor musculature. (**B**) Flexibility testing of the wrist flexor musculature.

Results. Pain in the region of the medial epicondyle is a positive result. It is impossible clinically to identify the specific flexor muscle involved because of the common origin.

Method 2

Indication. Method 2 is used to identify inflammation of the common flexor tendons about the elbow by imposing stress through stretching.

Method. The subject's forearm is fully supinated while the examiner places the elbow and wrist in maximal extension (see Fig. 6-42*B*).

Results. Pain over the medial epicondyle indicates a positive test result. As in method 1, localization of the specific flexor tendon involved is not possible. This position may be used in flexibility training of the affected structures.

JOINT PLAY (ACCESSORY MOVEMENTS)

Humeroulnar Joint

Distraction (Fig. 6-43)

Restriction. General hypomobility.

Open-Packed Position. Seventy degrees of flexion; 10 degrees of forearm supination.

Positioning. Subject lies supine, with a stabilizing strap across the distal humerus. The therapist bends forward, using proper body mechanics, and rests the subject's distal forearm on the shoulder. The therapist then grips the proximal forearm close to the joint space.

Movement. The therapist leans backward creating a distraction force on the joint.

Medial Glide (Fig. 6-44)

Restriction. Flexion and extension.

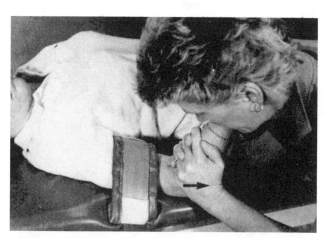

▲ **Figure 6.43** Distraction of the humeroulnar joint.

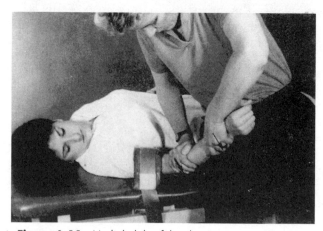

▲ **Figure 6.44** Medial glide of the ulna.

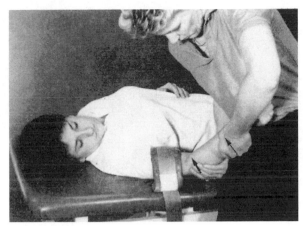

▲ **Figure 6.45** Lateral glide of the ulna.

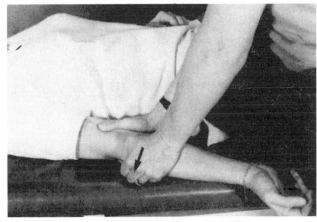

▲ **Figure 6.46** Posterior glide of the radius.

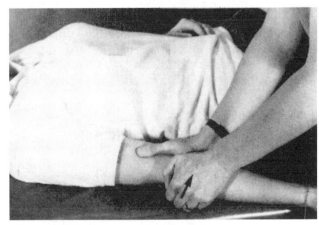

▲ **Figure 6.47** Anterior glide of the radius.

Positioning. Subject lies supine with a strap stabilizing the distal humerus. The therapist places the mobilizing hand proximally on the radial side of the forearm and supports the subject's forearm by holding the distal forearm.

Movement. The therapist delivers a medially directed force through the radial side of the proximal forearm.

Lateral Glide (Fig. 6-45)

Restriction. Flexion and extension.

Positioning. Subject lies supine, with a strap stabilizing the distal humerus. The therapist places the mobilizing hand proximally on the ulnar side of the forearm and supports the subject's forearm by holding the distal forearm.

Movement. The therapist delivers a laterally directed force through the ulnar side of the proximal forearm.

Radiohumeral Joint

Anterior Glide (Fig. 6-46)

Restriction. Extension.

Open-Packed Position. Full elbow extension; full forearm supination.

Positioning. Subject lies supine, with the upper limb stabilized by the table. The therapist grips the distal humerus and proximal ulna, thereby providing additional stabilization. The thenar eminence of the opposite hand is placed anteriorly on the proximal radius, close to the joint space.

Movement. The therapist imposes a posterior force on the anterior surface of the proximal radius.

Anterior Glide (Fig. 6-47)

Restriction. Flexion.

Positioning. Same as for dorsal glide, except the distal phalanges of digits two through five are placed posteriorly along the proximal radius.

Movement. The therapist imposes an anterior force to the posterior surface of the proximal radius.

Superior Radioulnar Joint

Posterior Medial Glide (Fig. 6-48)

Restriction. Forearm supination.

Open-Packed Position. Seventy degrees of elbow flexion; 35 degrees of forearm supination.

Positioning. Subject may be either seated or supine with the table stabilizing the limb. One hand of the therapist grips the distal humerus and proximal ulna, thereby providing additional stabilization. The

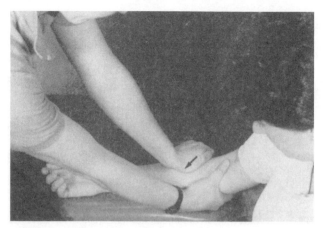

▲ **Figure 6.48** *Anterior medial glide of the radius.*

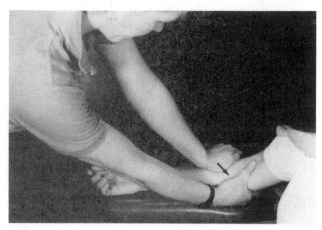

▲ **Figure 6.49** *Posterior lateral glide of the radius.*

thenar eminence of the opposite hand is placed anteriorly on the proximal radius, close to the joint space. The distal phalanges of digits two through five are placed posteriorly along the proximal radius.

Movement. The therapist imposes an anterior medial force to the posterior surface of the proximal radius.

Posterior Lateral Glide (Fig. 6-49)

Restriction. Forearm pronation.

Positioning. Same as for anterior medial glide.

Movement. The therapist imposes a posterior lateral force to the anterior surface of the proximal radius.

Distraction (Fig. 6-50)

Restriction. Proximal positional fault of the radius.

Positioning. Subject is supine or seated. One hand of the therapist stabilizes the distal humerus, while the other grasps the distal radius.

Movement. The therapist pulls the radius distally along its long axis, thereby creating a distraction force to the proximal radius. The positional fault is corrected not only at the superior radioulnar joint, but at the radiohumeral joint as well.

Compression (Fig. 6-51)

Restriction. Distal positional fault of the radius.

Positioning. Same as for distraction glide.

Movement. The therapist moves the radius proximally along its long axis, thereby creating a compression force to the proximal radius. The positional fault is corrected not only at the superior radioulnar joint, but at the radiohumeral joint as well.

Inferior Radioulnar Joint

Anterior Medial Glide (Fig. 6-52)

Restriction. Forearm pronation.

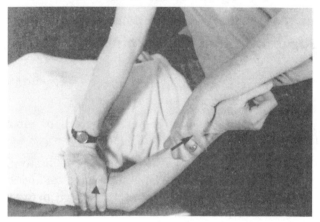

▲ **Figure 6.50** *Distraction or distal glide of the radius.*

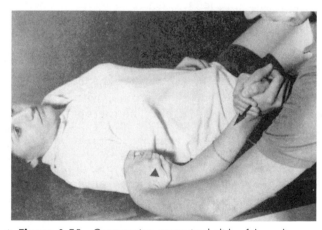

▲ **Figure 6.51** *Compression or proximal glide of the radius.*

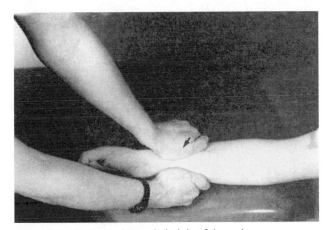

▲ **Figure 6.52** Anterior medial glide of the radius.

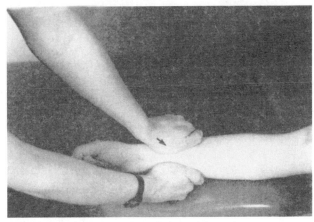

▲ **Figure 6.53** Posterior lateral glide of the radius.

TABLE 6.1	**Summary of Joint Play of the Elbow and Forearm Joints**		
GLIDE	RESTRICTION	FIXED BONE	MOVING BONE
Humeroulnar Joint			
Distraction	General hypomobility	Humerus	Ulna
Anterior	Flexion	Humerus	Ulna
Medial	Flexion-extension	Humerus	Ulna
Lateral	Flexion-extension	Humerus	Ulna
Radiohumeral Joint			
Distraction	General hypomobility	Humerus	Radius
Anterior	Flexion	Humerus	Radius
Posterior	Extension	Humerus	Radius
Superior Radioulnar Joint			
Anterior medial	Supination	Ulna	Radius
Posterior lateral	Pronation	Ulna	Radius
Distraction	Proximal positional fault	Ulna	Radius
Compression	Distal positional fault	Ulna	Radius
Inferior Radioulnar Joint			
Anterior medial	Pronation	Ulna	Radius
Posterior lateral	Supination	Ulna	Radius

Open-Packed Position. Ten degrees of forearm supination.

Positioning. Subject is either supine or seated. One hand of the therapist stabilizes the distal ulna. The mobilizing hand is placed with the thenar eminence on the anterior surface of the distal radius, and the distal phalanges of digits two through five on the posterior surface of the distal radius.

Movement. The therapist imparts ventral medial force to the posterior surface of the distal radius.

Posterior Lateral Glide (Fig. 6-53)

Restriction. Forearm supination.

Positioning. Same as for anterior medial glide.

Movement. The therapist produces a posterior lateral force on the anterior surface of the distal radius.

Table 6-1 provides a summary of joint play of the elbow and forearm joints.

REFERENCES

1. Andrews JA, Wilk KE, Satterwhite YE, Tedder JL: Physical examination of the thrower's elbow. JOSPT 17(6):296–304, 1993
2. Beals RK: The normal carrying angle of the elbow. Clin Orthop 119:194, 1976
3. Volz RC, Morrey BF: The physical examination of the elbow. In Morrey BF (ed): The Elbow and Its Disorders. Philadelphia, WB Saunders, 1985

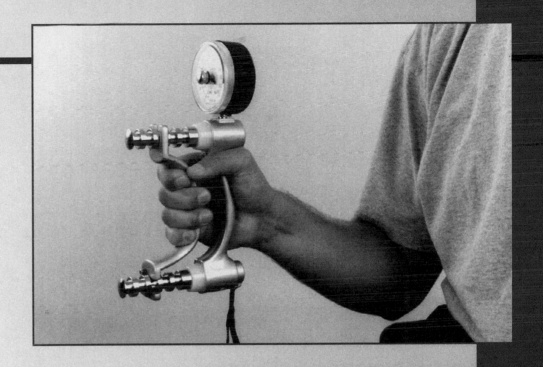

7

Wrist and
Hand

The wrist and hand are complex structures that are dependent on the entire upper limb. The hand is necessary for such delicate activities of daily living as sewing and painting and such powerful ones as hammering. Loss in the proximal upper limb may translate into diminished function of the hand.

The wrist joint is formed by the distal end of the radius, the proximal carpal bones (scaphoid and lunate), and the articular disk of the ulna and the triquetrum. The joint moves in two planes of motion and is called a condyloid synovial joint. Intercarpal motions occur during wrist joint flexion, extension, abduction, and adduction. The intercarpal joints are plane joints. The axis for flexion and extension is transverse (from medial to lateral) and is located at the level of the capitate bone. The axis for radial deviation (abduction) and ulnar deviation (adduction) is transverse anteriorly and posteriorly and through the capitate.

In the hand, the distal row of carpal bones articulates with the metacarpals. These joints, called saddle joints, have little or no movement except in the first and fifth digits. The base of the first metacarpal articulates with the trapezium and allows three degrees of freedom of motion. The joint is capable of flexion, extension, abduction, adduction, and opposition. The metacarpophalangeal (MCP) joints of the medial four digits are condyloid joints and permit flexion, extension, abduction, and adduction motions. The first digit's MCP joint is like an interphalangeal (IP) joint of the medial four digits, which are hinge joints, permitting only flexion and extension.

GONIOMETRY

Wrist

WRIST FLEXION

The majority of wrist flexion occurs at the radiocarpal joint in the sagittal plane between the radius and the scaphoid and lunate bones. Movement of wrist flexion also occurs between the intercarpals and the head of the ulna and the articular disk. As the wrist joint flexes, the proximal row of carpal bones glides in a posterior direction on the distal end of the radius. The fingers are held loosely in extension to allow complete range of motion at the wrist joint.

Motion. From 0 to 90 degrees from the anatomical wrist position into flexion.

Position

• Preferred: Subject sits with the forearm supported on the table in pronation. The elbow

joint is flexed 90 degrees, the wrist is in the neutral position, and the fingers are extended.
• Alternate:
1. Subject sits with the elbow flexed. The forearm is in a position between supination and pronation. Fingers are held loosely in extension.
2. Subject lies supine with the elbow flexed. The forearm and wrist are positioned as above.

Goniometric Alignment (Figs. 7-1 to 7-3)

Axis

• Preferred: Placed distal to the styloid process of the ulna, the axis shifts slightly distally following movement.

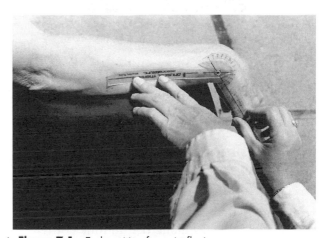

▲ **Figure 7.1**   End position for wrist flexion.

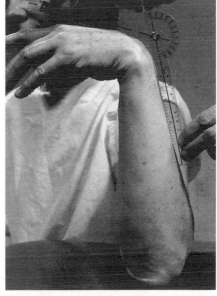

▲ **Figure 7.2**   Alternate end position for wrist flexion with the goniometer placed on the posterior surface of the joint.

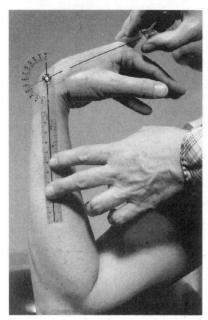

▲ **Figure 7.3** Alternate end position for wrist flexion with the placement of the goniometer on the lateral aspect of the joint.

- Alternate: Placed over the capitate bone.
- Alternate: Placed on the styloid process of the radius (see Fig. 7-3).

Stationary Arm

- Preferred: Placed parallel to and over the lateral midline of the ulna, in line with the olecranon process.
- Alternate: Placed along the midline of the dorsal surface of the forearm.
- Alternate: Placed along the radial shaft in line with the head.

Moving Arm

- Preferred: Placed along the lateral midline of the fifth metacarpal.
- Alternate: Placed on the midline of the dorsal surface of the third metacarpal.
- Alternate: Placed on the midline of the second metacarpal.

Stabilization. The forearm is stabilized.

Precautions

- Make sure fingers stay relaxed during measurement.
- Avoid radial and ulnar deviation of the wrist joint.
- Avoid depression of the fifth metacarpal.

WRIST EXTENSION AND HYPEREXTENSION

Wrist extension and hyperextension occur in the sagittal plane at the radiocarpal and intercarpal joints. As the wrist moves into extension, the proximal row of carpal bones glides anteriorly. Wrist extension is the return from flexion. Wrist flexion and extension can be measured on the radial or ulnar side of the hand, but the measurements of the two sides will vary because of anatomical structure of the wrist and the cupping of the hand on the ulnar side. If measured on the radial side, the second metacarpal is used as the distal landmark.

Motion. From 90 to 0 degrees of extension and about 70 degrees of hyperextension.

Position. Same as for wrist flexion, with the fingers held loosely in flexion.

Goniometric alignment and stabilization are the same as for wrist flexion (Figs. 7-4 to 7-6).

Precautions

- Avoid extension of the fingers.
- Avoid radial and ulnar deviation at the wrist joint.
- Prevent cupping of the fifth metacarpal.
- Range of motion will vary according to the position of the goniometer. Always place consistently on each subject.

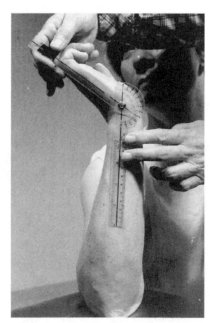

▲ **Figure 7.4** End position for wrist joint extension and hyperextension.

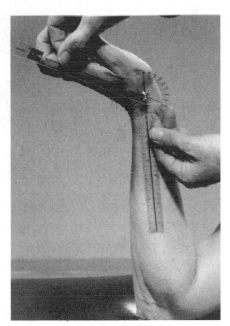

▲ **Figure 7.5** Alternate end position for wrist extension and hyperextension with the goniometer placed on the lateral aspect of the joint.

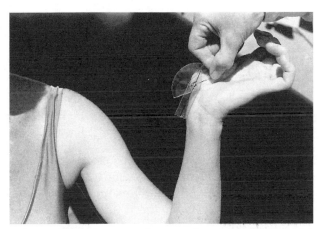

▲ **Figure 7.6** Alternate end position for wrist extension and hyperextension with the goniometer placed on the anterior surface of the joint.

WRIST RADIAL DEVIATION (ABDUCTION)

In the anatomical position, the motion of radial deviation at the wrist occurs in the coronal plane. The motion occurs between the radius and the proximal row of carpal bones and between the intercarpals. The distal row of carpals moves radially, and the proximal row glides ulnarly on the distal end of the radius during wrist abduction.

Motion. From 0 to 25 degrees of radial deviation.

Position

• Preferred: Subject sits with the elbow flexed and forearm pronated on the table. The fore-

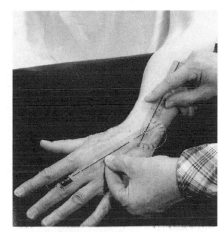

▲ **Figure 7.7** End position for radial deviation (abduction) of the wrist.

arm and hand are supported on the table top with the wrist in a neutral position.
• Alternate: The subject lies supine.

Goniometric Alignment (Fig. 7-7)

Axis. Placed on the dorsal surface of the wrist over the capitate bone.

Stationary Arm. Placed along the dorsal midline surface of the forearm.

Moving Arm. Placed on the midline of the dorsal surface of the third metacarpal bone.

Stabilization. The forearm is stabilized.

Precautions

• Avoid flexion or extension of the wrist.
• Avoid pronation or supination of the forearm.
• Do not use the third digit as a point of reference.

WRIST ULNAR DEVIATION (ADDUCTION)

In the test position, the motion occurs in the coronal plane. The motion occurs between the intercarpal bones and the radiocarpal joint. When ulnar deviation occurs, the distal carpal bones move in an ulnar direction, and at the end of the range, the proximal row of carpal bones glides radially on the distal end of the radius.

Motion. From 0 to 35 degrees of ulnar deviation from the neutral position of the wrist joint.

Position. Subject sits with the elbow flexed to 90 degrees, the forearm pronated on the table, and the hand supported.

Goniometric alignment, stabilization, and precautions are the same as for wrist radial deviation (Fig. 7-8).

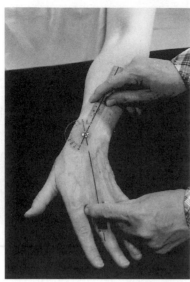

▲ **Figure 7.8** End position for ulnar deviation (adduction) of the wrist.

Metacarpophalangeal (MCP) Joints (Digits Two to Five)

METACARPOPHALANGEAL JOINT FLEXION

The hand is in a neutral position with the forearm in midposition between supination and pronation. In the anatomical position, the motion occurs in the sagittal plane. The motion occurs between the metacarpals and the proximal phalanx of each of the fingers. As the motion occurs, the base of the phalanx glides in an anterior direction.

If the subject has edema or bony joint changes and the arms of the goniometer cannot be placed accurately, alternate measurements may be made. A ruler measurement may be made from the tip of each finger to the distal carpal crease. Tracings, x-rays, or photographs may also be used. A goniometer with short arms or a goniometer designed for the digits is recommended for measurements.

Motion. From 0 to 90 degrees of flexion while maintaining the IP joints in extension.

Position. Subject is sitting, with the elbow flexed to 90 degrees, the forearm supported in the midposition, and the wrist and fingers in the anatomical position.

Goniometric Alignment (Fig. 7-9)

Axis. Placed on the dorsal surface of the MCP joint.

Stationary Arm. Placed on the midline of the dorsal surface of the metacarpal of the joint being measured.

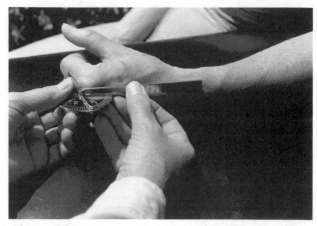

▲ **Figure 7.9** End position for metacarpophalangeal joint flexion.

Moving Arm. Placed on the midline of the dorsal surface of the proximal phalanx of the joint being measured.

Stabilization. The metacarpals are stabilized.

Precautions

- Hold the fingers loosely in extension.
- Hyperextend the wrist slightly.
- Avoid MCP joint abduction and adduction.

METACARPOPHALANGEAL JOINT EXTENSION AND HYPEREXTENSION

Extension of the MCP joint is the return of flexion, and hyperextension occurs beyond the neutral (0) position. As the proximal phalanx moves into extension and hyperextension, the base glides in a posterior direction.

Motion. From 90 to 0 degrees for extension and 0 to 30 degrees for hyperextension, with the IP joints held loosely in flexion.

Position. Subject sits with elbow and shoulder flexed and forearm in midposition between supination and pronation. The wrist remains in the anatomical position.

Goniometric Alignment (Fig. 7-10)

Axis. Placed over the palmar aspect of the MCP joint being measured.

Stationary Arm. Placed along the palmar midline shaft of the metacarpal being measured.

Moving Arm. Placed along the palmar midline shaft of the proximal phalanx being measured.

Stabilization. The metacarpals are stabilized.

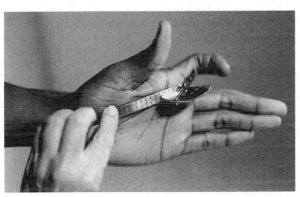

▲ **Figure 7.10** End position for metacarpophalangeal joint extension and hyperextension.

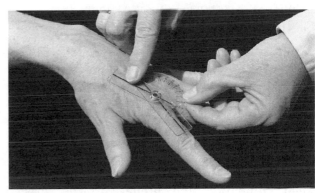

▲ **Figure 7.11** End position for metacarpophalangeal joint abduction.

Precautions

- Keep the fingers relaxed in a flexed position.
- Keep the wrist in the anatomical position.

METACARPOPHALANGEAL JOINT ABDUCTION

In the test position, MCP joint abduction motion occurs in the coronal plane. The MCP joints are maintained in an extended position. The second digit (index finger) moves in a radial direction from the third digit (middle finger), and the fourth and fifth digits (ring and little fingers) move in an ulnar direction from the middle finger. The proximal phalanx glides in the same direction on the head of the metacarpal. The third digit abducts both radially and ulnarly.

Motion. From 0 to 20 degrees of MCP joint abduction (movement away from the middle finger).

Position. Subject sits with the elbow joint flexed and the wrist joint in a neutral position. The forearm and hand are supported in a pronated position.

Goniometric Alignment (Fig. 7-11)

Axis. Placed over the dorsal midline of the MCP joint to be tested.

Stationary Arm. Placed over the dorsal midline of the metacarpal being tested.

Moving Arm. Placed over the dorsal midline of the proximal phalanx of the joint being tested.

Stabilization. The metacarpal is stabilized.

Precautions

- Prevent wrist motions.
- Avoid flexion at the MCP joint.

METACARPOPHALANGEAL JOINT ADDUCTION

Adduction at the MCP joints is the return from abduction. The test position is in the coronal plane. The second digit (index finger) moves in an ulnar direction, and the fourth and fifth digits (ring and little fingers) move radially toward the third digit. The base of the proximal phalanx adducts on the head of the metacarpal and glides in the same direction as the motion.

Motion. From 0 to 20 degrees at the MCP joints.

Position. Subject sits with the elbow joint flexed, the forearm pronated, and the wrist and fingers in a neutral position. The forearm and hand are supported. The third digit (middle finger) is positioned to allow 20 degrees of motion to occur from the anatomical position.

Goniometric alignment, stabilization, and precautions are the same as for MCP abduction (Fig. 7-12).

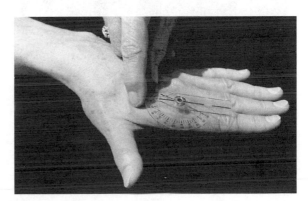

▲ **Figure 7.12** End position for metacarpophalangeal joint adduction.

PROXIMAL INTERPHALANGEAL (PIP) JOINT FLEXION

Flexion at the proximal intercarpophalangeal joints occurs in the sagittal plane in the anatomical position. As the middle phalanx flexes on the proximal one, it glides in an anterior direction.

Motion. From 0 to 120 degrees for flexion.

Position. Subject sits, with elbow flexed and forearm supported on the table in the midposition between supination and pronation. The wrist is slightly hyperextended.

Goniometric Alignment (Fig. 7-13)

Axis

- Preferred: Placed over the dorsal aspect of the proximal interphalangeal (PIP) joints.
- Alternate: Placed over the radial aspect of the joint.

Stationary Arm

- Preferred: Placed along the dorsal midline of the proximal phalanx.
- Alternate: Placed along the radial midline of the proximal phalanx.

Moving Arm

- Preferred: Placed along the dorsal midline of the middle phalanx.
- Alternate: Placed along the radial midline of the middle phalanx

Stabilization. The proximal phalanx is stabilized.

Precaution

- Prevent wrist flexion.

PROXIMAL INTERPHALANGEAL JOINT EXTENSION AND HYPEREXTENSION

Extension motion of the PIP joint is the return from flexion. The base of the middle phalanx glides in a posterior direction as the joint moves into extension.

Motion. From 120 to 0 degrees for extension and 0 to 10 degrees for hyperextension.

Position. Subject sits, with elbow flexed and forearm supported on the table in the midposition between supination and pronation. The wrist joint is in the anatomical position, and the digits are relaxed in flexion.

Goniometric Alignment (Fig. 7-14)

Axis

- Preferred: Placed over the palmar aspect of the joint being measured.
- Alternate: Refer to alternate placement for PIP flexion.

Stationary Arm. Placed over the midline of the palmar aspect of the proximal phalanx.

Moving Arm. Placed over the midline of the palmar aspect of the middle phalanx.

Stabilization. The proximal phalanx is stabilized.

Precaution

- Prevent wrist hyperextension.

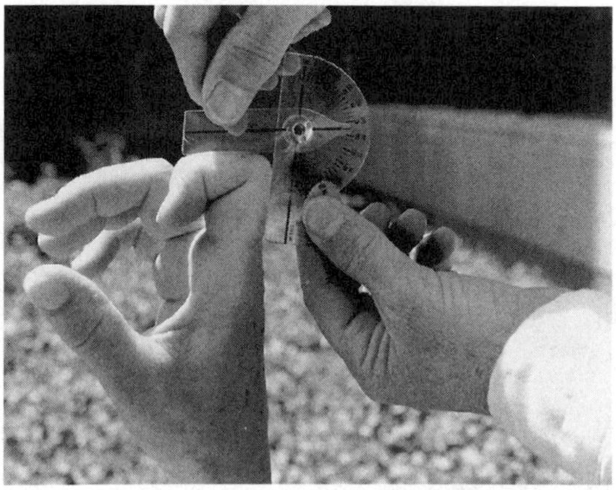

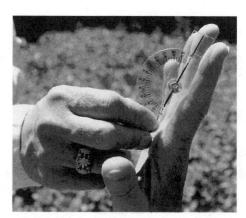

▲ **Figure 7.13** End position for proximal interphalangeal joint flexion.

▲ **Figure 7.14** End position for proximal interphalangeal joint extension.

DISTAL INTERPHALANGEAL JOINT FLEXION

Distal interphalangeal (DIP) flexion occurs between the middle and distal phalanges. As flexion of the DIP joint occurs, the base of the distal phalanx glides in an anterior direction.

Motion. From 0 to 80 degrees of DIP joint flexion with the PIP joint positioned in slight flexion.

Position. Subject sits with elbow flexed and forearm in midposition between supination and pronation. The forearm and hand are supported on the table. The wrist is slightly hyperextended.

Goniometric Alignment (Fig. 7-15)

Axis

- Preferred: Placed over the dorsal surface of the joint being measured.
- Alternate: Placed over the radial midline of the DIP.

Stationary Arm

- Preferred: Placed over the dorsal midline shaft of the middle phalanx of each digit.
- Alternate: Place over radial side of middle phalanx.

Moving Arm

- Preferred: Placed over the dorsal midline shaft of each distal phalanx.
- Alternate: Placed over radial side of distal phalanx.

Stabilization. The middle phalanx of each digit is stabilized.

Precaution

- Allow the wrist to remain slightly hyperextended.

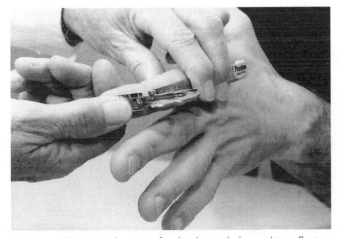

▲ **Figure 7.15**   End position for distal interphalangeal joint flexion.

DISTAL INTERPHALANGEAL JOINT EXTENSION

Extension motion of the DIP joint is the return from flexion of the DIP joints. During the motion, the base of the distal phalanx glides in a posterior direction on the head of the middle phalanx.

Motion. From 80 to 0 degrees of extension, and 0 to 10 degrees of hyperextension at the DIP joints.

Position, goniometeric alignment, and stabilization are the same as for DIP flexion (Fig. 7-16).

Precaution

- Keep wrist and MCP joints properly aligned.

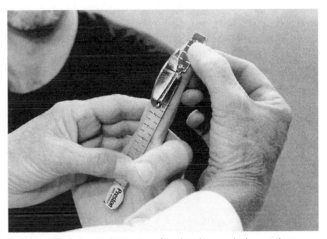

▲ **Figure 7.16**   End position for distal interphalangeal joint extension.

THUMB CARPOMETACARPAL JOINT FLEXION

In the test position, flexion at the carpometacarpal (CMC) joint occurs in the coronal plane between the first metacarpal and the trapezium. The first metacarpal moves across the palm of the hand, and the base glides ulnarly.

Motion. From 0 to 15 degrees at the CMC joint (allow the first metacarpal to slide over the second metacarpal).

Position. Subject sits with the elbow joint flexed and the forearm supinated and supported. The wrist, fingers, and thumb joints are in the anatomical position.

Goniometric Alignment (Fig. 7-17)

Axis. Placed over the palmar surface of the first CMC joint.

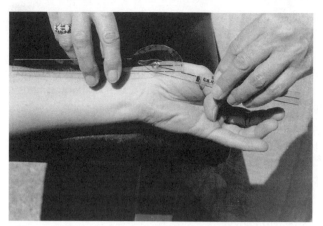

▲ **Figure 7.17** End position for first digit carpometacarpal joint flexion.

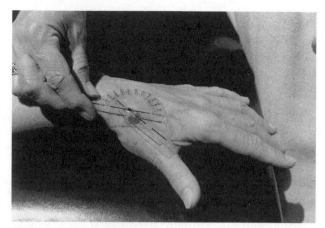

▲ **Figure 7.18** End position for carpometacarpal joint extension.

Stationary Arm. Placed along the long axis of the radial shaft.

Moving Arm. Placed along the long axis of the first metacarpal shaft.

Stabilization. The carpal bones are stabilized.

Precautions

- Prevent wrist flexion and ulnar deviation.
- Prevent thumb opposition.

THUMB CARPOMETACARPAL JOINT EXTENSION AND HYPEREXTENSION (RADIAL ABDUCTION)

In the anatomical position, extension at the CMC joint occurs in the coronal plane. During the motion, the base of the first metacarpal glides radially in the same direction as the motion on the trapezium bone.

Motion. From 0 to 70 degrees of extension at the metacarpal joint. The thumb is extended in the plane of the palm.

Position. Subject sits with the elbow flexed and the forearm pronated and supported. The wrist and fingers remain in the anatomical position.

Goniometric Alignment (Figs. 7-18 and 7-19)

Axis

- Preferred: Placed over the dorsal aspect of the CMC joint of the thumb.
- Alternate: Placed over the palmar aspect of the CMC joint of the thumb.

Stationary Arm

- Preferred: Placed dorsally on the midline of the radius.

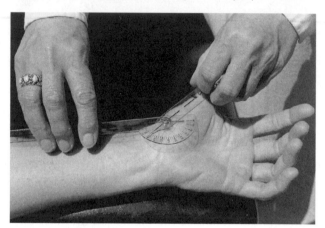

▲ **Figure 7.19** Alternate end position for carpometacarpal joint extension.

- Alternate: Placed over the anterior midline of the radius.

Moving Arm

- Preferred: Placed on the midline of the dorsal surface of the first metacarpal bone.
- Alternate: Placed over the anterior midline of the first metacarpal bone.

Stabilization. The carpal bones are stabilized.

Precautions

- Prevent thumb flexion or abduction.
- Prevent radial deviation of the wrist joint.

THUMB CARPOMETACARPAL JOINT OPPOSITION

The motion of opposition is a combination of flexion, abduction, and medial rotation between the first metacarpal and the trapezium. The movement of rotation occurs as the thumb moves toward the base or tip of the fifth finger. A ruler or tape measure is used to determine the distance between the fifth finger and the thumb when complete motion is not obtained. Normally the thumb pad touches the fifth finger and the thumbnail faces away from the palm.

Motion. The distance is between the tip of the fifth finger and the thumb. The pad of the thumb approaches the base of the fifth finger.

Position. Subject sits with elbow flexed and forearm supported in supination. The wrist and finger joints are in the anatomical position.

Measurement. When motion is limited, the ruler is placed from the tip of the thumb to the tip or base of the fifth finger. The distance recorded is the deficit in complete range of motion (Figs. 7-20 and 7-21).

Stabilization. The metacarpal and fingers not involved in the motion are stabilized.

Precautions

- Prevent wrist flexion.
- Allow the three motions of flexion, abduction, and medial rotation at the first CMC joint.

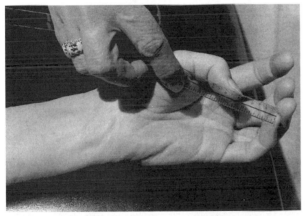

▲ **Figure 7.20** Measuring opposition with a ruler or measuring tape.

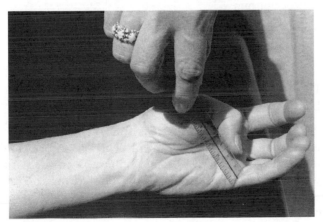

▲ **Figure 7.21** Alternate end position for measuring opposition.

THUMB CARPOMETACARPAL JOINT ABDUCTION (PALMAR ABDUCTION)

In the anatomical position, thumb CMC joint abduction occurs in the sagittal plane. The thumb moves at right angles to the palm of the hand. The first metacarpal abducts on the trapezium bone, and its base glides dorsally on the trapezium bone.

Motion. From 0 to 60 degrees of abduction at the first CMC joint.

Position. Subject sits with the elbow flexed and the forearm in midposition between supination and pronation. The hand is supported and resting on the ulnar border. The wrist and fingers are in the anatomical position.

Goniometric Alignment (Fig. 7-22)

Axis. Placed between the first and second CMC joints on the dorsal surface.

Stationary Arm. Placed on the lateral midline of the second metacarpal bone.

Moving Arm. Placed on the midline of the dorsal surface of the first metacarpal bone.

Stabilization. The carpal and second metacarpal are stabilized.

Precautions

- Prevent medial rotation of the thumb.
- Observe web space for skin tightness.
- Prevent flexion or extension of the thumb.
- Avoid wrist joint motions.

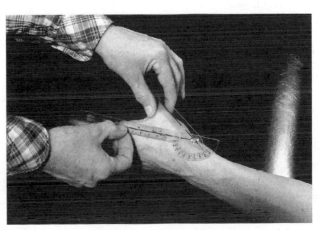

▲ **Figure 7.22** End position for carpometacarpal joint abduction.

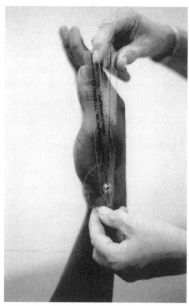

▲ **Figure 7.23** End position for carpometacarpal joint adduction.

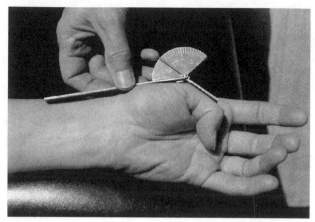

▲ **Figure 7.24** End position for metacarpophalangeal joint flexion.

THUMB CARPOMETACARPAL JOINT ADDUCTION

Adduction of the CMC joint of the first digit is the return from CMC joint abduction. It is also the anatomical position for the first CMC joint. As the first metacarpal moves toward adduction, its base glides anteriorly in the opposite direction over the trapezium.

Motion. From 60 to 0 degrees of adduction at the first CMC joint into the anatomical position.

Position, goniometric alignment, stabilization, and precautions are the same as for thumb CMC abduction (Fig. 7-23).

THUMB METACARPOPHALANGEAL JOINT FLEXION

In the anatomical position, flexion of the thumb MCP joint occurs in the coronal plane. The proximal phalanx flexes on the first metacarpal as the base glides in a radial direction on the head of the first metacarpal.

Motion. From 0 to 50 degrees of flexion, maintaining the IP joint in extension.

Position. Subject sits with elbow flexed and forearm and hand supported in a supinated position. The wrist, thumb, and finger joints are in the anatomical position.

Goniometric Alignment (Fig. 7-24)

Axis

- Preferred: Placed over the dorsal aspect of the MCP joint.
- Alternate: Placed over the anterior surface of the MCP joint.

Stationary Arm

- Preferred: Placed over the dorsal midline shaft of the first metacarpal bone.
- Alternate: Placed over the anterior surface of the first metacarpal.

Moving Arm

- Preferred: Placed over the dorsal midline shaft of the proximal phalanx.
- Alternate: Placed over the anterior surface of the proximal phalanx.

Stabilization. The metacarpal bones are stabilized.

Precautions

- Prevent wrist joint motion.
- Avoid CMC joint flexion and opposition.

THUMB METACARPOPHALANGEAL JOINT EXTENSION AND HYPEREXTENSION

Extension of the MCP joint is the return from MCP joint flexion to the anatomical position and beyond into hyperextension. The motion occurs in the coronal plane in the anatomical position. During the motion of extension and hyperextension, the first metacarpal bone glides ulnarly on the trapezium.

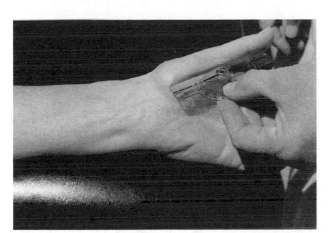

▲ **Figure 7.25** End position for metacarpophalangeal joint extension and hyperextension.

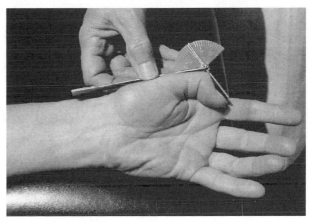

▲ **Figure 7.26** End position for first digit interphalangeal joint flexion.

Motion. From 50 to 0 degrees for extension and 0 to 10 degrees for hyperextension. The IP joint remains extended.

Position, goniometeric alignment, stabilization, and precautions are the same as for thumb MCP flexion (Fig. 7-25).

THUMB INTERPHALANGEAL JOINT FLEXION

IP joint flexion of the first digit occurs in the coronal plane. As the base of the distal phalanx flexes on the head of the proximal phalanx, it glides in a radial direction.

Motion. 0 to 80 or 90 degrees of flexion at the IP joint of the thumb.

Position. Subject sits with elbow flexed and forearm supinated and supported. The wrist, fingers, and thumb are in the anatomical position.

Goniometric Alignment (Fig. 7-26)

Axis

- Preferred: Placed over the dorsal surface of the IP joint.
- Alternate: Placed over the anterior aspect of the IP joint.

Stationary Arm

- Preferred: Placed along the dorsal midline surface of the proximal phalanx.
- Alternate: Placed over the anterior aspect of the proximal phalanx.

Moving Arm

- Preferred: Placed along the dorsal midline surface of the distal phalanx.

- Alternate: Placed over the anterior aspect of the distal phalanx.

Stabilization. The proximal phalanx is stabilized.

Precautions

- Prevent wrist motions.
- Prevent MCP joint flexion or extension.

THUMB INTERPHALANGEAL JOINT EXTENSION AND HYPEREXTENSION

Extension of the IP joint occurs in the coronal plane in the test position and is the return from flexion. The base of the distal phalanx of the thumb glides ulnarly on the head of the proximal phalanx during the extension and hyperextension motion. The range of motion varies from person to person.

Motion. From 90 to 0 degrees for extension and 0 toward 90 degrees for hyperextension.

Position, goniometric alignment, stabilization, and precautions are the same as for thumb IP joint flexion.

Goniometric Alignment (Fig. 7-27)

Axis. Placed over the dorsal aspect of the IP joint. For the motion of hyperextension, the axis is over the IP joint on the palmar surface.

Stationary Arm. Placed along the dorsal midline surface of the proximal phalanx. For hyperextension motion, the stationary arm is along the midline palmar surface of the proximal phalanx.

Moving Arm. Placed along the midline dorsal surface of the distal phalanx. For hyperextension, the

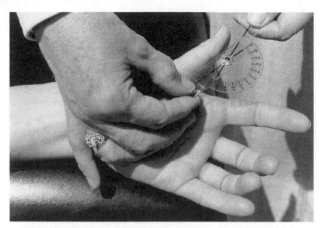

▲ **Figure 7.27** End position for first digit interphalangeal joint extension and hyperextension.

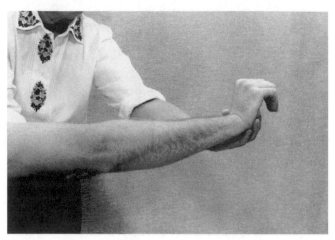

▲ **Figure 7.28** Muscle length testing for wrist flexor muscles.

moving arm is placed on the palmar midline surface of the distal phalanx.

Stabilization. The proximal phalanx is stabilized.

Precautions

- Prevent wrist movements.
- Prevent MCP and CMC joint motion.

MUSCLE LENGTH TESTING

Wrist

The wrist joint allows the hand to assume various positions. Changes in the position of the elbow affect the length of the forearm muscles and the function of the muscles of the wrist and hand. The position of the wrist is a determining factor in the strength of the hand muscles. Its major contribution to upper limb function is to provide a stable base for hand function. The wrist flexor muscles act synergistically with finger extension. The wrist flexor muscles cross the elbow and wrist joints anteriorly. Functionally, wrist extensor muscles are important in maintaining the length-tension relationship for gripping objects. The wrist extensor muscles cross the elbow and wrist joints posteriorly. They act synergistically with the finger flexor muscles.

FLEXOR CARPI ULNARIS, FLEXOR CARPI RADIALIS, AND PALMARIS LONGUS MUSCLES

Position. The subject is supine or sitting with the elbow joint extended.

Movement. The examiner extends the wrist joint while the elbow is maintained in extension.

Measurement. Wrist joint extension is measured with a goniometer aligned with bony landmarks as discussed in goniometry (Fig. 7-28).

Considerations

1. The fingers and thumb are relaxed and in slight flexion to minimize the tension of the extrinsic hand flexor tendons.
2. Radial and ulnar deviation are avoided.
3. Anterior joint capsular structures also will limit wrist extension range of motion.

EXTENSOR CARPI RADIALIS LONGUS AND BREVIS, EXTENSOR CARPI ULNARIS MUSCLES

Position. The subject is either in a supine or sitting position with the elbow extended.

Movement. The examiner flexes the wrist joint, allowing the fingers and thumb to remain relaxed (Fig. 7-29).

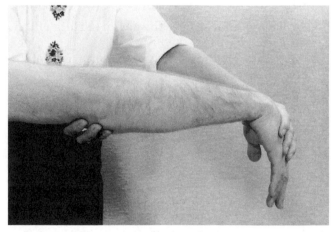

▲ **Figure 7.29** Muscle length testing for the wrist extensor muscle group.

Measurement. Refer to goniometeric measurements for the wrist joint.

Considerations

1. The elbow joint is extended to place the wrist extensor muscles at their greatest length because they cross anterior to the joint.
2. The fingers and thumb are relaxed to eliminate the effect of the extrinsic hand tendons and the wrist joint.
3. Posterior joint capsular structures also will limit wrist flexion range of motion.

Fingers

The extrinsic hand muscles are considered multijoint muscles crossing the elbow joint proximally and the wrist and phalangeal joints distally. The flexor digitorum profundus, extensor indices, extensor pollicis longus and brevis, flexor pollicis longus, and abductor pollicis longus muscles lie deep in the forearm and do not cross the elbow joint, but they do influence the wrist and phalangeal joints. The synergistic action of the wrist is critical for finger and thumb function. Wrist extension always accompanies finger and thumb flexion.

FLEXOR DIGITORUM SUPERFICIALIS MUSCLE

Position. The subject is sitting or supine with the elbow and wrist joints extended completely (hyperextended).

Movement. The examiner extends the metacarpal joints completely, maintaining the elbow, wrist, and IP joints in complete extension (hyperextendcd).

Measurement. The limitation is measured using a finger goniometer as illustrated in the goniometry section (Fig. 7-30).

Considerations

1. Elbow joint position has no effect on the flexor digitorum profundus but does affect extension of wrist and finger joints. If the limitation in the fingers exists regardless of elbow joint position, then the flexor digitorum superficialis is not tight.
2. The intrinsic hand muscles may demonstrate limitation in length but would not be influenced by wrist or elbow joint position. The intrinsic hand muscles that flex the MCP joints are the dorsal and palmar interossei and the lumbrical muscles.

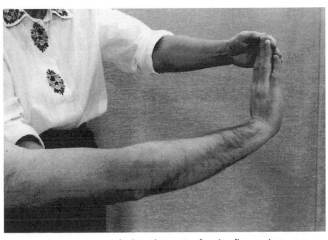

▲ **Figure 7.30** Muscle length testing for the flexor digitorum superficialis muscle.

EXTENSOR DIGITORUM AND EXTENSOR DIGITI MINIMI MUSCLES

Position. The subject is sitting or supine with the elbow joint extended and wrist and IP joints flexed.

Movement. The examiner flexes the MCP joints with the wrist joint flexed and elbow joint extended.

Measurement. The limitation is measured using a goniometer as illustrated in the goniometry section (Fig. 7-31).

Considerations

1. The extensor indices, extensor pollicis longus and brevis, and abductor pollicis tendons cross the wrist and MCP joint posteriorly but do not cross the elbow joint. If the elbow joint position makes no difference in the range of motion at the MCP joints, then the extensor digi-

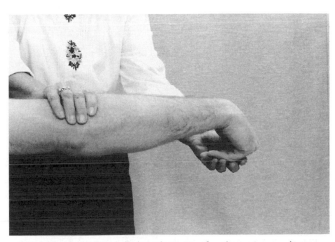

▲ **Figure 7.31** Muscle length testing for the extensor digitorum and extensor digiti minimi muscles.

torum and extensor digiti minimi muscles are not tight.

2. Limitation in MCP flexion range of motion may be produced by the extrinsic muscles that cross the wrist and not the elbow joints.

3. The intrinsic muscles that contribute to the extensor hood covering the posterior aspect of the fingers may not allow complete IP joint flexion.

4. The posterior capsular structures, if not at optimal length, will limit flexion of the MCP joints.

MANUAL MUSCLE TESTING

Wrist

FLEXOR CARPI RADIALIS MUSCLE

The flexor carpi radialis muscle produces the motion of wrist flexion from a starting position of extension. All grades are tested with the subject in the sitting or supine position with the forearm resting on a table. The fingers should remain relaxed.

Palpation. The tendon is superficial at the level of the carpal creases. It is palpated slightly lateral to the midline of the wrist (Fig. 7-32).

Position

Against gravity (AG): The dorsal surface of the hand rests on the table with the fingers in slight flexion (Fig. 7-33).

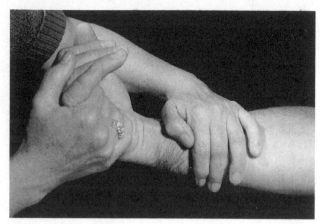

▲ **Figure 7.33** Testing the flexor carpi radialis muscle in the AG position.

Gravity minimized (GM): The subject is positioned with the ulnar border of the hand resting on the table. Fingers are relaxed in flexion (Fig. 7-34).

Movement. Flexion of the wrist with radial deviation.

Resistance. Applied to palm of the hand into extension and ulnar deviation.

Stabilization. Forearm is stabilized.

Substitutions

• Subject may hyperextend the wrist, then relax, giving the appearance of flexion.
• Keep fingers relaxed to prevent substitution by finger flexors.
• Palpate to determine the functions of each muscle.

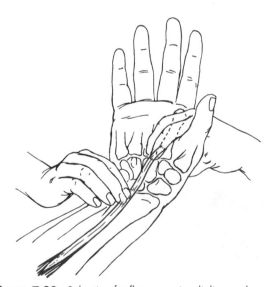

▲ **Figure 7.32** Palpation for flexor carpi radialis muscle.

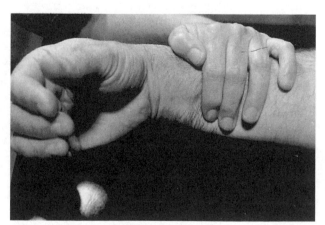

▲ **Figure 7.34** Testing the flexor carpi radialis muscle in the GM position.

▼ Attachments of Flexor Carpi Radialis Muscle

Muscle	Proximal	Distal	Innervation
Flexor carpi radialis	Common flexor tendon from medial epicondyle of humerus	Base of second and third metacarpal palmar surface	Median C7 (C6)

FLEXOR CARPI ULNARIS MUSCLE

The flexor carpi ulnaris muscle produces the motions of wrist flexion and adduction, or ulnar deviation. The test motion is wrist flexion to 90 degrees with accompanying ulnar deviation from the anatomical starting position.

Palpation. Flexor carpi ulnaris tendon is superficial and palpable immediately proximal to the pisiform (Fig. 7-35).

Position

AG: Subject sits or lies supine with the forearm supinated and the dorsal surface of the hand resting on a table, with the fingers in slight flexion.
GM: Subject is positioned as above but with the ulnar border of the hand not resting on the table. The fingers are relaxed in slight flexion (see Figs. 7-33 and 7-34).

Movement. Flexion of the wrist joint through the test range accompanied by ulnar deviation.

Resistance. Applied to the palm of the hand into extension and radial deviation.

Stabilization. The forearm is stabilized.

Substitutions

- Subject may hyperextend the wrist then relax, giving the appearance of flexion. Keep the fingers relaxed to prevent substitution by the finger flexors.
- Palpate to determine the function of ulnar deviation.

PALMARIS LONGUS MUSCLE

The palmaris longus muscle may or may not be present. It is absent in 15% to 20% of the population. When present, it is located in the midline of the wrist and performs wrist flexion without deviations into abduction or adduction. It does not have a bony attachment distally but rather pulls on the palmar fascia during wrist flexion.

Palpation. If present, the tendon is superficial at the level of the carpal creases in the midline of the wrist. The tendon is more prominent if the hand is cupped during the motion of wrist flexion (Fig. 7-36).

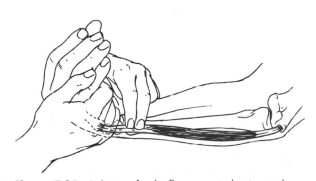

▲ **Figure 7.35** Palpation for the flexor carpi ulnaris muscle.

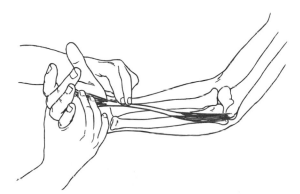

▲ **Figure 7.36** Palpation for the palmaris longus muscle.

▼ Attachments of Flexor Carpi Ulnaris Muscle

Muscle	Proximal	Distal	Innervation
Flexor carpi ulnaris	Common flexor tendon from humeral medial epicondyle, medial aspect of olecranon, and proximal border of ulna	Pisiform bone, hamate, and base of fifth metacarpal	Ulnar C8 (C7)

▼ Attachments of Palmaris Longus Muscle

Muscle	Proximal	Distal	Innervation
Palmaris longus	Common flexor tendon from medial epicondyle	Palmar fascia	Median C8 (C7)

Position

AG: Subject sits with the dorsal surface of the hand resting on the table and the fingers relaxed.

GM: Subject sits with the hand resting on the ulnar border and the fingers relaxed (see Figs. 7-33 and 7-34).

Movement. Flexion of the wrist.

Resistance. Applied to the palm of the hand into extension.

Stabilization. The forearm is stabilized.

Substitutions

- The superficial finger flexors may be palpated instead of the palmaris longus.
- Hyperextension of the wrist may give the appearance of wrist joint flexion.
- Prevent substitution by finger flexors by keeping them relaxed.

EXTENSOR CARPI RADIALIS LONGUS MUSCLE

The extensor carpi radialis longus muscle produces the movement of wrist hyperextension and radial deviation from a starting position of flexion. For all grades of testing, the subject is either sitting or supine. The fingers must be relaxed.

Palpation. With the forearm pronated, the examiner palpates on the radiodorsal aspect of the wrist proximal to the second metacarpal (Fig. 7-37).

Position

AG: The hand rests on the palmar surface on the table with the fingers relaxed in flexion (Fig. 7-38).

GM: The hand rests on the ulnar border and the table with the fingers relaxed (Fig. 7-39).

Movement. Extend the wrist, with radial deviation.

Resistance. Applied to the dorsum of the hand into flexion and ulnar deviation.

Stabilization. Forearm is stabilized.

Substitutions

- The subject may flex the wrist, then relax.
- Keep the fingers relaxed in flexion to prevent substitution by extensor digitorum.

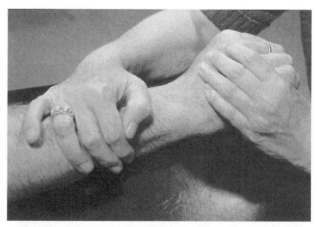

▲ **Figure 7.38** Testing the extensor carpi radialis longus muscle in the AG position.

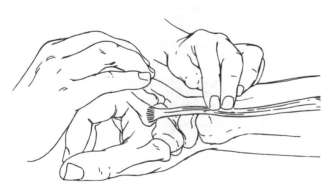

▲ **Figure 7.37** Palpation for the extensor carpi radialis longus muscle.

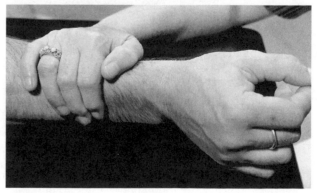

▲ **Figure 7.39** Testing the extensor carpi radialis longus muscle in the GM position.

▼ Attachments of Extensor Carpi Radialis Longus Muscle			
Muscle	**Proximal**	**Distal**	**Innervation**
Extensor carpi radialis longus	Distal third of lateral supracondylar ridge of humerus	Base of second metacarpal, dorsal surface	Radial C6 and C7

EXTENSOR CARPI RADIALIS BREVIS MUSCLE

The extensor carpi radialis brevis tendon is located over the axis for the wrist joint; it participates in the extension of the wrist joint with no deviation.

Palpation. The extensor carpi radialis brevis is somewhat difficult to palpate. With the subject's forearm pronated and the hand off the table, the examiner places a finger in the depression over the capitate bone. The subject is asked to abduct the thumb in the sagittal plane. The extensor carpi radialis brevis contracts as a synergist to stabilize the wrist (Fig. 7-40).

Position

AG: Subject sits with the palmar surface of the hand resting on a table, keeping the fingers relaxed in flexion.
GM: Subject's hand rests on the ulnar border, with the fingers relaxed in flexion (see Figs. 7-38 and 7-39).

Movement. Extend the wrist.

Resistance. Applied to the dorsum of the hand into flexion.

Stabilization. The forearm is stabilized.

Substitutions

- Subject may flex the wrist, then relax.
- Keep the fingers relaxed in flexion.

EXTENSOR CARPI ULNARIS MUSCLE

The extensor carpi ulnaris muscle produces the movements of wrist hyperextension and ulnar deviation. The muscle is tested as a wrist extensor muscle working in synergy with the extensor carpi radialis longus and brevis muscles.

Palpation. The extensor carpi ulnaris is palpated between the head of the ulna and the tubercle of the fifth metacarpal (Fig. 7-41).

Position

AG: Subject sits with the hand on its palmar surface and the fingers relaxed.
GM: Subject sits with the hand resting on its ulnar border, with the fingers relaxed (see Figs. 7-38 and 7-39).

Movement. Extend and deviate the wrist toward the ulna.

Resistance. Applied to the dorsum of the hand into flexion and radial deviation.

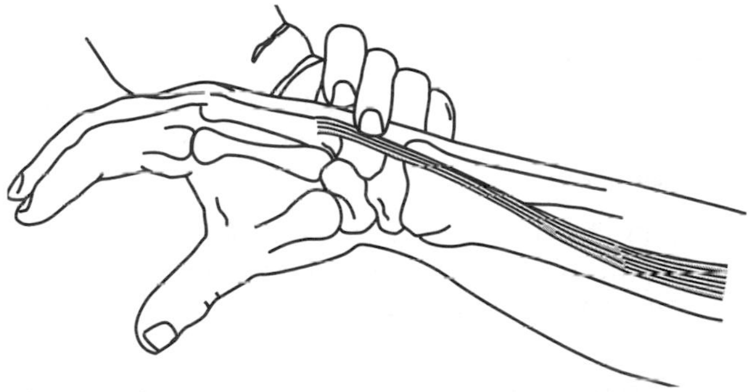

▲ **Figure 7.40** Palpation for the extensor carpi radialis brevis muscle.

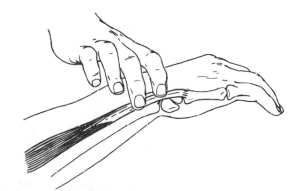

▲ **Figure 7.41** Palpation for the extensor carpi ulnaris muscle.

▼ Attachments of Extensor Carpi Radialis Brevis Muscle			
Muscle	**Proximal**	**Distal**	**Innervation**
Extensor carpi radialis brevis	Common extensor tendon from lateral epicondyle and radial collateral ligament	Base of third metacarpal	Radial C7 and C8

▼ Attachments of Extensor Carpi Ulnaris Muscle

Muscle	Proximal	Distal	Innervation
Extensor carpi ulnaris	Common extensor tendon from lateral epicondyle of humerus and posterior aspect of ulna	Base of fifth metacarpal, medial side	Radial C8 (C7)

Stabilization. The forearm is stabilized.

Substitutions

- Subject may flex the wrist, then relax.
- Keep the fingers relaxed.

Fingers

Each finger is tested separately. Gravity has little effect on the fingers or thumb; therefore, the test position may be any comfortable position, usually sitting or supine. The grading key differs for the fingers and thumb (see Chap. 2). No half grades are given.

FLEXOR DIGITORUM SUPERFICIALIS MUSCLE

The flexor digitorum superficialis muscle is a flexor of the PIP joints of the second through the fifth digits. The muscle assists in wrist and MCP joint flexion. The movement is 120 degrees of flexion of the PIP joints with the MCP joints in extension. All grades are determined with the forearm in supination; each finger is evaluated independently.

Palpation. The flexor digitorum superficialis muscle or tendon is palpated where it crosses the palmar surface of each proximal phalanx (Fig. 7-42).

Position. The hand rests on a table on its dorsal surface. Both the wrist and metacarpal joints are in a neutral position (Fig. 7-43).

Movement. Flexion of the PIP joint without flexion of the DIP joint. To test the flexor digitorum superficialis, the distal joint must remain inactive.

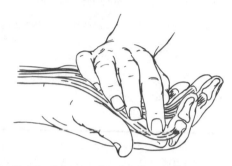

▲ **Figure 7.42** Palpation for the flexor digitorum superficialis muscle.

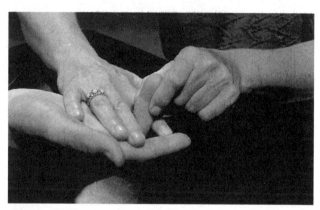

▲ **Figure 7.43** Testing position for the flexor digitorum superficialis muscle.

Resistance. Applied to the palmar surface of the middle phalanx.

Stabilization. Proximal phalanx and palm of the hand are stabilized; tips of the fingers are relaxed.

Substitutions

- Subject may quickly extend the PIP joint.
- The flexor digitorum profundus can cause substitute motion, flexing the DIP joints.

▼ Attachments of Flexor Digitorum Superficialis Muscle

Muscle	Proximal	Distal	Innervation
Flexor digitorum superficialis	Common flexor tendon from medial epicondyle of humerus, ulnar collateral ligament, coronoid process of ulna, and oblique line on radius	Four tendon slips to each side of middle phalanx of medial four fingers	Median C8 (C7 and T1)

FLEXOR DIGITORUM PROFUNDUS MUSCLE

The movement produced by the flexor digitorum profundus muscle is flexion of the DIP joints of the second through the fifth digits, with the other finger joints remaining in extension. The muscle may assist in PIP joint and MCP joint flexion. The flexor digitorum profundus muscle is the only muscle that flexes the DIP joint. All grades are determined with the forearm in supination; each finger is evaluated independently.

Palpation. Palpate each tendon where it crosses the palmar surface of each middle phalanx of the medial four digits (Fig. 7-44).

Position. The hand rests on its dorsal surface on a table. Both the wrist and metacarpal joints are in a neutral position (Fig. 7-45).

Movement. Flexion of the DIP joints; fingers not being tested are allowed to flex.

Resistance. Applied to the palmar surface of the distal phalanx.

Stabilization. The middle phalanx and PIP joint are stabilized.

Substitution

• Subject may quickly extend the DIP joint, then relax.

EXTENSOR DIGITORUM, EXTENSOR INDICIS, EXTENSOR DIGITI MINIMI MUSCLES

The test movement for the extensor digitorum, extensor indicis, and extensor digiti minimi is extension at the MCP joints from a starting position of flexion. Motion occurs at each of the medial MCP joints simultaneously. The upper limb rests on the table with the forearm pronated. All grades are tested in the sitting position.

Palpation

Extensor Digitorum. Palpate each tendon where it crosses the dorsal aspect of the palm (Fig. 7-46).

Extensor Indicis. Palpate over the dorsal aspect of the second metacarpal, close to the head. It is the tendon closer to the ulna (Fig. 7-47).

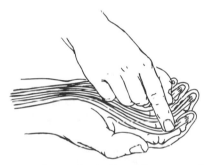

▲ **Figure 7.44** Palpation for the flexor digitorum profundus muscle.

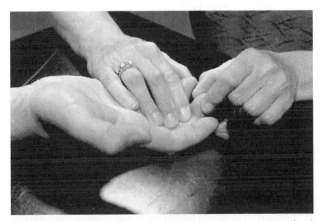

▲ **Figure 7.45** Testing position for the flexor digitorum profundus muscle.

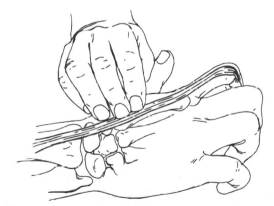

▲ **Figure 7.46** Palpation for the extensor digitorum muscle.

▼ Attachments of Flexor Digitorum Profundus Muscle			
Muscle	**Proximal**	**Distal**	**Innervation**
Flexor digitorum profundus	Anterior and medial surfaces of proximal three quarters of ulna	Four tendon slips to base of each distal phalanx of the medial four fingers	Radial two—median; ulnar two—ulnar C8 (T1)

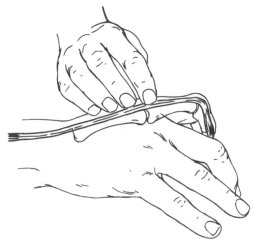

▲ **Figure 7.47** Palpation for the extensor indicis muscle.

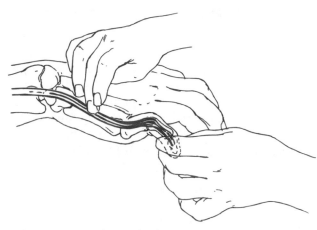

▲ **Figure 7.48** Palpation for the extensor digiti minimi muscle.

Extensor Digiti Minimi. Palpate over the dorsal aspect of the fifth metacarpal, close to the head of the ulna (Fig. 7-48).

Position. The hand rests on its palmar surface on a table with the wrist in a neutral position. The MCP joints are flexed 90 degrees off the edge of the table (Fig. 7-49).

Movement. Extension of the metacarpal joints, with IP joints flexed.

Resistance. Applied to the distal end of the proximal phalanx on the dorsal aspect.

Stabilization. Stabilize the hand and wrist.

Substitutions

- Subject may quickly flex the MCP joints, then relax.
- Wrist flexion puts tension on the extensor tendons.
- Lumbrical muscles can cause extension of the IP joints.

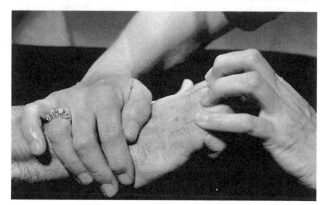

▲ **Figure 7.49** Testing position for the extensor digitorum, extensor indicis, and extensor digiti minimi muscles.

LUMBRICAL MUSCLES

The lumbrical muscles perform the motion of IP joint extension with the MCP joints held in extension. The forearm is pronated and the wrist extended. Other authors state that the lumbrical muscles produce MCP joint flexion simultaneously with IP joint extension.

Palpation. Because of their size and position, the lumbrical muscles usually cannot be palpated. Therefore, a "1" or "T" grade cannot be given.

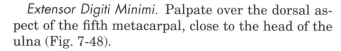

▼ **Attachments of Extensor Digitorum, Extensor Indicis, and Extensor Digiti Minimi Muscles**			
Muscle	**Proximal**	**Distal**	**Innervation**
Extensor digitorum	Common extensor tendon on lateral epicondyle of humerus	Four tendons, from second to fifth digit through extensor hood to base of distal phalanx	Radial C7 (C8)
Extensor indicis	Distal posterior surface of ulna	Into extensor hood of index finger with extensor digitorum	Radial C8 (C7)
Extensor digiti minimi	Common extensor tendon of lateral epicondyle of humerus	Into extensor hood of fifth finger with extensor digitorum	Radial C7 (C8)

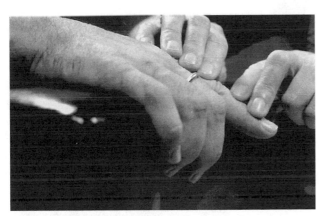

▲ **Figure 7.50** Testing position for the lumbrical muscles.

Position

- Preferred: The hand rests on its palmar surface with the middle and distal phalanges flexed over the edge of the table. The MCP joints are supported in extension by the table (Fig. 7-50).
- Alternate: Hand rests on palmar surface with the proximal, middle, and distal phalanges extended off the table.

Movement

- Preferred: Extension of the proximal and DIP joints.
- Alternate: Flexion of the MCP joint with the proximal and DIP joints maintained in extension.

Resistance

- Preferred: Applied to the dorsal surface of the middle and distal phalanges. The medial four fingers may be resisted simultaneously or separately.
- Alternate: Apply resistance to the palmar surface of the proximal phalanx.

Stabilization. Stabilize under the proximal phalanx of the fingers being tested. With the other hand, stabilize the wrist and MCP joint in the neutral position.

Substitions

- Extensor digitorum can cause hyperextension of the MCP joints.
- Flexion of the IP joints followed by relaxation can substitute.
- Maintain the MCP joints in extension.

DORSAL INTEROSSEI, ABDUCTOR DIGITI MINIMI MUSCLES

The dorsal interossei and the abductor digiti minimi muscles produce the test motion of abduction, with the fingers in extension. The forearm is pronated and the wrist extended.

Palpation

Dorsal Interossei. Palpate the first dorsal interossei on the radial side of the second metacarpal; palpate the tendon of the second on the radial side of the proximal phalanx of the middle finger; palpate the tendon of the third on the ulnar side of the proximal phalanx of the middle finger; and palpate the tendon of the fourth on the ulnar side of the proximal phalanx of the ring finger (Fig. 7-51).

Abductor Digiti Minimi. Palpate along the ulnar border of the fifth metacarpal (Fig. 7-52).

Position. The hand rests on its palmar surface on a table, with the wrist in a neutral position and the fingers extended (Figs. 7-53 and 7-54).

Movement. Move the index, ring, and little fingers away from the middle finger; the middle finger moves toward the index and ring fingers.

Resistance. Applied to the side of the distal end of the proximal phalanx of each of the four fingers.

Stabilization. Hand and fingers not being tested are stabilized.

▼ Attachments of Lumbrical Muscles			
Muscle	**Proximal**	**Distal**	**Innervation**
First and second lumbrical muscles	Radial side of flexor digitorum profundus tendon to index and middle fingers	Radial side of extensor expansion of the medial four fingers	Median T1 (C8)
Third and fourth lumbrical muscles	Adjacent sides of flexor digitorum tendon to ring and little fingers	Radial side of extensor expansion of the medial four fingers	Ulnar T1 (C8)

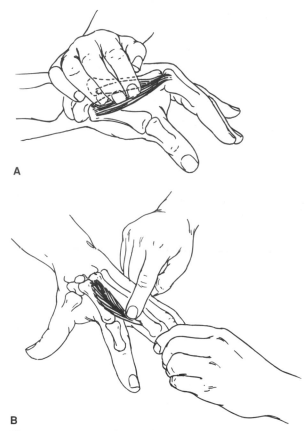

A

B

▲ **Figure 7.51** **(A)** Palpation for the first dorsal interosseous muscle. **(B)** Palpation for the second dorsal interosseous muscle.

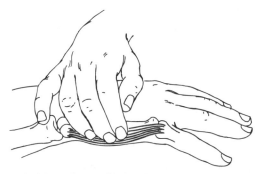

▲ **Figure 7.52** Palpation for the abductor digiti minimi muscle.

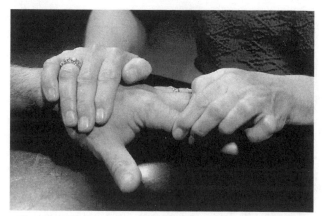

▲ **Figure 7.53** Testing position for the first dorsal interosseous muscle.

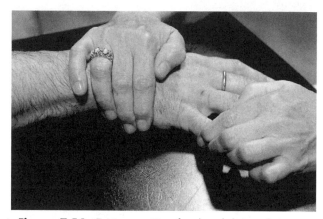

▲ **Figure 7.54** Testing position for the abductor digiti minimi muscle.

Substitutions

- When the MCP joints hyperextend, they also abduct.
- Wrist flexors put extensor tendons on a stretch, which produces abduction by tendon action. Do not allow subject to push down onto the table.
- Lumbrical muscles may assist in abduction.

▼ Attachments of Dorsal Interossei and Abductor Digiti Minimi Muscles			
Muscle	**Proximal**	**Distal**	**Innervation**
Dorsal interossei:	Between each metacarpal on adjacent sides		Ulnar T1 (C8)
First and second		Radial side of extensor expansion of index and middle fingers	
Third and fourth		Ulnar side of extensor expansion of middle and ring fingers	
Abductor digiti minimi	Pisiform bone and tendon of flexor carpi ulnaris muscle	Base of proximal phalanx of fifth finger and ulnar aspect of extensor expansion	Ulnar T1 (C8)

PALMAR INTEROSSEI MUSCLES

The palmar interossei muscles produce the motion of adduction of the fingers from a starting position of abduction. The forearm is pronated, and the wrist and fingers are extended.

Palpation. The three tendons cross the MCP joints (Fig. 7-55). Palpate the first interosseous on the ulnar side of the proximal phalanx of the index finger. Palpate the second interosseous on the radial side of the proximal phalanx of the ring finger. Palpate the third interosseous on the radial side of the proximal phalanx of the little finger.

Position. The hand rests on its palmar surface, with the wrist and fingers in an extended position (Fig. 7-56).

Movement. Move index, ring, and little fingers toward the middle finger from the starting position of abduction.

Resistance. Applied to the side of the distal end of the proximal phalanx.

Stabilization. The hand and fingers that are not being tested are stabilized.

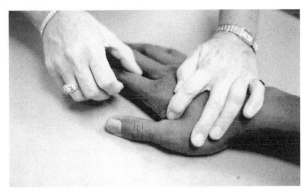

▲ **Figure 7.56** Testing position for the first palmar interosseous muscle.

Substitutions

- Finger flexors will cause the MCP joints to flex. Do not let the fingers press down onto table.
- If the wrist is allowed to extend, the MCP joints will passively flex and adduct.
- Extensor digitorum and extensor indicis may cause adduction of the index finger.
- The lumbrical muscles may assist in adduction.

FLEXOR POLLICIS LONGUS, FLEXOR POLLICIS BREVIS MUSCLES

The flexor pollicis longus and the flexor pollicis brevis muscles produce the flexion motion at the MCP and IP joints. During the test, the forearm is placed in supination and is supported by the table.

Palpation. Palpate the tendon of the flexor pollicis longus where it crosses the palmar surface of the proximal phalanx of the thumb (Fig. 7-57).

Palpate the muscle belly of the flexor pollicis brevis on the ulnar side of the first metacarpal (Fig. 7-58).

Position. The hand is resting on its dorsal surface on a table; the wrist is in a neutral position, and the thumb is adducted (Figs. 7-59 and 7-60).

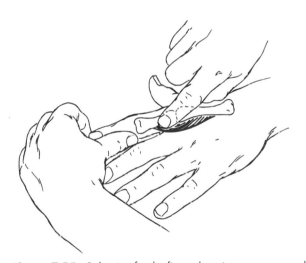

▲ **Figure 7.55** Palpation for the first palmar interosseous muscle.

▼ Attachments of Palmar Interossei Muscles			
Muscle	**Proximal**	**Distal**	**Innervation**
Palmar interossei: First	Length of ulnar side of second metacarpal	Ulnar side of extensor expansion and proximal phalanx of index finger	Ulnar T1 (C8)
Second	Length of radial side of fourth metacarpal	Radial side of extensor expansion and proximal phalanx of ring finger	
Third	Length of radial side of fifth metacarpal	Radial side of extensor expansion and proximal phalanx of little finger	

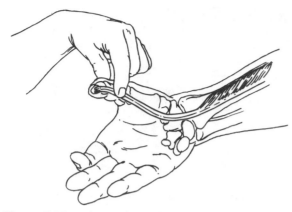

▲ **Figure 7.57** Palpation for the flexor pollicis longus muscle.

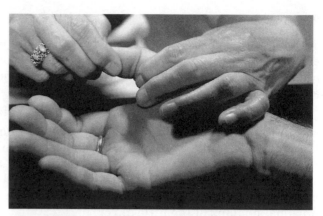

▲ **Figure 7.59** Testing position for the flexor pollicis longus muscle.

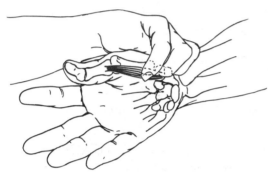

▲ **Figure 7.58** Palpation for the flexor pollicis brevis muscle.

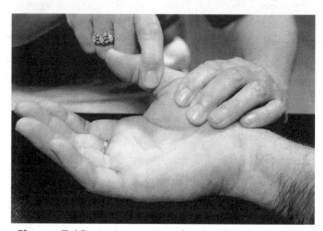

▲ **Figure 7.60** Testing position for the flexor pollicis brevis muscle.

Movement. Flexion of the MCP and IP joints in the coronal plane.

Resistance. Applied to the proximal phalanx for the flexor pollicis brevis and the distal phalanx for the flexor pollicis longus.

Stabilization. The first metacarpal is stabilized for the flexor pollicis brevis and the proximal phalanx for the flexor pollicis longus.

Substitutions

- The flexor pollicis longus instead of the brevis flexes the IP joint.

- The abductor pollicis brevis and adductor pollicis together may flex the MCP joint.
- Quick extension and relaxation of the IP joint may give the appearance of IP flexion.

EXTENSOR POLLICIS LONGUS, EXTENSOR POLLICIS BREVIS MUSCLES

The extensor pollicis longus and brevis muscles produce the motion of extension at the MCP and IP joints from a starting position of complete flexion.

Palpation. Palpate the tendon of the extensor pollicis longus where it crosses the dorsal aspect at the base of the first MCP joint directed toward the distal phalanx (Fig. 7-61).

▼ **Attachments of Flexor Pollicis Longus and Flexor Pollicis Brevis Muscles**			
Muscle	**Proximal**	**Distal**	**Innervation**
Flexor pollicis longus	Anterior shaft of radius, interosseous membrane, and coronoid process of ulna	Base of distal phalanx of thumb, palmar surface	Median C8 (T1)
Flexor pollicis brevis	Trapezium bone, trapezoid, capitate, and flexor retinaculum	Base of proximal phalanx of thumb on radial side	Median and ulnar C8 (T1)

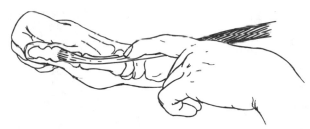

▲ **Figure 7.61** Palpation for the extensor pollicis longus muscle.

Palpate the tendon of the extensor pollicis brevis where it crosses the lateral aspect of the base of the first MCP joint directed toward the proximal phalanx (Fig. 7-62).

Position. The hand rests with the ulnar border on the table. With the extensor pollicis brevis, the MCP joint is flexed and abducted. With the extensor pollicis longus, the MCP joint is abducted and the IP joint flexed (Figs. 7-63 and 7-64).

Movement. Extension of the MCP and IP joints individually.

Resistance. Applied to the dorsal surface of the proximal phalanx for the extensor pollicis brevis and to the dorsal surface of the distal phalanx for the extensor pollicis longus.

Stabilization. The first metacarpal is stabilized for the brevis muscle and the proximal phalanx and metacarpal for the longus muscle.

Substitutions

• The extensor pollicis longus may extend the MCP joint.

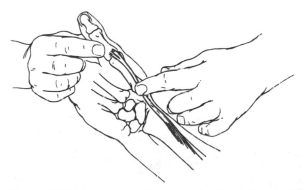

▲ **Figure 7.62** Palpation for the extensor pollicis brevis muscle.

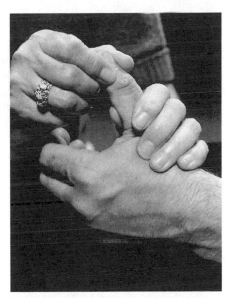

▲ **Figure 7.63** Testing position for the extensor pollicis longus muscle.

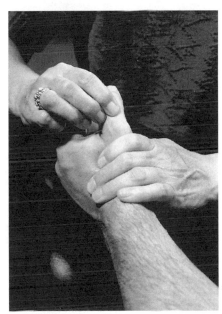

▲ **Figure 7.64** Testing position for the extensor pollicis brevis muscle.

• Quick flexion and relaxation of the MCP joint may substitute.
• Quick flexion and relaxation of the IP joint may substitute.

▼ Attachments of Extensor Pollicis Longus and Extensor Pollicis Brevis Muscles			
Muscle	**Proximal**	**Distal**	**Innervation**
Extensor pollicis longus	Middle third posterior aspect of ulna	Base of distal phalanx of thumb posteriorly	Radial C8 (C7)
Extensor pollicis brevis	Posterior surface distally on radius	Base of proximal phalanx of thumb posteriorly	Radial C8 (C7)

ABDUCTOR POLLICIS LONGUS, ABDUCTOR POLLICIS BREVIS MUSCLES

The abductor pollicis longus and brevis muscles produce the movement of abduction at the CMC joint. The test movements occur in the sagittal plane through a range of 75 degrees for the abductor pollicis brevis muscle and in the frontal plane for the abductor pollicis longus muscle. The MCP and IP joints should remain flexed when one examines the abductor pollicis longus muscle to lessen the effect of the thumb extensors. The forearm is positioned midway between supination and pronation or is completely supinated.

Palpation

Abductor Pollicis Longus. Palpate its tendon immediately proximal to the first CMC joint. It is the most anterior of the three tendons at the base of the CMC joint (Fig. 7-65).

Abductor Pollicis Brevis. Palpate along the anterior surface of the shaft of the first metacarpal (Fig. 7-66).

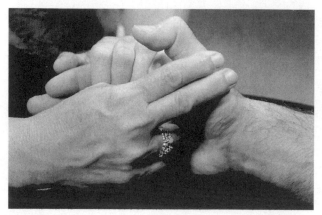

▲ **Figure 7.67** Testing position for the abductor pollicis longus muscle.

Position. The hand rests on the ulnar border, or the forearm is in supination with the wrist in a neutral position and the thumb adducted (Figs. 7-67 and 7-68).

Movement

Abductor Pollicis Longus. The thumb abducts in the plane of the palm in the frontal plane.

Abductor Pollicis Brevis. The thumb abducts at a right angle from the palm in the sagittal plane.

Resistance. Applied into adduction to the distal end of the first metacarpal to test the abductor pollicis longus and on the proximal phalanx for the abductor pollicis brevis.

Stabilization. The palm of the hand is stabilized.

Substitutions

- Lift the metacarpal toward the midline of the hand for the abductor pollicis brevis only to prevent substitution.

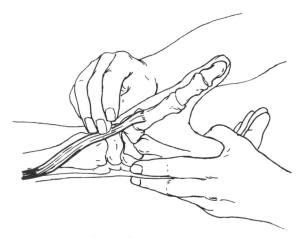

▲ **Figure 7.65** Palpation for the abductor pollicis longus muscle.

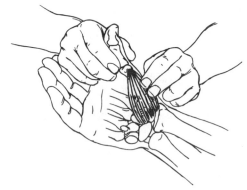

▲ **Figure 7.66** Palpation for the abductor pollicis brevis muscle.

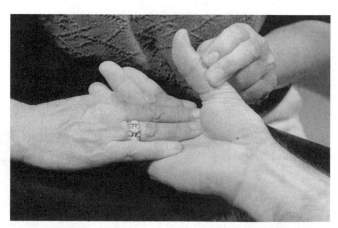

▲ **Figure 7.68** Testing position for the abductor pollicis brevis muscle.

▼ Attachments of Abductor Pollicis Longus and Abductor Pollicis Brevis Muscles

Muscle	Proximal	Distal	Innervation
Abductor pollicis longus	Posterior aspect of shaft of distal ulna and midradius	Base of first metacarpal, radial side	Radial C8 (C7)
Abductor pollicis brevis	Anterior aspect of scaphoid, trapezium bones, and flexor retinaculum	Base of proximal phalanx, radial side	Median C8 (T1)

- The extensor pollicis longus and brevis may extend and contribute to abduction of the first metacarpal.
- The abductor pollicis longus abducts the thumb to the radial side of the hand.
- The opponens pollicis tends to rotate thumb.
- The flexor pollicis brevis and longus are accessory muscles to the motion of abduction.

ADDUCTOR POLLICIS MUSCLE

The adductor pollicis muscle produces the motion of adduction of the thumb from a starting position of radial abduction in the sagittal plane through a range of 75 degrees. The forearm may be supinated, the hand resting on its ulnar border or pronated. The thumb remains in the plane of the palm.

Palpation. Palpate in the first web space; push the finger and thumb deep to the first dorsal interossei (Fig. 7-69).

Position. The hand rests on a table with the thumb abducted from the palm in the sagittal plane (Fig. 7-70).

Movement. Adduction of the first CMC joint.

Resistance. Apply resistance to the proximal phalanx into radial abduction.

Stabilization. Stabilize the palm of the hand.

Substitutions

- The flexor pollicis brevis muscle flexes the MCP joint.
- The flexor pollicis longus muscle flexes the IP joint.

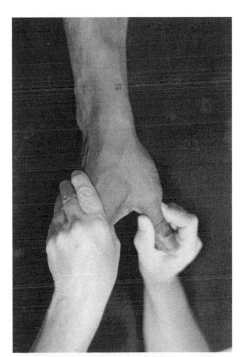

▲ **Figure 7.70** Testing position for the adductor pollicis muscle.

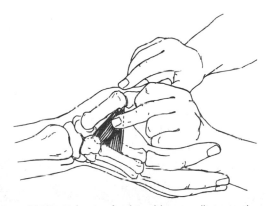

▲ **Figure 7.69** Palpation for the adductor pollicis muscle.

▼ Attachments of Adductor Pollicis Muscle

Muscle	Proximal	Distal	Innervation
Adductor pollicis	Capitate and base of second and third metacarpal bones; also palmar surface of shaft of third metacarpal	Base of proximal phalanx of thumb	Ulnar T1 (C8)

OPPONENS POLLICIS MUSCLE

The opponens pollicis muscle produces the motion of opposition of the thumb at the first CMC joint. The movement is complex, initiated by palmar abduction at the first CMC joint followed by ulnar adduction, which continues to the final position with slight flexion and rotation of the CMC joint.

Palpation. Palpate along the lateral shaft of the first metacarpal. Push the abductor pollicis brevis toward the ulna and palpate deep to it (Fig. 7-71).

Position. The hand rests on its dorsal surface with the forearm supinated (Fig. 7-72).

Movement. Roll the head of the first metacarpal toward the ulnar side of the hand while keeping the tip of the thumb against the pad of the tip or base of the fifth finger.

Resistance. Applied to distal end of first and fifth metacarpals into derotation.

Stabilization. First and fifth metacarpals and palm of hand are stabilized.

Substitutions

- The abductor pollicis brevis can abduct the thumb without rotation.
- Motion should only occur at the CMC joints.

OPPONENS DIGITI MINIMI MUSCLE

The opponens digiti minimi muscle produces its action at the fifth CMC joint. The movement is rotation followed by flexion. It helps to cup the palm.

Palpation. Palpate along the shaft of the fifth metacarpal deep to the abductor digiti minimi (Fig. 7-73).

Position. The hand rests on the dorsal surface with the forearm supinated (Fig. 7-74).

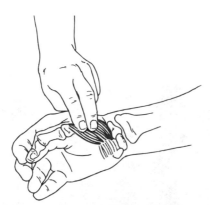

▲ **Figure 7.71** Palpation for the opponens pollicis muscle.

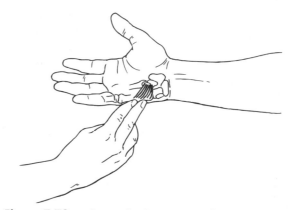

▲ **Figure 7.73** Palpation for the opponens digiti minimi muscle.

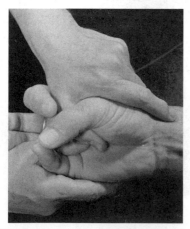

▲ **Figure 7.72** Testing for the opponens pollicis muscle.

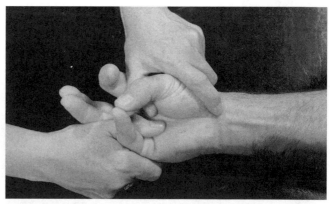

▲ **Figure 7.74** Testing position for the opponens digiti minimi muscle.

▼ **Attachments of Opponens Pollicis Muscle**			
Muscle	**Proximal**	**Distal**	**Innervation**
Opponens pollicis	Trapezium and flexor retinaculum	Entire lateral shaft of first metacarpal	Median C8 (T1)

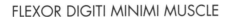

▼ Attachments of Opponens Digiti Minimi Muscle			
Muscle	**Proximal**	**Distal**	**Innervation**
Opponens digiti minimi	Hook of hamate and flexor retinaculum	Entire shaft of fifth metacarpal	Ulnar T1 (C8)

Movement. Roll the fifth metacarpal toward the radial side of the hand, attempting to touch the pad of the thumb.

Resistance. Applied to the distal end of the fifth metacarpal into derotation.

Stabilization. Stabilize the palm of the hand.

Substitutions

- For the little finger flexors, motion should occur only at the CMC joint.
- The abductor digiti minimi can abduct the little finger without rotation.

FLEXOR DIGITI MINIMI MUSCLE

The flexor digiti minimi muscle performs the motion of MCP joint flexion for the fifth digit and assists in opposition.

Palpation. Palpate laterally along the shaft of the fifth metacarpal (Fig. 7-75).

Position. The hand rests on its dorsal surface, with the forearm supinated (Fig. 7-76).

Movement. Flexion of the fifth MCP joint with the IP joints remaining extended.

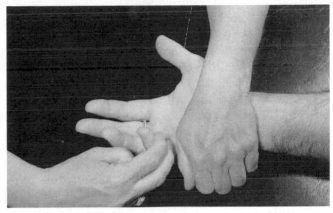

▲ **Figure 7.76** Testing position for the flexor digiti minimi muscle.

Resistance. Applied to the palmar surface of the proximal phalanx.

Stabilization. The fifth metacarpal and the palm are stabilized.

Substitutions

- The opponens digiti minimi may rotate the fifth metacarpal.
- The flexor digitorum superficialis and profundus to the fifth finger can cause flexion of the IP joints.

CLINICAL ASSESSMENT

Observation and Screening

The wrist and hand should be observed for integrity of the skin, both volarly and dorsally. The skin on the volar surface should be moist and thick with little mobility over the deeper structures of the hand and the palmar creases clearly delineated. The presence of Dupuytren's contracture, a contracture of the palmar fascia, often creates dense fibrous bands across the palm of the hand. These fibrous bands often re-

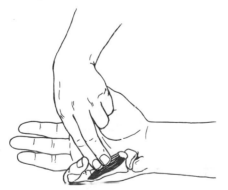

▲ **Figure 7.75** Palpation for the flexor digiti minimi muscle.

▼ Attachments of Flexor Digiti Minimi Muscle			
Muscle	**Proximal**	**Distal**	**Innervation**
Flexor digiti minimi	Hook of hamate, flexor retinaculum	Proximal phalanx of fifth digit	Ulnar T1 (C8)

sult in a loss of extension mobility of the fourth and fifth fingers, with observable flexion deformities of the MCP and PIP joints.[14] Dorsally, the skin should be thin and very mobile with no abnormalities of the nail beds of the digits. Any changes in skin texture or sweating patterns may indicate vasomotor abnormalities, such as Raynaud's disease, diabetes, peripheral vascular disease, or neurovascular problems.

Nail beds may be checked for capillary refill by applying direct pressure to the nail, resulting in a blanched appearance, which is followed by a return of color once the pressure is removed. Additionally, nails should be examined for ridging, discoloration, or other abnormalities. Clubbing of nails is commonly associated with respiratory or cardiac problems.

The presence of Heberden's nodes on the dorsal aspect of the DIP joint is commonly associated with osteoarthritis whereas Bouchard's nodes located on the PIP dorsal surface can be associated with rheumatoid arthritis or gastrectasis. Deformities of the joints of the hands may indicate rheumatoid arthritis, past trauma, or neurological involvement. A swan neck deformity, seen in patients with rheumatoid arthritis, is identified by flexion of the MCP and DIP joints with hyperextension of the PIP joint. Other rheumatoid arthritis deformities of the hand include ulnar drift at the MCP joints and boutonniere deformities. A boutonniere deformity is characterized by extension of the MCP joint, PIP joint flexion, and hyperextension of the DIP joint.

The hand should be observed for evidence of muscular atrophy involving the thenar and hypothenar muscle groups, indicating median and ulnar nerve involvement, respectively. Further, wasting of the first dorsal interosseous muscle may be associated with involvement of the C7 nerve or nerve root. Specific hand deformities observed with peripheral nerve injuries include the following:

1. Claw hand, associated with a loss of intrinsics and characterized by MCP hyperextension and PIP and DIP joint flexion. This deformity is also referred to as an intrinsic minus hand.
2. Ape hand, resulting from median nerve palsy in which the thumb falls back in line with the plane of the fingers. The subject is unable to oppose or flex the thumb and demonstrates atrophy of the thenar eminence.
3. Benediction hand, associated with ulnar nerve palsy, in which the medial two fingers assume a flexed position due to involvement of the interossei and medial two lumbrical muscles. Muscular wasting is also evident over the hypothenal muscle group.
4. Wrist drop, resulting from a radial nerve palsy. The subject is unable to extend the

wrist and fingers because of involvement of the extensor muscles.

Palpation and Surface Anatomy

The skeletal anatomy of the wrist and hand is presented in Fig. 7-77. The structures and landmarks of the wrist and hand that should be palpated or observed as part of the examination process include the following (Fig. 7-78):

1. Individual carpal bones
2. Radial styloid process
3. Anatomical snuff-box boundaries and radial artery within
4. Ulnar styloid process
5. Ulnar artery at wrist, lateral to the tendon of the flexor carpi ulnaris muscle
6. Radial artery at wrist, between the tendons of the flexor carpi radialis longus and abductor pollicis longus muscles
7. Flexor tendons where they cross the wrist
8. Hook of the hamate where the flexor carpi ulnaris muscle inserts
9. Carpal tunnel and components
10. Thenar eminence
11. Hypothenar eminence
12. MCP and IP joints

Active and Passive Movements

The following motions should be assessed during active and passive testing of the wrist and hand:

1. Wrist flexion
2. Wrist extension
3. Wrist radial deviation
4. Wrist ulnar deviation
5. MCP flexion of digits one to five
6. MCP extension of digits one to five
7. IP flexion of digits one to five
8. IP extension of digits one to five
9. Abduction of the thumb
10. Adduction of the thumb
11. Opposition of the thumb and little finger

Contractile Testing

Contractile testing of the wrist and hand should include the following:

1. Wrist flexion
2. Wrist extension
3. Wrist radial deviation
4. Wrist ulnar deviation

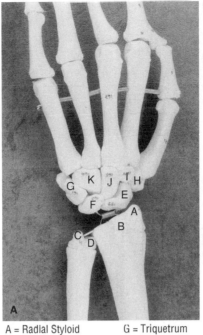

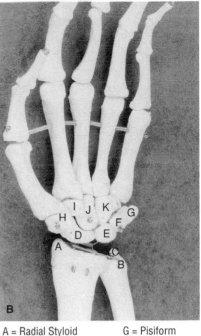

A = Radial Styloid	G = Triquetrum
B = Lister's Tubercle	H = Trapezium
C = Ulnar Styloid	I = Trapezoid
D = Ulnar Head	J = Capitate
E = Scaphoid	K = Hamate
F = Lunate	

A = Radial Styloid	G = Pisiform
B = Ulnar Head	H = Trapezium
C = Ulnar Styloid	I = Trapezoid
D = Scaphoid	J = Capitate
E = Lunate	K = Hamate
F = Triquetrum	

▲ **Figure 7.77** Skeletal anatomy of the wrist and hand. **(A)** Dorsal view. **(B)** Volar view.

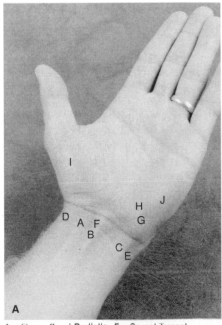

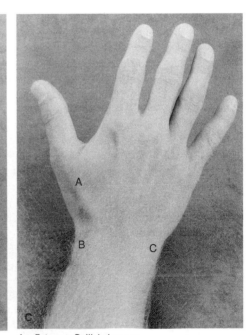

A = Flexor Carpi Radialis	F = Carpal Tunnel
B = Palmaris Longus	G = Pisiform
C = Flexor Carpi Ulnaris	H = Hook of Hamate
D = Radial Styloid	I = Thenar Eminence
E = Ulnar Head	J = Hypothenar Eminence

| A = Abductor Pollicis Longus |
| B = Extensor Pollicis Longus |
| C = Anatomical Snuff Box |

| A = Extensor Pollicis Longus |
| B = Radial Styloid |
| C = Ulnar Styloid |

▲ **Figure 7.78** Surface anatomy of the wrist and hand. **(A)** Volar view. **(B)** Radial view. **(C)** Dorsal view.

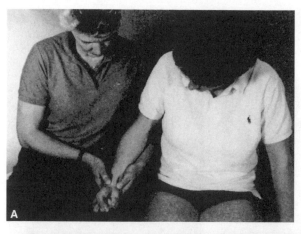

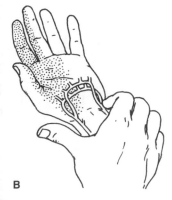

▲ **Figure 7.79** (**A**) In Allen's test, radial and ulnar arteries are compressed at the wrist, while the subject keeps the hand maintained in a tightly clenched fist. (**B**) With the hand opened, each artery is released separately. Note the flushing pattern.

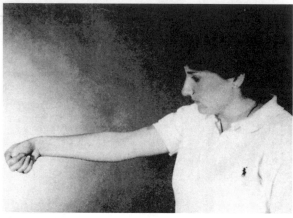

▲ **Figure 7.80** Finkelstein's test.

5. MCP flexion of digits one to five
6. MCP extension of digits one to five
7. IP flexion of digits one to five
8. IP extension of digits one to five
9. Abduction of the thumb
10. Adduction of the thumb
11. Opposition of the thumb and little finger

SPECIAL CLINICAL TESTS

ALLEN'S TEST

Indication. Allen's test[2] is performed to determine the integrity of the radial and ulnar arteries supplying the hand.

Method. The subject is instructed to open and close the hand aggressively several times as quickly as possible and to terminate the cycle with the hand tightly clenched into a fist. The examiner places the thumb and index finger over the radial and ulnar arteries where they cross the wrist. The examiner presses down on these two points to occlude blood flow distally (Fig. 7-79*A*). The subject is then asked to open the hand. The examiner releases one of the

arteries and watches for flushing of the portion of the hand supplied by that particular artery (see Fig. 7-79*B*). Finally, the remaining artery is released, and again the flushing pattern is observed. This process is repeated with the opposite hand and comparisons are made.

Results. Midway through the test, when the subject opens the hand that was clenched into a fist, the hand should appear whitish or pale because of poor blood flow distal to the points of compression. Normally as each artery is released, a flushing pattern is seen as blood flow returns to the hand. If there is an absence or diminution of blood flow to the hand because of pathology, the hand will remain whitish, indicating a positive result.

FINKELSTEIN'S TEST

Indication. An indication for Finkelstein's test[12] would be suspected de Quervain's tenosynovitis.

Method. The subject is asked to make a fist of the test hand while enclosing the thumb within the flexed fingers. The examiner stabilizes the forearm while the wrist is passively or actively moved into ulnar deviation (Fig. 7-80).

Results. A positive result is indicated by pain laterally over the wrist. Stretching of the tendons of the abductor pollicis longus and the extensor pollicis brevis tendons where they cross the wrist is responsible for the pain. Because normal people notice some discomfort during this test, it is recommended that testing be carried out bilaterally to detect a difference.

BRUNNEL-LITTLER TEST

Indication. The Brunnel-Littler test[1] is useful in distinguishing tightness of the intrinsic hand muscles from restriction of the capsule of the MCP joint as the cause of loss of flexion at the MCP joint.

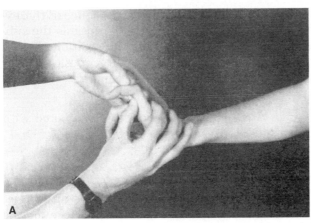

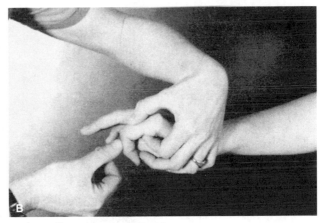

▲ **Figure 7.81** (**A**) In the Brunnel-Littler test, proximal interphalangeal joint flexion is assessed with the metacarpophalangeal joint maintained in extension. (**B**) Proximal interphalangeal joint flexion is assessed with the metacarpophalangeal joint in slight flexion.

Method. The examiner stabilizes the MCP joint in slight extension, thereby stretching the lumbrical muscles. While maintaining the MCP extension, the PIP joint is flexed and the quantity of motion is noted (Fig. 7-81*A*). Next, the MCP joint is slightly flexed, decreasing tension on the lumbrical muscles. While the MCP joint is in flexion, the PIP joint is again flexed while the examiner observes the amount of flexion obtained (see Fig. 7-81*B*).

Results. If there is restriction of PIP flexion while the MCP joint is maintained in extension, the restriction may be due to either tight intrinsics or capsular involvement at the PIP joint.

When PIP flexion is attempted while the MCP joint is flexed, ability to move into full flexion represents tightness of the intrinsics responsible for limitation in motion. If, during flexion of the PIP joint with the MCP joint flexed, the motion of the PIP joint remains incomplete, capsular restrictions must be considered as the primary cause.

OBLIQUE RETINACULAR LIGAMENT TEST

Indication. This test differentiates between tightness of the oblique retinacular ligament and restrictions in the capsule of the PIP joint as causes of restriction of DIP joint flexion.

Method. The examiner positions the PIP joint in a neutral position while attempting to flex the DIP joint. The degree of flexion is noted, and the process is repeated while the PIP joint is held in slight flexion (Fig. 7-82).

Results. The oblique retinacular ligaments are slack when the PIP joint is slightly flexed. A compromise in DIP joint flexion in that position probably is a result of capsular involvement of that joint. If the retinacular ligaments are relaxed by PIP flexion, thereby allowing full range of DIP joint flexion, the initial limitation most likely was a result of retinacular ligament tightness.

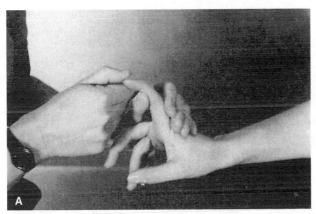

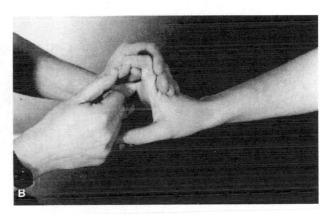

▲ **Figure 7.82** (**A**) In the retinacular test, distal interphalangeal joint flexion is assessed with the proximal joint maintained in an extended position. (**B**) Distal interphalangeal joint flexion is assessed with the proximal joint in slight flexion.

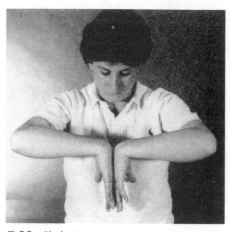

▲ **Figure 7.83** Phalen's test.

CLINICAL TESTS FOR CARPAL TUNNEL SYNDROME

Phalen's Test

Indication. Phalen's test[17] is used to aid in the diagnosis of carpal tunnel syndrome.

Method. The subject is instructed to flex both wrists maximally and simultaneously approximate the dorsal surfaces of both hands to assist in maintaining the flexed posture (Fig. 7-83). This position is held for 1 minute.

Results. Tingling of the palmar surface of the thumb, index, middle, and lateral half of the ring finger is a positive result.

Reverse Phalen's test

Indication. The reverse Phalen's test[1] may be used in conjunction with Phalen's test in the assessment of carpal tunnel syndrome.

Method. The subject is asked to squeeze the examiner's hand while the examiner extends the subject's wrist. While maintaining the position of wrist extension, the examiner applies direct pressure over the carpal tunnel and maintains that pressure for 1 minute (Fig. 7-84).

Results. Reproduction of symptoms as noted with Phalen's test represents a positive test.

Tinel's Sign

Indication. The test for Tinel's sign[15] is an adjunct to the diagnosis of carpal tunnel syndrome for the median nerve.

Method. The subject's forearm is positioned in supination so that the examiner has easier access to the area over the carpal tunnel. The examiner taps the wrist over the carpal tunnel (Fig. 7-85).

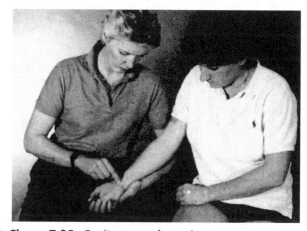

▲ **Figure 7.85** Tinel's sign test for median nerve entrapment.

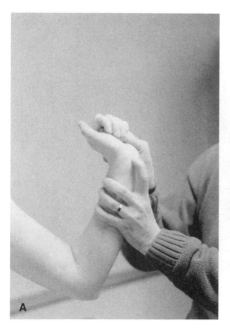

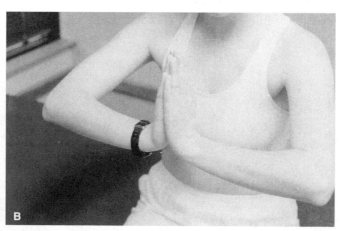

▲ **Figure 7.84** (**A**) Reverse Phalen's test. (**B**) Alternate method for reverse Phalen's test.

Results. A positive test result is confirmed when the sensory changes noted for Phalen's test occur.

Three-Jaw Chuck Test

Indication. The three-jaw chuck test is useful in assessing carpal tunnel syndrome.

Method. The subject places the hand being examined in the posture of a three-jaw chuck pinch, then flexes the wrist (Fig. 7-86). This combined posture is maintained for at least 1 minute.

Results. Reproduction of symptoms as noted in the previous two tests represents a positive result.

TESTS OF INSTABILITY

Murphy's Sign

Indication. Murphy's sign[7] may be used to assist the clinician in determining the presence of a dislocation of the lunate carpal bone.

Method. The subject is asked to form a fist, and the relationship of the metacarpal heads is examined in that position.

Results. Normally, the third metacarpal head extends more distally than the second or fourth metacarpal heads when the hand is positioned in a fist (Fig. 7-87). In the presence of a lunate dislocation, the third metacarpal head will lie in the same plane as the second and fourth metacarpal heads, indicating a positive test.

Watson Test

Indication. This test is designed to help in determining instability or subluxation of the scaphoid carpal bone.[19]

Method. The subject is seated with the forearm supported on the treatment table or examiner's lap. The examiner stabilizes the distal forearm (radius and ulna) with one hand. The thumb and index or

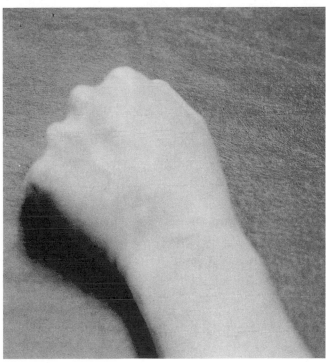

▲ **Figure 7.87** Negative Murphy's sign.

middle finger of the other hand grips the scaphoid dorsally and volarly (Fig. 7-88). The examiner then passively moves the scaphoid in dorsal and volar direction to determine the amount of mobility present.

Results. Excessive mobility of the scaphoid relative to that found on the uninvolved side indicates a positive test.

Lunatotriquetral Ballottment Test

Indication. This test is designed to assess instability of the articulation between the triquetrum and lunate carpal bones.

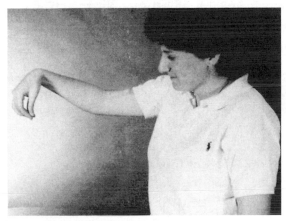

▲ **Figure 7.86** Three-jaw chuck test.

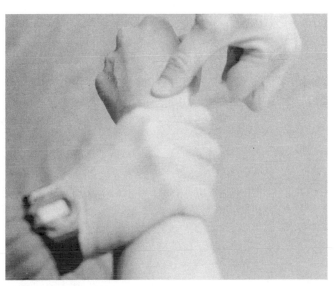

▲ **Figure 7.88** Watson test.

Method. The subject is seated with the forearm supported on the table or examiner's lap. The examiner uses a thumb and index or middle finger to grip the lunate on its dorsal and volar surfaces, while that same grip on the triquetrum is maintained with the examiner's other hand. As the triquetrum is stabilized, the examiner passively moves the lunate in a dorsal and volar direction (Fig 7-89).

Results. Excessive mobility of the lunate compared to the uninvolved side indicates a positive test. Additionally, the presence of pain or crepitus may indicate a positive test.

Collateral Ligament Test

Indication. The collateral ligament test is helpful in the diagnosis of collateral ligament involvement of the MCP joint.

Method. The subject can be positioned standing, seated, or supine for this test. The examiner stabilizes the distal metacarpal with the thumb and index finger of one hand. The thumb and index finger of the other hand are placed along the radial and ulnar aspects of the subject's proximal phalanx. The examiner applies a valgus/varus force to the MCP joint by way of the proximal phalanx to stress the medial and lateral collateral ligaments, respectively (Fig. 7-90).

Results. Pain or excessive gapping of the MCP joint indicates a positive test.

NEUROLOGICAL TESTS

Froment Sign

Indication. This test is used to assess ulnar nerve compromise in the hand by evaluating thumb adduction.[15]

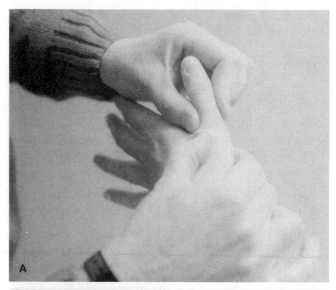

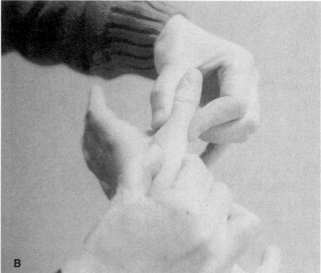

▲ **Figure 7.90** (**A**) Lateral collateral stress test. (**B**) Medial collateral stress test.

Method. A piece of paper is placed between the subject's thumb and index finger, and the subject is instructed to grip the paper as the examiner attempts to pull it from between the thumb and finger (Fig. 7-91).

Results. The test is positive if the subject tries to maintain a grip on the paper by flexing the DIP joint of the thumb to compensate for adductor pollicis weakness due to ulnar nerve injury. Further, simultaneous thumb MCP hyperextension during this test is identified as Jeanne's sign.[2]

GRIP AND PINCH TESTS

Grip Strength

Indication. Grip strength is used to assess functional grip strength.

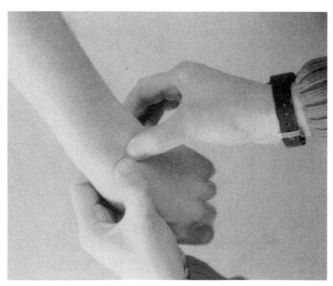

▲ **Figure 7.89** Lunatotriquetral ballottment test.

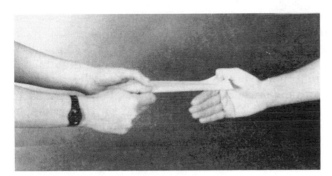

▲ **Figure 7.91** Froment's sign.

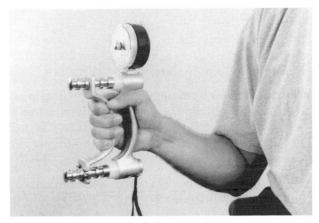

▲ **Figure 7.92** Grip strength dynamometer.

Method. A handheld dynamometer, such as the Jamar Grip Dynamometer (Asimov Engineering, Los Angeles, CA), is used for objective testing. Grip strength is assessed using five separate handle positions in ½-in increments from 1 to 3 in. The subject may be seated or standing with the arm adducted against the side, the elbow flexed 90 degrees, and the forearm in the midposition. The subject is instructed to squeeze the handle with maximal force. Testing is performed alternately between the right and left hands, and the average of three trials is the value recorded (Fig. 7-92).

Results. Grip strength values obtained are compared to normative values, based on gender and age, as noted in Table 7-1.[2,4,11,13,18] A 5% to 10% difference between dominant and nondominant hands is accepted as normal. Plotting of the values obtained in each of the five handle positions should represent a bell curve, because the middle handle positions are the strongest and the terminal handle positions weakest. Plotted values that do not form a bell curve are representative of maximal effort during testing.

TABLE 7.1 Average Performance of All Subjects on Grip Strength (pounds)

AGE (Y)	HAND	MEN					WOMEN				
		MEAN	SD	SE	LOW	HIGH	MEAN	SD	SE	LOW	HIGH
20–24	R	121.0	20.6	3.8	91	167	70.4	14.5	2.8	46	95
	L	104.5	21.8	4.0	71	150	61.0	13.1	2.6	33	88
25–29	R	120.8	23.0	4.4	78	158	74.5	13.9	2.7	48	97
	L	110.5	16.2	3.1	77	139	63.5	12.2	2.4	48	97
30–34	R	121.8	22.4	4.3	70	170	78.7	19.2	3.8	46	137
	L	110.4	21.7	4.2	64	145	68.0	17.7	3.5	36	115
35–39	R	119.7	24.0	4.8	76	176	74.1	10.8	2.2	50	99
	L	112.9	21.7	4.4	73	157	66.3	11.7	2.3	49	91
40–44	R	116.8	20.7	4.1	84	165	70.4	13.5	2.4	38	103
	L	112.8	18.7	3.7	73	157	62.3	13.8	2.5	35	94
45–49	R	109.9	23.0	4.3	65	155	62.2	15.1	3.0	39	100
	L	100.8	22.8	4.3	58	160	56.0	12.7	2.5	37	83
50–54	R	113.6	18.1	3.6	79	151	65.8	11.6	2.3	38	87
	L	101.9	17.0	3.4	70	143	57.3	10.7	2.1	35	76
55–59	R	101.1	26.7	5.8	59	154	57.3	12.5	2.5	33	86
	L	83.2	23.4	5.1	43	128	47.3	11.9	2.4	31	76
60–64	R	89.7	20.4	4.2	51	137	55.1	10.1	2.0	37	77
	L	76.8	20.3	4.1	27	116	45.7	10.1	2.0	29	66
65–69	R	91.1	20.6	4.0	56	131	49.6	9.7	1.8	35	74
	L	76.8	19.8	3.8	43	117	41.0	8.2	1.5	29	63
70–74	R	75.3	21.5	4.2	32	108	49.6	11.7	2.2	33	78
	L	64.8	18.1	3.7	32	93	41.5	10.2	1.9	23	67
75+	R	65.7	21.0	4.2	40	135	42.6	11.0	2.2	25	65
	L	55.0	17.0	3.4	31	119	37.6	8.9	1.7	24	61
All subjects	R	104.3	28.3	1.6	32	176	62.8	17.0	0.96	25	137
	L	93.1	27.6	1.6	27	160	53.9	15.7	0.88	23	115

(From Mathiowetz B, Kashman N, Volland G, et al: Grip and pinch strength: Normative data for adults. Arch Phys Med Rehabil 66:71–72, 1995)

Pinch Grip

Indication. Pinch grip is used to assess the strength of three different types of functional pinch, including pulp to pulp, lateral, and three jaw chuck.

Method. A pinch meter is used for testing in which each pinch type is assessed, alternating between right and left hands. Three trials of each pinch are performed with the average value of each recorded (Fig. 7-93).

Results. Pinch values obtained are compared to normative values (Tables 7-2 and 7-3).[6,11,13]

SENSORY-PERCEPTUAL TESTS

Weber's Two-Point Discrimination Test

Indication. This test is designed to evaluate the slowly adapting fiber receptor system.

Method. The subject is seated with the forearm supported on a firm surface or by the examiner's hand. An instrument such as a Boley Gauge (Research Designs, Houston, TX) or Disk-Criminator (Disk-Criminator, Baltimore, MD) is used for this test. If such instruments are unavailable, a paper clip may be used as a substitute. The two points of the instrument are placed simultaneously in a longitudinal manner moving proximal to distal along the radial or ulnar aspect of the finger being tested. The distance between the two points is increased or decreased according to the subject's response. Further trials are performed with the two points being progressively moved closer to one another, until the subject is unable to distinguish two separate points.[6,8,9,16]

Results. A normal discrimination distance is reported to be less than 6 mm. See Table 7-4 for two-point discrimination values associated with various functional activities.

Dellon's Moving Two-Point Discrimination

Indication. This test assesses the quickly adapting fiber receptor system and helps in the prediction of functional recovery.

Method. The subject is positioned as in the previous test. Two points are moved from proximal to distal in a longitudinal manner along the radial or ulnar side of the digit tested. Initial testing is per-

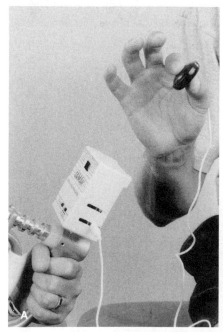 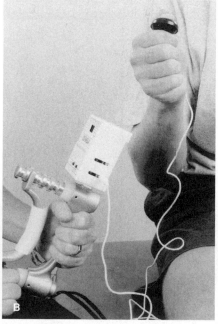 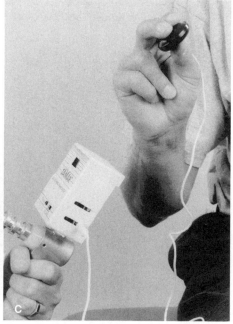

▲ **Figure 7.93** Pinch grip assessment. **(A)** Pulp to pulp pinch. **(B)** Lateral pinch. **(C)** Three jaw chuck pinch.

TABLE 7.2 Average Performance of All Subjects on Tip Pinch (pounds)

AGE (Y)	HAND	MEN					WOMEN				
		MEAN	SD	SE	LOW	HIGH	MEAN	SD	SE	LOW	HIGH
20–24	R	18.0	3.0	.57	11	23	11.1	2.1	.42	8	16
	L	17.0	2.3	.43	12	33	10.5	1.7	.34	8	14
25–29	R	18.3	4.4	.84	10	34	11.9	1.8	.35	8	16
	L	17.5	5.2	.99	12	36	11.3	1.8	.35	9	18
30–34	R	17.6	6.7	.71	12	25	12.6	3.0	.58	8	20
	L	17.6	4.8	.93	10	27	11.7	2.8	.54	7	17
35–39	R	18.0	3.6	.73	12	27	11.6	2.5	.50	8	19
	L	17.7	3.8	.76	10	24	11.9	2.4	.47	8	16
40–44	R	17.8	4.0	.78	11	25	11.5	2.7	.49	5	15
	L	17.7	3.5	.68	12	25	11.1	3.0	.54	6	17
45–49	R	18.7	4.9	.92	12	30	13.2	3.0	.60	9	19
	L	17.6	4.1	.77	12	28	12.1	2.7	.55	7	18
50–54	R	18.3	4.0	.80	11	24	12.5	2.2	.44	9	18
	L	17.8	3.9	.77	12	26	11.4	2.4	.49	7	16
55–59	R	16.6	3.3	.73	11	24	11.7	1.7	.34	9	16
	L	15.0	3.7	.81	10	26	10.4	1.4	.29	8	13
60–64	R	15.8	3.9	.80	9	22	10.1	2.1	.43	7	17
	L	15.3	3.7	.76	9	23	9.9	2.0	.39	6	15
65–69	R	17.0	4.2	.81	11	27	10.6	2.0	.39	7	15
	L	15.4	2.9	.55	10	21	10.5	2.4	.45	7	17
70–74	R	13.8	2.6	.52	11	21	10.1	2.6	.48	7	15
	L	13.3	2.6	.51	10	21	9.8	2.3	.43	6	17
75+	R	14.0	3.4	.68	7	21	9.6	2.8	.54	4	16
	L	13.9	3.7	.75	8	25	9.3	2.4	.47	4	13
All subjects	R	17.0	4.1	.23	7	34	11.3	2.6	.15	4	20
	L	16.4	4.0	.23	8	36	10.8	2.4	.14	4	18

(From Mathiowetz B, Kashman N, Volland G, et al: Grip and pinch strength: Normative data for adults.
Arch Phys Med Rehabil 66:71–72, 1995)

TABLE 7.3 Average Performance of All Subjects on Key Pinch (pounds)

AGE (Y)	HAND	MEN					WOMEN				
		MEAN	SD	SE	LOW	HIGH	MEAN	SD	SE	LOW	HIGH
20–24	R	26.0	3.5	.65	21	34	17.6	2.0	.39	14	23
	L	24.8	3.4	.64	19	31	16.2	2.1	.41	13	23
25–29	R	26.7	4.9	.94	19	41	17.7	2.1	.41	14	22
	L	25.0	4.4	.85	19	39	16.6	2.1	.41	13	22
30–34	R	26.4	4.8	.93	20	36	18.7	3.0	.60	13	25
	L	26.2	5.1	.98	17	36	17.8	3.6	.70	12	26
35–39	R	26.1	3.2	.65	21	32	16.6	2.0	.40	12	21
	L	25.6	3.9	.77	18	32	16.0	2.7	.53	12	22
40–44	R	25.6	2.6	.50	21	31	16.7	3.1	.56	10	24
	L	25.1	4.0	.79	19	31	15.8	3.1	.55	8	22
45–49	R	25.8	3.9	.73	19	35	17.6	3.2	.65	13	24
	L	24.8	4.4	.84	18	42	16.6	2.9	.58	12	24
50–54	R	26.7	4.4	.88	20	34	16.7	2.5	.50	12	22
	L	26.1	4.2	.84	20	37	16.1	2.7	.53	12	22
55–59	R	24.2	4.2	.92	18	34	15.7	2.5	.50	11	21
	L	23.0	4.7	1.02	13	31	14.7	2.2	.44	12	19
60–64	R	23.2	5.4	1.13	14	37	15.5	2.7	.55	10	20
	L	22.2	4.1	.84	16	33	14.1	2.5	.50	10	19
65–69	R	23.4	3.9	.75	17	32	15.0	2.6	.49	10	21
	L	22.0	3.6	.70	17	28	14.3	2.8	.53	10	20
70–74	R	19.3	2.4	.47	16	25	14.5	2.9	.54	8	22
	L	19.2	3.0	.59	13	28	13.8	3.0	.56	9	22
75+	R	20.5	4.6	.91	9	31	12.6	2.3	.45	8	17
	L	19.1	3.0	.59	13	24	11.4	2.6	.50	7	16
All subjects	R	24.5	4.6	.26	9	41	16.2	3.0	.17	8	25
	L	23.6	4.6	.26	11	42	15.3	3.1	.18	7	26

(From Mathiowetz B, Kashman N, Volland G, et al: Grip and pinch strength: Normative data for adults.
Arch Phys Med Rehabil 66:71–72, 1995)

TABLE 7.4	**Two-Point Discrimination Normal Values and Discrimination Distances Required for Certain Tasks**
Normal	Less than 6 mm
Fair	6–10 mm
Poor	11–15 mm
Protective	1 point perceived
Anesthetic	0 points perceived
Winding a watch	6 mm
Sewing	6–8 mm
Handling precision tools	12 mm
Gross tool handling	>15 mm

(Adapted from Callahan AD: Sensibility testing. In Hunter J, et al (eds): Rehabilitation of the Hand: Surgery and Therapy, p. 605. St. Louis, C V Mosby, 1990)

formed with the two points placed 8 mm apart. Distance between points is increased or decreased depending on the subject's response. Subsequent testing is performed with the distance between the two points progressively decreased until the subject is unable to distinguish two separate points.[8,9,16]

Results. The normal distance for discrimination is 2 to 5 mm.

FUNCTIONAL TESTS

Box and Block Test

Indication. The block and box test[5] is used to assess gross manual dexterity.

Method. A box divided in half is used in the transfer of blocks from one side of the box to the other. Each block is 2.5 cm^2, and 150 blocks are included. A short practice trial of 15 seconds is permitted prior to actual testing.

Results. The number of blocks successfully transferred from one side to the other indicates the score.

Minnesota Rate of Manipulation Test

Indication. This test is designed to assess gross coordination and dexterity.[11]

Method. Activities involving fine motor activities are assessed, including placing, turning, and displacement of objects and one- and two-handed turning and placing.

Results. The subject is timed for each activity and compared to normal values.

Nine-Hole Peg Test

Indication. This test is used in the assessment of finger dexterity.[5]

Method. The subject is instructed first to place 3.2 cm^2 pegs into a 12.7 cm^2 hole and then remove them. The test is performed with one hand and then the other.

Results. A score is obtained by the amount of time required to complete the test.

Purdue Pegboard Test

Indication. The Purdue pegboard[3,11] is designed to assess fine motor coordination.

Method. The subject places small objects, such as collars and washers, onto pegs placed into holes on a board. Testing is completed using the right hand, left hand, and both hands.

Results. Times for each category of testing are compared to normative values based on occupation and gender.

Moberg Pickup Test

Indication. This test is used in the evaluation of median or combined median and ulnar nerve lesions.[8]

Method. Nine or ten small objects, including screws, pins, paper clips, and keys, are used in testing. The subject is instructed to place the objects into a box using first the affected hand, then the unaffected hand, and finally the affected hand with eyes closed.

Results. Time of task completion is the score for this test. Subjects with paresthesias in certain digits will tend to use those digits less during the performance of this test.

JOINT PLAY (ACCESSORY MOVEMENTS)

Radiocarpal Joint

Distraction (Fig. 7-94)

Restriction. General hypomobility.

Open-Packed Position. Ten degrees of wrist flexion and slight ulnar deviation.

Positioning. Subject sits beside treatment table with forearm pronated. Stabilization may be accomplished with the use of a wedge beneath the distal radius and ulna or by stabilizing the distal forearm against the body. The stabilizing hand of the therapist holds the distal radius and ulna as close to the joint space as possible. The other hand grasps the proximal row of carpal bones.

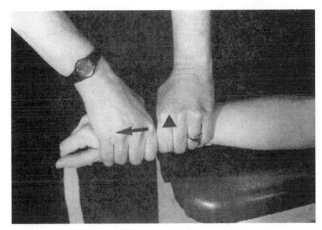

▲ **Figure 7.94** Distraction of the radiocarpal joint.

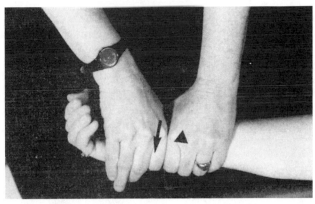

▲ **Figure 7.96** Dorsal glide of the proximal carpal bones.

Movement. The therapist delivers a distracting force to the proximal row of carpal bones.

Ventral Glide (Fig. 7-95)

Restriction. Wrist extension.

Positioning. Same as for distraction glide.

Movement. The therapist delivers a ventral force to the proximal row of carpal bones, with the focus of the application through the radial side of the index finger, the web space, and the ulnar side of the thumb.

Dorsal Glide (Fig. 7-96)

Restriction. Wrist flexion.

Positioning. Same as for distraction glide, except that the forearm is supine.

Movement. The therapist delivers a dorsal force to the proximal row of carpal bones, with the focus of the application through the radial side of the index

finger, the web space, and the ulnar side of the thumb.

Radial Glide (Fig. 7-97)

Restriction. Wrist ulnar deviation.

Positioning. Subject sits beside treatment table with forearm in the midposition. Stabilization may be accomplished with the use of a wedge beneath the distal ulna or by stabilizing the distal forearm against the therapist's body. The stabilizing hand of the therapist holds the distal radius and ulna as close to the joint space as possible. The other hand grasps the proximal row of carpal bones.

Movement. The therapist delivers a radial force to the proximal row of carpal bones, with the focus of the application through the palmar surface of the index finger to the medial side of the ulna.

Ulnar Glide (Fig. 7-98)

Restriction. Wrist radial deviation.

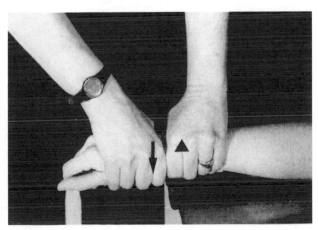

▲ **Figure 7.95** Ventral glide of the proximal carpal bones.

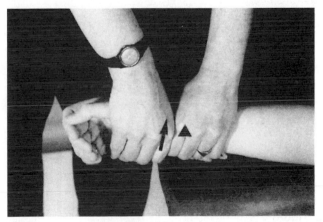

▲ **Figure 7.97** Radial glide of the proximal carpal bones.

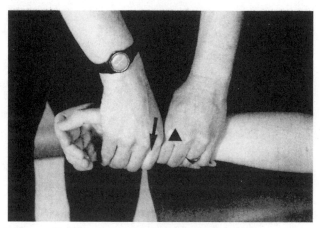

▲ **Figure 7.98** Ulnar glide of the proximal carpal bones.

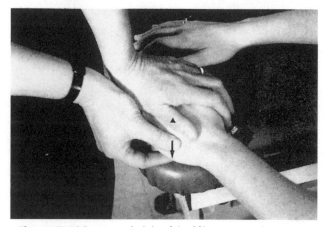

▲ **Figure 7.100** Ventral glide of the fifth metacarpal.

Positioning. Same as for radial glide.

Movement. The therapist delivers an ulnar force to the proximal row of carpal bones, with the focus of the application through the web space to the lateral side of the distal radius.

SECOND THROUGH FIFTH CARPOMETACARPAL JOINTS

Distraction (Fig. 7-99)

Restriction. General hypomobility.

Open-Packed Position. Resting.

Positioning. Subject sits beside a table with the forearm pronated. The distal carpal row, which articulates with the proximal metacarpal bases, is stabilized on the wedge. One hand of the therapist provides additional stabilization by grasping the specific carpal bone with the index finger and thumb. The other hand grips the corresponding metacarpal as close to the base as possible.

Movement. The therapist creates a distraction force to the proximal metacarpal.

Ventral Glide (Fig. 7-100)

Restriction. General hypomobility.

Positioning. Subject sits beside a table with forearm pronated. The metacarpal adjacent to the one being mobilized is stabilized on a wedge. One hand of the therapist rests on the dorsum of the stabilized metacarpal, providing additional support. The thenar eminence of the other hand is placed on the metacarpal to be mobilized.

Movement. Using the radial aspect of the thenar eminence, the therapist imposes a ventral force to the metacarpal being mobilized. This technique applies not only to CMC joint mobilization, but also to intermetacarpal mobilization.

CARPOMETACARPAL JOINT OF THE THUMB

Distraction (Fig. 7-101)

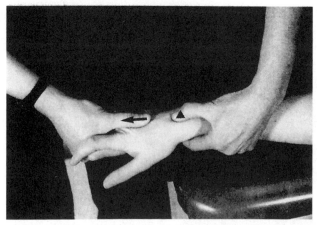

▲ **Figure 7.99** Distraction of the second to the fifth carpometacarpal joints.

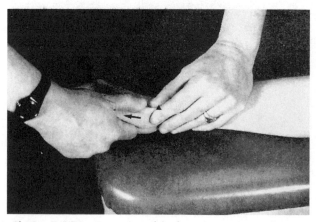

▲ **Figure 7.101** Distraction of the first carpometacarpal joint.

Restriction. General hypomobility.

Open-Packed Position. Midway between flexion and extension and between abduction and adduction.

Positioning. Subject sits beside a table with forearm in midposition. The therapist stabilizes the trapezium and trapezoid as a unit, with the thumb and index finger of one hand. The thumb and index finger of the other hand are placed on the dorsal and palmar surfaces, respectively, of the subject's first metacarpal.

Movement. The therapist applies a distraction force to the subject's first metacarpal.

Ulnar Glide (Fig. 7-102)

Restriction. Flexion of the thumb.

Positioning. Subject sits beside a table with the forearm in midposition. The therapist stabilizes the trapezium and trapezoid as a unit with the thumb and index finger of one hand. The thenar eminence of the other hand is placed on the first metacarpal of the subject's thumb, and the fingers wrap around the thumb to assist in maintaining the resting position.

Movement. The therapist applies an ulnarly directed force through the thenar eminence to the radial aspect of the subject's metacarpal.

Radial Glide (Fig. 7-103)

Restriction. Extension of the thumb.

Positioning. Same as for ulnar glide.

Movement. The therapist applies a radially directed force through the thenar eminence to the ulnar aspect of the subject's first metacarpal.

Dorsal Glide (Fig. 7-104)

Restriction. Abduction of the thumb.

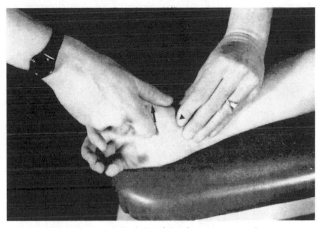

▲ **Figure 7.103**   Radial glide of the first metacarpal.

Positioning. Same as for ulnar glide, except with the forearm fully supinated.

Movement. The therapist applies a dorsally directed force through the thenar eminence to the anterior aspect of the subject's first metacarpal.

Ventral Glide (Fig. 7-105)

Restriction. Adduction of the thumb.

Positioning. Same as for dorsal glide.

Movement. The therapist applies a ventrally directed force to the posterior aspect of the subject's first metacarpal.

FIRST THROUGH FIFTH METACARPOPHALANGEAL AND INTERPHALANGEAL JOINTS

Distraction, Ventral, and Dorsal Glide (Fig 7-106)

Restriction. General hypomobility, flexion, extension.

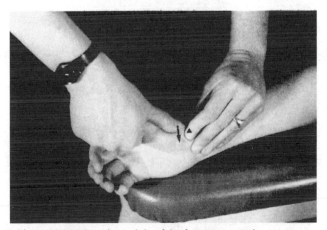

▲ **Figure 7.102**   Ulnar glide of the first metacarpal.

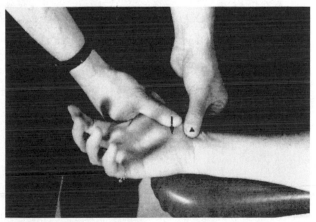

▲ **Figure 7.104**   Dorsal glide of the first metacarpal.

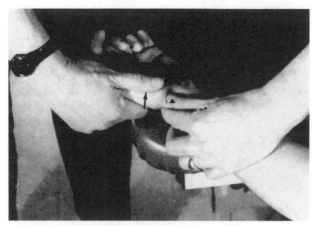

▲ **Figure 7.105** Ventral glide of the first metacarpal.

Open-Packed Position. Slight flexion.

Positioning. Subject is seated with the proximal articulating partner stabilized on the wedge. The therapist's one hand is placed on the dorsal surface of the stabilized bone to provide additional support. The thumb and index finger of the other hand are placed on the dorsal and palmar surfaces of the subject's distal articulating partner as close to the joint space as possible.

Movement. The therapist applies a distraction force to the distal articulating segment for general-ized hypomobility restrictions. A ventral or palmar glide is performed for restrictions in flexion, and a dorsal glide is used for limitations in extension.

Carpal Bone Mobility Testing

Kaltenborn has developed a systematic approach to examination of joint play of the individual carpal bones (Fig. 7-107). The suggested format is as follows:

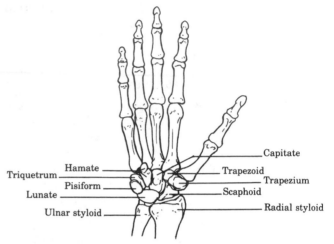

▲ **Figure 7.107** Anterior view of the anatomical relationship of the distal forearm and carpal bones.

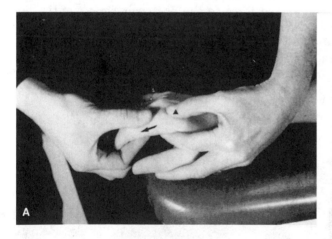

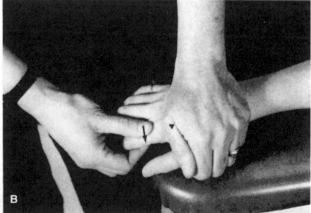

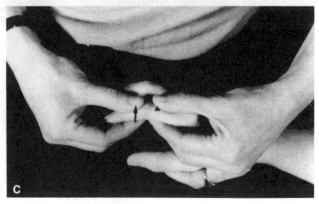

▲ **Figure 7.106** (**A**) Mobilization of metacarpophalangeal and interphalangeal joints. Distraction of the metacarpophalangeal joint. (**B**) Ventral glide of the proximal phalanx. (**C**) Dorsal glide of the middle phalanx.

TABLE 7.5 Summary of Joint Play in the Wrist and Hand

Glide	Restriction	Fixed Bone	Moving Bone
Radiocarpal Joint			
Distraction	General hypomobility	Radius	Scaphoid/lunate/disk
Ventral	Extension	Radius	Scaphoid/lunate/disk
Dorsal	Flexion	Radius	Scaphoid/lunate/disk
Radial	Ulnar deviation	Radius	Scaphoid/lunate/disk
Ulnar	Radial deviation	Radius	Scaphoid/lunate/disk
Second Through Fifth Carpometacarpal Joints			
Distraction	General hypomobility	Carpal	Metacarpal
Dorsal	Flexion	Carpal	Metacarpal
Ventral	Extension	Carpal	Metacarpal
Carpometacarpal Joint of Thumb			
Distraction	General hypomobility	Carpal	Metacarpal
Ulnar	Flexion	Carpal	Metacarpal
Radial	Extension	Carpal	Metacarpal
Dorsal	Abduction	Carpal	Metacarpal
Ventral	Adduction	Carpal	Metacarpal
First Through Fifth Metacarpophalangeal Joints			
Distraction	General hypomobility	Metacarpal	Proximal phalanx
Ventral	Flexion	Metacarpal	Proximal phalanx
Dorsal	Extension	Metacarpal	Proximal phalanx
First Through Fifth Interphalangeal Joints			
Distraction	General hypomobility	Proximal phalanx	Distal phalanx
Ventral	Flexion	Proximal phalanx	Distal phalanx
Dorsal	Extension	Proximal phalanx	Distal phalanx

1. Stabilize the capitate and move the trapezium and trapezoid as a unit.
2. Stabilize the capitate and move the scaphoid.
3. Stabilize the capitate and move the lunate.
4. Stabilize the capitate and move the hamate.
5. Stabilize the scaphoid and move the trapezium and trapezoid as a unit.
6. Stabilize the radius and move the scaphoid.
7. Stabilize the radius and move the lunate.
8. Stabilize the ulna with the articular disk and move the triquetrum.
9. Stabilize the triquetrum and move the hamate.
10. Stabilize the triquetrum and move the pisiform.

Table 7-5 provides a summary of joint play in the wrist and hand.

REFERENCES

1. American Society for Surgery of the Hand: The Hand Examination and Diagnosis. Aurora, CO, 1978
2. Aulicino PL, DuPuy TE: Clinical examination of the hand. In Hunter JM, Schneider LH, Mackin EJ, et al (eds): Rehabilitation of the Hand: Surgery and Therapy, 3rd ed, pp. 31–52. St. Louis, CV Mosby, 1990
3. Baxter-Petralia PL, Blackmore SM, McEntee PM: Physical capacity evaluation. In Hunter J, et al: Rehabilitation of the Hand: Surgery and Therapy. St. Louis, CV Mosby, 1990
4. Bechtal CD: Grip test: The use of a dynamometer with adjustable handle spacings. J Bone Joint Surg 36A:820–832, 1954
5. Beckenbaugh RD, Shives TCC, Dobyns JH, Linschied RL: Kienbockis disease: The natural history of Keinbockis disease and consideration of lunate fractures. Clin Orthop 149–198, 1980
6. Bell-Krotoski JA: Sensibility testing: State of the art. In Hunter JM, Schneider LH, Mackin EJ, et al (eds): Rehabilitation of the Hand: Surgery and Therapy, 3rd ed, pp. 575–584. St. Louis, CV Mosby, 1990
7. Booher JM, Thibodeau GA: Athletic Injury Assessment. St. Louis, CV Mosby, 1989
8. Callahan AD: Sensibility testing. In Hunter JM, Schneider LH, Mackin EJ, et al (eds): Rehabilitation of the Hand: Surgery and Therapy, 3rd ed. St. Louis, CV Mosby, 1990
9. Dellon AL, Kallman CH: Evaluation of functional sensation in the hand. J Hand Surg 8:865–870, 1983
10. Eversmann WW: Entrapment and compression neuropathies. In Green DP (ed): Operative Hand Surgery, pp. 957–1009. New York, Churchill Livingstone, 1982
11. Fess EE: Documentation: Essential elements of an upper extremity assessment batter. In Hunter JM, Schneider LH, Mackin EJ, et al (eds): Rehabilitation of the Hand: Surgery and Therapy, 3rd ed. St. Louis, CV Mosby, 1990
12. Finkelstein H: Stenosing tendovaginitis at the radial styloid process. J Bone Joint Surg 12:509, 1930
13. Mathiowetz V, Weber K, Volland G, Kashman N: Reliability and validity of grip and pinch strength evaluations. J Hand Surg 9A:222–226, 1984
14. McFarlane RM: Dupuytrenis contracture. In Green DP (ed): Operative Hand Surgery, pp. 463–498. New York, Churchill-Livingstone, 1982
15. Moldaver J: Tinel's sign—Its characteristics and significance. J Bone Joint Surg 60A:412, 1978
16. Omer GE: Report to the Committee for Evaluation of the Clinical Result in Peripheral Nerve Injury. J Hand Surg 8:754–759, 1983
17. Phalen GS: The carpal tunnel syndrome. Clinical evaluation of 598 hands. Clin Orthop 83:29, 1972
18. Spinner M: Injuries to the Major Branches of the Peripheral Nerves in the Forearm, 2nd ed. Philadelphia, WB Saunders, 1978
19. Taleisnik J: Carpal instability. J Bone Joint Surg 70A:1262–1268, 1988

8

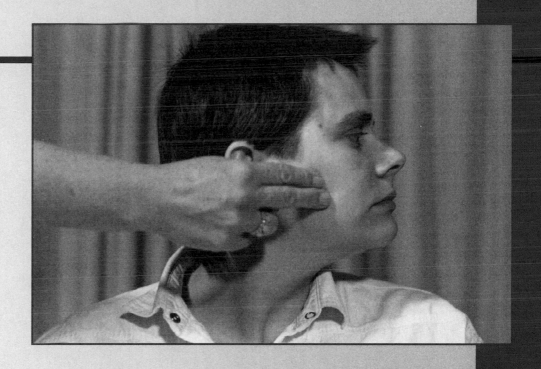

Face and Temporomandibular Joint

MANUAL MUSCLE TESTING

All facial muscle testing is performed in the sitting or supine position. Gravity is not considered a factor for muscle assessment of the face. The grades are therefore altered from the standard format:

Zero: No contraction
Trace: Minimal contraction
Fair: Movement with difficulty
Normal: Completion of movement with ease

Resistance is usually given only to the muscles of mastication. Stabilization is not applied by the examiner, as long as the neck is stable.

It is difficult for a person with weak facial muscles to use substitution movements or synergistic muscles. The examiner should observe motion for symmetry, although many of the muscles of facial expression may be asymmetrical. The muscles of the face are divided into two types. Those that lie in the subcutaneous tissue and function by moving the skin are called the muscles of facial expression (Fig. 8-1). The other type of facial muscle have a bony attachment and affect motion at the temporomandibular joint (TMJ). These muscles are termed muscles of mastication.

MUSCLES OF FACIAL EXPRESSION

Muscles of the Forehead and Nose

OCCIPITOFRONTALIS MUSCLE

The occipitofrontalis is a two-headed muscle and is part of the scalp with a large intervening aponeurosis. The muscle is named for its location on the occipital and frontal bones of the skull. Its function is to produce transverse wrinkles in the skin on the forehead and to move the scalp without raising the head. The frontal portion elevates the eyebrows (Fig. 8-2).

Palpation. Palpate on both sides of the midline above the eyebrows. The occipital portion is posterior on the skull over the occipital bone.

Movement. Wrinkles the forehead by raising the eyebrows.

Innervation. Facial nerve, temporalis branch.

CORRUGATOR MUSCLE

The corrugator muscle lies medial to the eyebrows and produces frowns (Fig. 8-3).

Palpation. Palpate the medial end of each eyebrow.

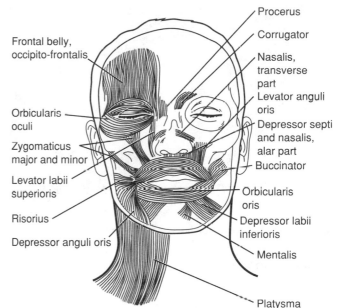

▲ **Figure 8.1** Muscles of facial expression.

Procerus
Corrugator
Nasalis, transverse part
Levator anguli oris
Depressor septi and nasalis, alar part
Buccinator
Orbicularis oris
Depressor labii inferioris
Mentalis
Platysma
Frontal belly, occipito-frontalis
Orbicularis oculi
Zygomaticus major and minor
Levator labii superioris
Risorius
Depressor anguli oris

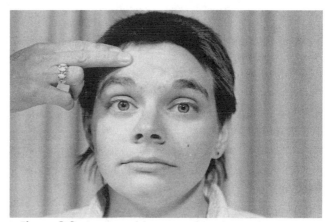

▲ **Figure 8.2** Location of the occipitofrontalis muscle.

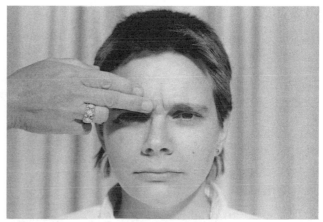

▲ **Figure 8.3** Location of the corrugator muscle.

Movement. Draw the eyebrows together, forming vertical wrinkles between the eyebrows, as in frowning.

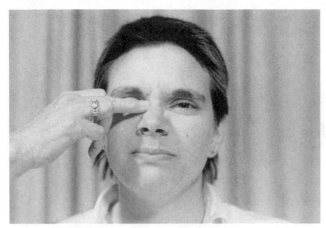

▲ **Figure 8.4** Location of the procerus muscle.

Innervation. Facial nerve, temporal and zygomatic branches.

PROCERUS MUSCLES

The procerus muscles are located along the lateral side of the nose and extend superiorly between the eyebrows. They produce the facial expression of distaste by wrinkling the skin on the nose, and they draw the eyebrows medially and inferiorly, as in a squint (Fig. 8-4).

Palpation. Palpate along the lateral portion of each side of the nose.

Movement. Draw the skin on the lateral nose upward, forming transverse wrinkles over the bridge of the nose.

Innervation. Facial nerve, buccal branches.

NASALIS (ALAR AND TRANSVERSE) MUSCLES

The nasalis muscles have an alar portion over the alar cartilage that flares the nostrils and a depressor septi and transverse portion, horizontal fibers, that compress the nostrils (Fig. 8-5).

Palpation. Palpate over the alar portion of the nose.

Movement. Dilate and compress the nostrils, changing the aperture of the nostrils.

Innervation. Facial nerve, buccal branches.

Muscles of the Eye

ORBICULARIS OCULI MUSCLE

The orbicularis oculi is an expansive sphincter muscle that encircles the eye, extending down over the cheek area. Two portions of the muscle, orbital and palpebral, are tested together. The starting position is with the eyes open wide. Contraction of the muscle fibers narrows the orbital opening and encourages the flow of tears by helping to empty the lacrimal gland (Fig. 8-6).

Palpation. Palpate as close to the upper and lower eyelids as possible without interfering with the motion.

Movement. Close the eyes tightly.

Resistance. Following the movement, resistance can be applied to lift the eyelids.

Innervation. Facial nerve, temporal and zygomatic branches.

SUPERIOR LEVATOR PALPEBRAE MUSCLE

The levator palpebrae muscle is located deep to the skin of the upper eyelid. The starting position is with the eyes slightly open.

Palpation. Palpate the upper eyelid (Fig. 8-7).

Movement. Lift the upper eyelids.

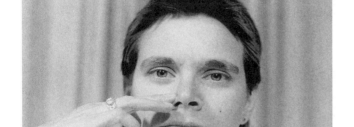

▲ **Figure 8.5** Location of the nasalis muscle.

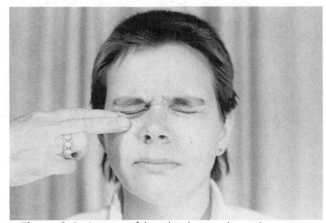

▲ **Figure 8.6** Location of the orbicularis oculi muscle.

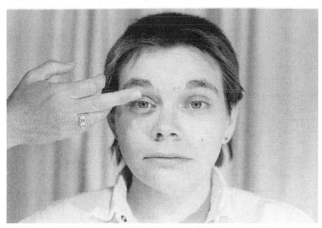

▲ **Figure 8.7** Location of the levator palpebrae muscle.

Innervation. Oculomotor nerve.

EXTRINSIC EYE MUSCLES: SUPERIOR, INFERIOR, MEDIAL, AND LATERAL RECTUS, AND SUPERIOR AND INFERIOR OBLIQUE

The extrinsic eye muscles are tested bilaterally and simultaneously because they usually do not function independently. All these muscles attach to the sclera of the eye from a cartilaginous ring around the optic nerve posteriorly in the orbit. The muscles are tested as the examiner is looking at the subject; the subject's left eye is to the examiner's right. The eye muscles are not palpated; instead, the movements are observed for symmetry. The six extrinsic eye muscles rotate the eyeball in the orbit about three axes (Figs. 8-8 and 8-9).

Movement

Subject moves eyes up and right; examiner observes the right superior rectus and left inferior oblique muscles (Fig. 8-10).

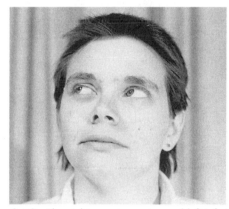

▲ **Figure 8.9** Extrinsic muscles of the eye.

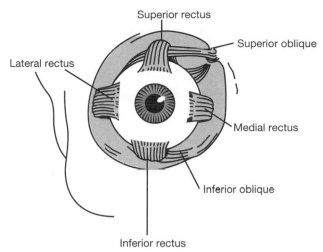

▲ **Figure 8.10** The right superior rectus and left inferior oblique muscles control this eye movement.

Subject moves eyes up and left; examiner observes the left superior rectus and right inferior oblique muscles (Fig. 8-11).
Subject moves eyes left; examiner observes the left lateral rectus and right medial rectus muscles (Fig. 8-12).

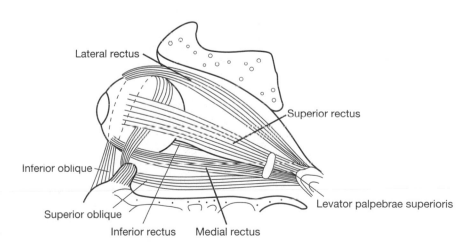

▲ **Figure 8.8** Extrinsic muscles of the eye.

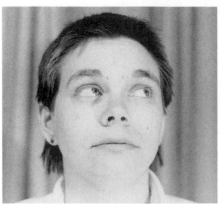

▲ **Figure 8.11** The left superior rectus and right inferior oblique muscles control this eye movement.

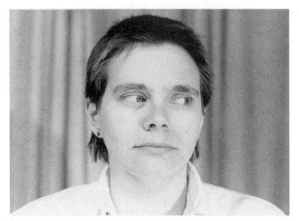

▲ **Figure 8.12** The left lateral rectus and right medial rectus muscles control this eye movement.

Subject moves eyes right; examiner observes the right lateral rectus and left medial rectus muscles (Fig. 8-13).

Subject moves eyes down and right; examiner observes the right inferior rectus and left superior oblique muscles (Fig. 8-14).

Subject moves eyes down and left; examiner observes the left inferior rectus and right superior oblique muscles (Fig. 8-15).

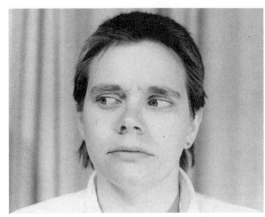

▲ **Figure 8.13** The right lateral rectus and left medial rectus muscles control this eye movement.

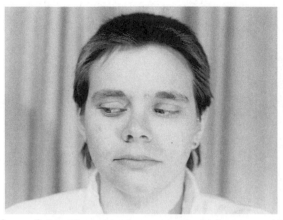

▲ **Figure 8.14** The right inferior rectus and left superior oblique muscles control this eye movement.

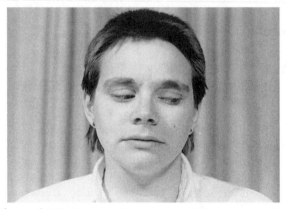

▲ **Figure 8.15** The left inferior rectus and right superior oblique muscles control this eye movement.

Subject moves eyes up; examiner observes the left superior rectus and right superior rectus muscles (Fig. 8-16).

Subject moves eyes down; examiner observes the left inferior rectus and right inferior rectus muscles (Fig. 8-17).

Innervation. Lateral rectus, abducens; superior oblique, trochlear; superior rectus, oculomotor; infe-

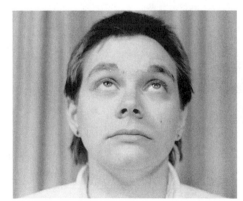

▲ **Figure 8.16** The left and right superior rectus muscles control this eye movement.

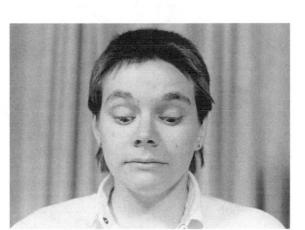

▲ **Figure 8.17** The left and right inferior rectus muscles control this eye movement.

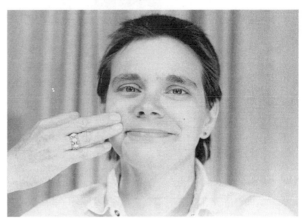

▲ **Figure 8.19** Location of the major and minor zygomatic muscles.

rior rectus, oculomotor; medial rectus, oculomotor; inferior oblique, oculomotor.

Muscles of the Mouth

ORBICULARIS ORIS

The orbicularis oris muscle is a sphincter with a wide distribution of muscle fibers that encircle the mouth extending onto the cheeks. The function of the muscle is to close the lips or pucker the lips as in kissing. It also helps to hold food between the teeth during mastication.

Palpation. Palpate above and below the lips (Fig. 8-18).

Movement. Close and protrude the lips.

Innervation. Facial nerve, buccal branches.

MAJOR AND MINOR ZYGOMATIC MUSCLES

The zygomatic muscles extend from the lateral angle of the mouth upward and laterally over the cheek.

Palpation. Palpate lateral to the angle of the mouth (Fig. 8-19).

Movement. Raise the corners of the mouth upward and laterally as in smiling.

Innervation. Facial nerve, buccal branches.

LEVATOR ANGULI ORIS MUSCLE

The levator anguli oris muscle is located at the angle of the mouth and extends superiorly, intermingling with other facial muscles. It lies deep to the zygomatic muscle and therefore is not easily palpated.

Palpation. Palpate on the upper lip at the angle of the mouth (Fig. 8-20).

Movement. Raise the upper border of the lip straight up as in sneering and showing the canine tooth.

Innervation. Facial nerve, buccal branches.

RISORIUS MUSCLE

The risorius muscle is extremely thin, extending laterally from the angle of the mouth. The function of the muscle is to produce the facial expression of grinning.

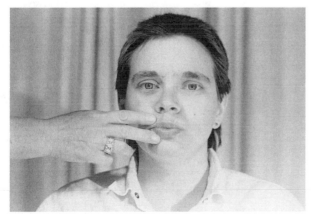

▲ **Figure 8.18** Location of the orbicularis oris muscle.

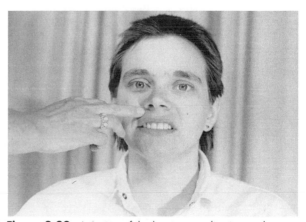

▲ **Figure 8.20** Location of the levator anguli oris muscle.

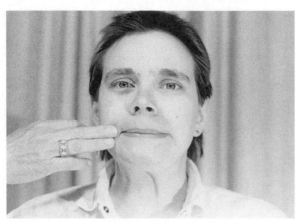

▲ **Figure 8.21** Location of the risorius muscle.

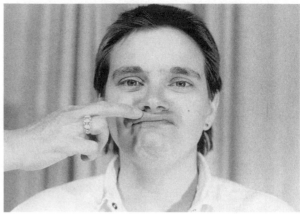

▲ **Figure 8.23** Location of the levator labii superioris muscle.

Palpation. Palpate the lateral angle of the mouth (Fig. 8-21).

Movement. Draw the corners of the mouth laterally.

Innervation. Facial nerve, mandibular and buccal branches.

BUCCINATOR MUSCLE

The buccinator muscle lies deep in the cheek region. A thin, flat muscle, it aids in mastication by pressing the cheeks against the teeth during chewing. The buccinator is also used in sucking or blowing when the cheeks are compressed against the teeth.

Palpation. Palpate lateral to the angle of the mouth (Fig. 8-22).

Movement. Press the cheeks firmly against the teeth.

Innervation. Facial nerve, buccal branches.

LEVATOR LABII SUPERIORIS MUSCLE

The levator labii superioris muscle extends from the superior border of the upper lip to the cheek lateral

to the nose. It functions to raise the upper lip. A few people are able to use this muscle to evert the upper lip as chimpanzees do.

Palpation. Palpate lateral to the midline of the upper lip (Fig. 8-23).

Movement. Protrude and elevate the upper lip.

Innervation. Facial nerve, buccal branches.

DEPRESSOR ANGULI ORIS AND PLATYSMA MUSCLES

The depressor anguli oris muscle is located inferior to the angle of the mouth extending onto the chin. The platysma muscle extends from the cheek area over the clavicle onto the anterior chest wall. These muscles tense the skin of the chin and neck as in shaving and draw down the corners of the mouth. The platysma assists in depressing the mandible.

Palpation. Palpate the anterior lateral neck and inferior lateral to the lower lip (Figs. 8-24 and 8-25).

Movement. Draw the corner of the mouth downward and tense the skin over the neck.

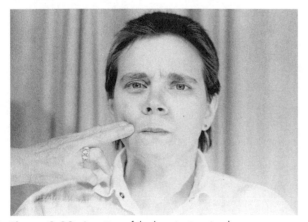

▲ **Figure 8.22** Location of the buccinator muscle.

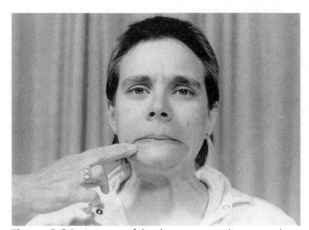

▲ **Figure 8.24** Location of the depressor anguli oris muscle.

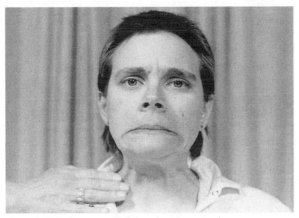

▲ **Figure 8.25** Location of the platysma muscle.

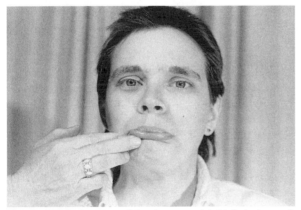

▲ **Figure 8.26** Location of the depressor labii inferioris muscle.

Innervation. Facial nerve, cervical for the platysma and buccal and mandibular for the depressor anguli oris.

DEPRESSOR LABII INFERIORIS MUSCLE

The depressor labii inferioris muscle protrudes the lower lip. It is located below the lower lip.

Palpation. Palpate below the lower lip and lateral to the midline (Fig. 8-26).

Movement. Protrude the lower lip, as in pouting.

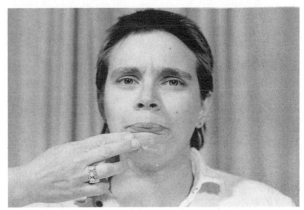

▲ **Figure 8.27** Location of the mentalis muscle.

Innervation. Facial nerve, buccal branches.

MENTALIS MUSCLE

The mentalis muscle is located in the midline of the chin. It wrinkles the skin on the chin, as when a person is about to cry.

Palpation. Midline of chin (Fig. 8-27).

Movement. Raise the skin on the chin.

Innervation. Facial nerve, mandibular branches.

Muscles of Mastication

TEMPORALIS MUSCLE

The temporalis muscle is thick and fan-shaped, covering the temporal region of the head. It performs the function of closing the jaw, moving the mandible to the same side as in chewing and grinding food. The starting position is with the mouth relaxed, partially open.

Palpation. Palpate the side of the head in the region over the temporal bone (Fig. 8-28).

Movement. Elevate and retract the mandible.

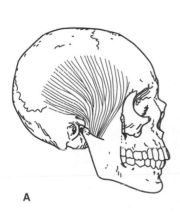

A

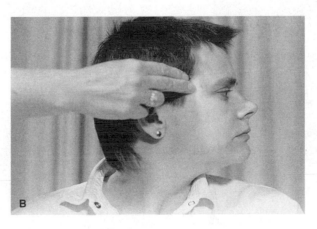

B

▲ **Figure 8.28 (A & B)** Location of the temporalis muscle.

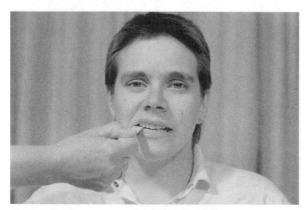

▲ **Figure 8.29** Resistance applied by pulling on a tongue depressor.

Resistance. Applied with a tongue depressor placed between the teeth and pulled out after the movement has occurred. Test both sides (Fig. 8-29).

MASSETER MUSCLE

The name of the masseter muscle comes from the Greek word meaning "masticator," or "chewer." The thick quadrate muscle is located on the side of the mandible. It elevates and helps to protract the mandible and clenches the teeth. The starting test position is with the mouth relaxed and partially open.

Palpation. Palpate the cheek above the angle of the mandible (Fig. 8-30).

Movement. Elevate the mandible, as in closing the jaw.

Resistance. Applied to the mandible using a tongue blade.

LATERAL PTERYGOID MUSCLE

The lateral pterygoid muscle has two short heads that have horizontal fibers. The muscle is deep. It lies on the medial side of the mandible and protracts the mandible and moves the jaw toward the opposite side, as in grinding and chewing.

Palpation. Palpate the pterygoid at its attachment to the neck of the mandible and joint capsule.

Movement. Acting together, the pterygoids protrude and depress the jaw (Figs. 8-31 to 8-33).

Resistance. Applied to the anterior surface of the chin.

MEDIAL PTERYGOID MUSCLE

The medial pterygoid muscle is thick and square, with two heads. The fibers run in a vertical plane. The muscle elevates the jaw.

▼ Attachments of Temporalis Muscle			
Muscle	**Proximal**	**Distal**	**Innervation**
Temporalis	Floor of temporal fossa	Coronoid process and anterior ramus of mandible	Mandibular division of trigeminal nerve

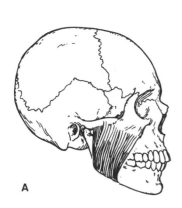

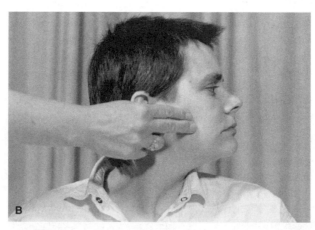

A **B**

▲ **Figure 8.30** **(A & B)** Location of the masseter muscle.

▼ Attachments of Masseter Muscle			
Muscle	**Proximal**	**Distal**	**Innervation**
Masseter	Inferior and deep surface of zygomatic arch	Lateral ramus and coronoid process of mandible	Mandibular division of trigeminal nerve

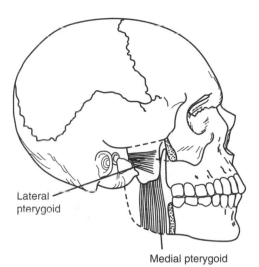

▲ **Figure 8.31** Pterygoid muscles.

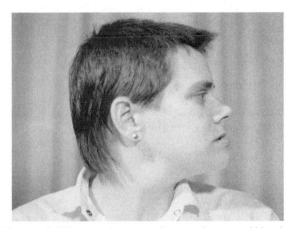

▲ **Figure 8.32** Lateral pterygoid protruding mandible—lateral view.

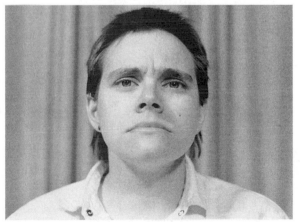

▲ **Figure 8.33** Lateral pterygoid protruding mandible—anterior view.

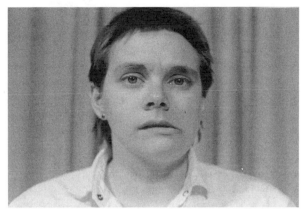

▲ **Figure 8.34** Right medial and lateral pterygoid muscles moving the mandible toward the left side.

Palpation. The medial pterygoid is deep; palpate inside the mouth.

Movement. Elevate and protrude the mandible (Fig. 8-34).

Resistance. Applied to the mandible.

SUPRAHYOID MUSCLES: MYLOHYOID, GENIOHYOID, STYLOHYOID, DIGASTRIC

The suprahyoid muscles lie superior to the hyoid bone and attach it to the skull. Their function is to elevate the hyoid bone and the larynx for swallowing and speaking. Collectively, the muscles also depress the mandible (Fig. 8-35).

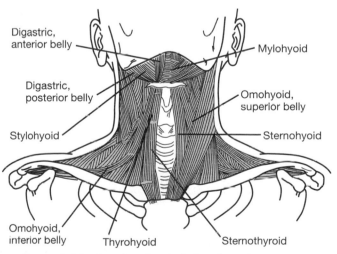

▲ **Figure 8.35** Suprahyoid and infrahyoid muscles.

▼ **Attachments of Lateral Pterygoid Muscle**			
Muscle	**Proximal**	**Distal**	**Innervation**
Lateral pterygoid	Greater wing of sphenoid and lateral pterygoid plate	Neck of mandible and articular cartilage	Mandibular division of trigeminal nerve

▼ Attachments of Medial Pterygoid Muscle

Muscle	Proximal	Distal	Innervation
Medial pterygoid	Medial surface of lateral pterygoid plate and tuberosity of maxilla	Medial surface of mandible close to angle	Mandibular division of trigeminal nerve

Palpation. Palpate the floor of the mouth (Fig. 8-36).

Movement. Press the tip of the tongue against the front teeth.

Resistance. Applied to the surface of the hyoid bone in an effort to protrude the tongue.

INFRAHYOID MUSCLES: STERNOHYOID, THYROHYOID, OMOHYOID, STERNOTHYROID

The infrahyoid muscles are often called strap muscles because of their thin, straplike appearance. As their name implies, they attach to the hyoid bone and stabilize it against the upward pull of the suprahyoid muscles and depress the hyoid bone and larynx during swallowing and speaking.

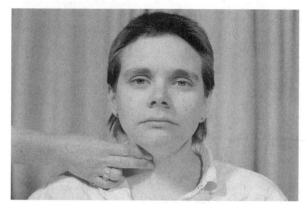

▲ **Figure 8.37** Infrahyoid muscle contraction during swallowing.

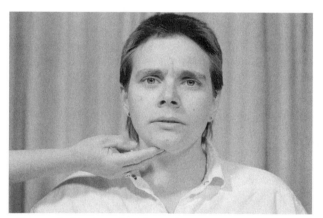

▲ **Figure 8.36** Suprahyoid muscle contraction during resisted tongue protrusion.

Palpation. Palpate below the hyoid bone immediately lateral to the midline (Fig. 8-37).

Movement. Depress the hyoid following swallowing or speaking.

Resistance. None is applied; the movement of the larynx and hyoid bone are observed.

CLINICAL ASSESSMENT

Observation and Screening

The biomechanical relationship between the TMJ and cervical spine, in addition to the effects of postural abnormalities on these regions, necessitates careful evaluation of all three components. Specific

▼ Attachments of Suprahyoid Muscles

Muscle	Proximal	Distal	Innervation
Mylohyoid	Medial surface of mandible	Body of hyoid bone	Mylohyoid branch of trigeminal nerve, mandibular division
Geniohyoid	Mental spine of mandible	Body of hyoid bone	Ventral ramus of C1 by way of hypoglossal nerve
Stylohyoid	Styloid process of temporal bone	Body of hyoid bone	Facial nerve
Anterior and posterior digastric	Internal surface of mandible and mastoid process of temporal bone	By intermediate tendon to hyoid bone	Anterior, mylohyoid branch of trigeminal nerve Posterior, facial

▼ **Attachments of Infrahyoid Muscles**

Muscle	Proximal	Distal	Innervation
Sternohyoid	Manubrium and medial end of clavicle	Body of hyoid bone	Ansa cervicalis
Omohyoid	Superior angle of scapula	Inferior body of hyoid bone	Ansa cervicalis
Sternothyroid	Posterior surface of manubrium	Thyroid cartilage	Ansa cervicalis
Thyrohyoid	Thyroid cartilage	Inferior body and greater horn of hyoid bone	C1 by way of hypoglossal

examination procedures of the cervical spine and posture analysis can be found in those chapters within this text.

Initial observation of the subject with suspected TMJ abnormalities should include analysis of facial symmetry. Both soft tissue and bony contours of the face should be examined for symmetry between left and right halves. Special attention should be given to evidence of muscular paralysis, such as ptosis of the eyelid or drooping of the mouth, which may be associated with Bell's palsy. Additionally, the face can be divided into three equal segments from top to bottom. The upper third of the face encompasses the area from the hairline (frontal crease) to the superior aspect of the nasal bone (bipupital line). The middle third extends from the superior border of the nasal bone to the inferior nose, while the lower third runs from the inferior nose to the chin (Fig. 8-38).

The tongue should be examined for the presence of bite marks or scalloping (tongue resting between teeth) resulting from the tongue not properly resting on the hard palate or from the tongue being excessively wide. Abnormalities of the tongue, including dryness or a whitish appearance, may indicate medical problems in the form of bacterial infections, dysfunction of the salivary glands, or adverse reaction to certain medications. The tongue should also be assessed for normal mobility (Fig. 8-39).

The teeth should be examined for orthodontic appliances, dentures, wear patterns, and evidence of bruxing. Missing teeth should also be identified as possibly contributing to alteration of biting and chewing patterns, and subsequent TMJ and muscular dysfunction. The examiner should also determine whether the upper and lower lip frenulums are properly aligned.

Abnormalities in occlusion (malocclusion) resulting in a faulty bite are sometimes present in people with TMJ dysfunction. An overbite occurs when the anterior maxillary teeth extend below the anterior mandibular teeth when the jaw is in centric occlusion. A crossbite is identified when the mandibular teeth protrude further anteriorly than the maxillary teeth.

The examiner can listen to the TMJ with a stethoscope placed over the joint, as the subject opens and closes the mouth. Normally, a single, solid occlusion sound is heard, but a slipping sound is heard when the teeth are not coming together simultaneously. Crepitus, usually heard during the end stage of opening, may be associated with arthritic changes, as apparent roughening of the condyle and articular eminence is present. Crepitus is also a finding in subjects with a hole in the disk. Subluxation of the disk commonly results in a simultaneous clicking sound. Clicking during opening or closing often represents pathomechanics involving the disk-condyle relationship but may also indicate muscular imbalances.

Other relevant information that can be provided by the subject includes the description of any painful or sensitive areas in the mouth that could result in the alteration of chewing and biting patterns. A history of pipe smoking, gum chewing, nail biting, or any other habit in which excessive or abnormal stresses are imposed to the TMJ may be relevant to determining the source of the subject's complaints.

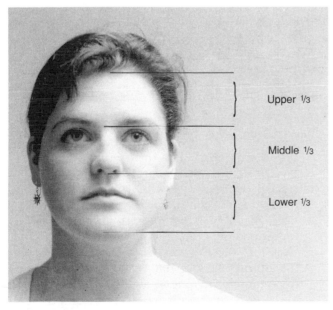

▲ **Figure 8.38** Facial thirds.

Upper ⅓

Middle ⅓

Lower ⅓

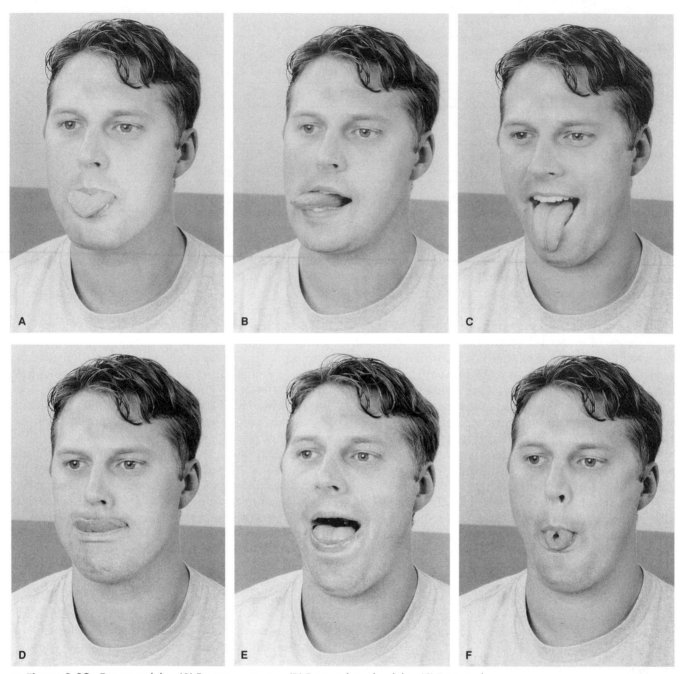

▲ **Figure 8.39** Tongue mobility. **(A)** Extrinsic protrusion. **(B)** Extrinsic lateral mobility. **(C)** Extrinsic depression. **(D)** Extrinsic elevation. **(E)** Intrinsic mobility. **(F)** Intrinsic protrusion.

Palpation and Surface Anatomy

The palpation of structures associated with the TMJ includes the temporomandibular ligament, the lateral capsule, and the retrodiscal tissue in the posterolateral aspect of the joint. Palpation is performed with the subject's mouth alternately closed and open, in the following manner:

1. With the subject's mouth open, place the index or fifth fingers bilaterally into the external auditory meati with the palmar portion of the fin-

ger forward (Fig. 8-40). Instruct the subject to close the mouth. When the examiner feels the condyle against the finger, the TMJ is in its resting, or "freeway space," position, in which the space between the upper and lower front teeth should be 2 to 4 mm. Anything greater represents hypermobility of both TMJs.

2. With the subject's mouth open, palpate around the lateral pole and along the line of the temporomandibular ligament, and include the tissues in the posterolateral portion of the joint cavity. The temporomandibular ligament originates at

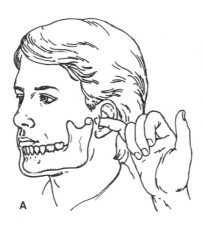

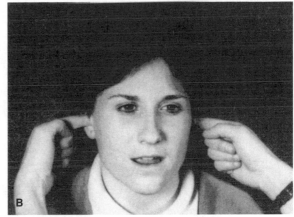

▲ **Figure 8.40** Palpation of the temporomandibular joint. **(A)** With little finger; **(B)** with index finger.

the inferior aspect of the zygomatic arch and travels obliquely and posteroinferiorly.

3. With the subject's mouth closed, palpate for joint effusion around the lateral pole and along the temporomandibular ligament.

Other structures that should be observed or palpated include the following:

1. Examine the mandible for left-to-right symmetry. Measure the distance between the posterior aspect of the TMJ and the notch of the chin for symmetry (Fig. 8-41).
2. Palpate the hyoid bone for normal, painless movement while the subject swallows. The hyoid can be found anterior to C2,3 vertebrae (Fig. 8-42).
3. The thyroid cartilage, located anterior to the C4,5 vertebrae, can be easily palpated and moved with the neck in a neutral position. Crepitation of this structure may be felt when the neck is in a backward-bending position and the thyroid cartilage becomes taut.
4. Palpate the mastoid processes for symmetry.
5. Palpate the bony landmarks of the cervical spine, including the spinous processes, transverse processes, and facet joints.

6. Palpate the musculature of the cervical region, including the suboccipital muscles, sternocleidomastoid, scalenes, and platysma.
7. Palpate the muscles of mastication for symmetry and function. These muscles include the lateral pterygoid, medial pterygoid, masseter, and temporalis muscles (Fig. 8-43).
8. Assess the tongue for resting position, movements, frenulum length, and size. A large tongue exerts excessive pressure against the teeth and may interfere with dental occlusion. A small tongue exerts too little pressure on the teeth. A short frenulum may interfere with tongue function.

Active and Passive Movements

ACTIVE MOVEMENTS

The active movements that should be assessed as part of the evaluation of the TMJ region include:

1. The opening and closing of the mouth
2. Lateral excursion of the mandible
3. Protrusion of the mandible

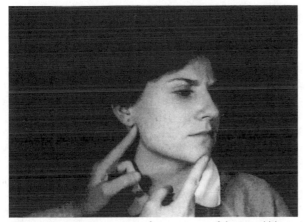

▲ **Figure 8.41** Measurement for symmetry of the mandible.

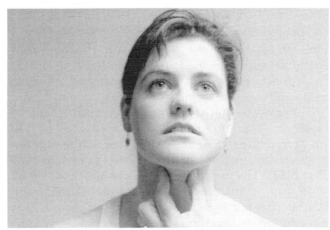

▲ **Figure 8.42** Palpation of the hyoid bone.

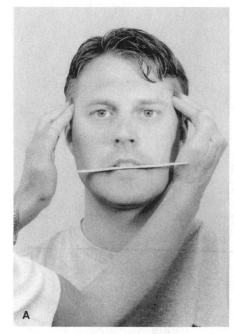
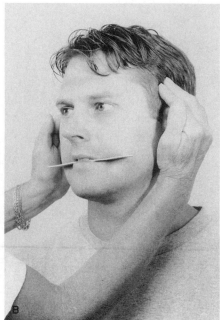
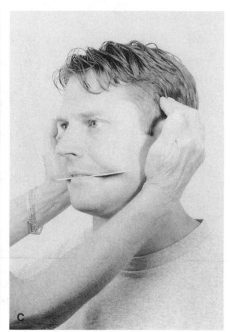

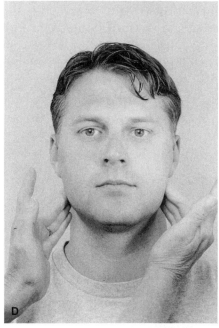

▲ **Figure 8.43** Palpation of muscles of mastication. (**A**) Anterior fibers of temporalis muscle. (**B**) Middle fibers of temporalis muscle. (**C**) Posterior fibers of temporalis muscle. (**D**) Posterior digastric muscle.

Opening and Closing the Mouth. Normally, when a person opens and closes the mouth, the movement of the mandible is fluid and smooth because both TMJs function symmetrically. The normal mandible opens and closes in a linear manner at the midline.

The subject's ability to open the mouth should be assessed. Mandibular opening is measured in millimeters, using a ruler or Boley gauge, as the distance between the incisors of the maxilla and mandible (Fig. 8-44). The normal range of opening is about 35 to 45 mm. A quick way to determine normal mandibular opening is to have the subject place two or three flexed proximal interphalangeal joints into the open mouth (Fig. 8-45).

If hypomobility of one TMJ is present, the mandible will deviate in a C to that side of the open mouth. The subject who demonstrates an S movement of the jaw while opening the mouth is probably suffering from a muscle imbalance. A subject's inability to open the mouth initially indicates a lack of rotation of the TMJ.

With the mouth closed, the mandible should remain in the midline, and the midpoints of the upper teeth should meet those of the lower teeth (Fig. 8-46).

Lateral Excursion of the Mandible. The subject is asked to move the mandible as far as possible to one side and then the other. Measurement of lateral ex-

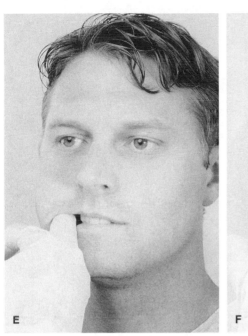
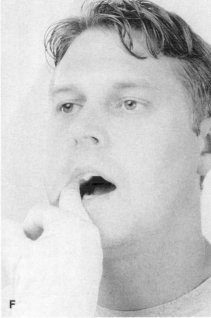
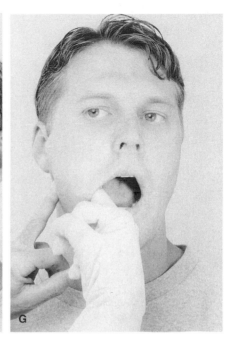

▲ **Figure 8.43** (continued) **(E)** Medial pterygoid muscle. **(F)** Lateral pterygoid muscle. **(G)** Simultaneous palpation of medial pterygoid and masseter muscles.

cursion is based on the distance from a midline point (zero position) located between the maxillary incisors to the most deviated mandibular point between the mandibular incisors (Fig. 8-47). If lateral excursion of the mandible is noted when the subject's mouth is open, the amount of excursion should be measured.

Contralateral structures that are implicated as a cause of lateral deviation include the disk; the masseter, temporalis, and lateral pterygoid muscles; and the temporomandibular ligament.

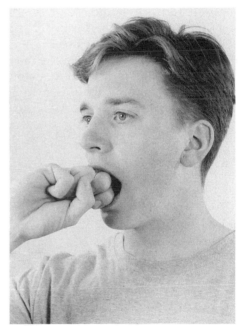

▲ **Figure 8.45** Functional measurement of mouth opening.

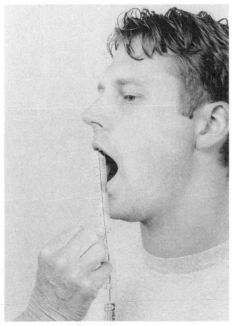

▲ **Figure 8.44** Measurement of mouth opening.

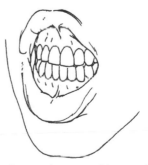

▲ **Figure 8.46** Correct alignment of the mandible and teeth.

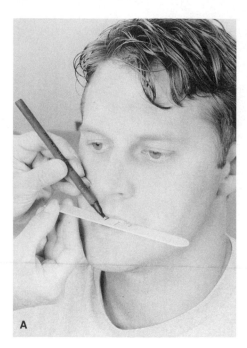
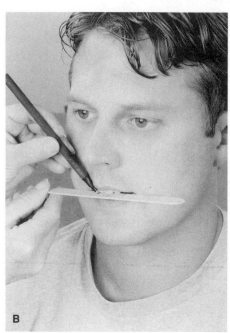

▲ **Figure 8.47** **(A)** Right lateral mandibular excursion measurement. **(B)** Left lateral mandibular excursion measurement.

Protrusion of the Mandible. The subject is directed to protrude the mandible, a motion that should be readily and easily performed. Normal protrusion, 5 mm, is determined by measuring the distance from the maxillary incisors to the mandibular incisors in the protruded position (Fig. 8-48). Abnormal protrusion to one side may also indicate involvement of the structures associated with lateral excursion (see above).

Retrusion, the close packed position of the TMJ, normally measures 3 to 4 mm.

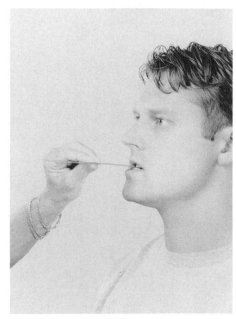

▲ **Figure 8.48** Measurement of mandibular protrusion.

PASSIVE MOVEMENTS

The usual indication for passive motion assessment is to determine the end feel in the open and closed positions. In the closed position, there should normally be a hard end feel as a result of the teeth coming together. The end feel with the mouth open is equivalent to a tissue stretch.

Contractile Tests

LOADING (FORCED BITING)

Loading may be accomplished by having the subject bite down with force onto a soft object, such as a cotton roll placed between the posterior teeth (Fig. 8-49). This motion causes compression of the condyle onto the articular eminence on the opposite side and

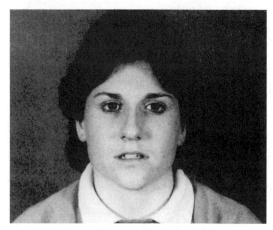

▲ **Figure 8.49** Forced biting.

a distraction of those structures on the same side. This maneuver can have two outcomes:

1. Complaints of increased pain on the side of forced biting indicate tension forces on the capsule and ligament.
2. No complaint of increased pain on the side of forced biting represents reduction of the load on retrodiscal tissue.

LOADING (FORCED RETRUSION)

The examiner pushes the anterior tip of the subject's mandible in a posterior and superior direction (Fig. 8-50). The initial force is delivered through the midline, the second to the right, and the third to the left. This test is used to assess retrodiscal tissues, but it may provide false-negative results (no pain) if the strong muscles of mastication inhibit mandibular motion.

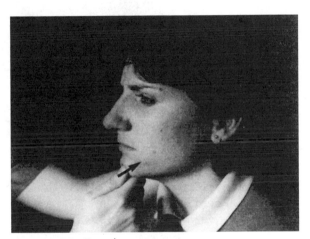

▲ **Figure 8.50** Forced retrusion.

SPECIAL CLINICAL TESTS

JAW REFLEX

Indication. The jaw reflex is tested to assess the integrity of the trigeminal nerve.

Method. The subject's mouth is relaxed and open in the resting posture. The examiner places a thumb on the mandible, then lightly taps the thumb with the pointed end of the reflex hammer (Fig. 8-51).

Results. A normal response is one in which the mouth closes.

CHVOSTEK TEST

Indication. This test is used to determine the integrity of the facial nerve (seventh cranial nerve).

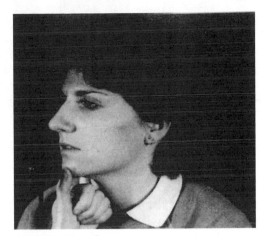

▲ **Figure 8.51** Jaw reflex.

Method. The examiner taps the parotid gland, which overlies the masseter muscle (Fig 8-52).

Results. A twitching of the facial muscles during tapping of the parotid gland indicates a positive test.

TESTS OF MUSCLES OF MASTICATION

Successful testing of the muscles of mastication requires that certain principles be observed.

1. The mouth must be open approximately 1 cm during the examination.
2. The head must be supported to prevent movement of the head and rotation of the neck.
3. The force imparted should be applied gradually to ensure a maximum buildup of tension by the subject.
4. Contact with the TMJ should be avoided during the examination so that the subject will not confuse pain associated with contact and pain arising from some dysfunction or pathology.

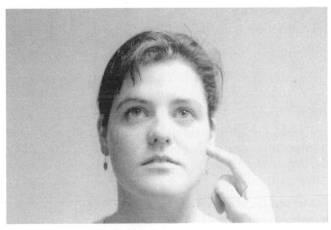

▲ **Figure 8.52** Chvostek test.

Testing the Lateral Pterygoid. The lateral pterygoid is important in opening the mouth. This structure is assessed by having the subject slightly open the mouth and then resist the therapist's attempt to close it forcefully. The musculature involved in closing the mouth is assessed by having the subject's mouth slightly open while the examiner attempts to open it further. The examiner places the thumbs on the lower anterior teeth and applies a downward force.

Testing the Medial and Lateral Pterygoid Muscles. Both the lateral and medial pterygoid muscles may be tested by assessing lateral excursion of the mandible. The medial pterygoid also elevates the mandible. The upper head of the lateral pterygoid influences the relationship between the condyle and the disk. The lower head of the lateral pterygoid protrudes and deviates the mandible to the opposite side. Protrusion of the mandible may also be accomplished by bilateral contraction of the lateral pterygoid.

Testing the Medial Pterygoid and Musculature Involved in Opening the Jaw. The subject is relaxed, with the mouth slightly open and the jaw slightly protruded. The examiner supports the head while attempting to move the jaw posteriorly as the subject resists. The medial pterygoid also elevates the mandible.

Testing the Digastric and Posterior Fibers of the Temporalis. The subject resists the attempt by the examiner to move the mandible forward by pushing anteriorly on the lingual surface of the lower anterior teeth. The anterior digastric muscle is also involved in the function of mandibular depression, while the temporalis also elevates the mandible.

JOINT PLAY (ACCESSORY MOVEMENT)

Distraction (Fig. 8-53)

Restriction. General hypomobility.

Open-Packed Position. The subject is seated with back and shoulders supported and mouth slightly open.

Fixed Segment. Examiner stabilizes subject's head (temporal bone) with one hand, placing the ulnar border of the little finger just superior to the joint space of the TMJ.

Moving Segment. With the other hand, the examiner holds the ramus of the mandible with the radial

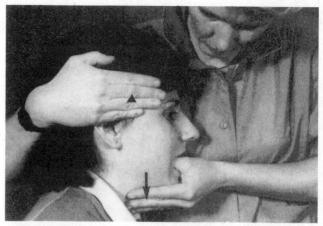

▲ **Figure 8.53** Distraction of the TMJ.

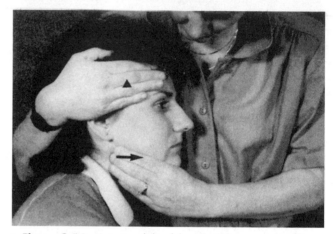

▲ **Figure 8.54** Anterior glide of the mandible.

side of the index finger while placing the thumb inside the mouth onto the lower molars.

Anterior Glide (Fig 8-54)

Restriction. Inability to open mouth fully.

Open-Packed Position. Subject is seated with back and shoulders supported and mouth slightly open.

Fixed Segment. Examiner holds subject's head (temporal bone) with one hand, placing the ulnar border of the little finger just superior to the joint space of the TMJ.

Moving Segment. Examiner grasps the subject's mandible with the other hand, with the fingers pointed posteriorly and gripping the angle of the mandible.

Medial-Lateral Glide (Fig. 8-55)

Restriction. Lateral excursion.

Open-Packed Position. Subject is supine with mouth slightly open.

TABLE 8.1	**Summary of TMJ Play**		
GLIDE	RESTRICTION	FIXED BONE	MOVING BONE
Distraction	General hypomobility	Temporal	Mandible
Anterior	Inability to open mouth fully	Temporal	Mandible
Medial-lateral	Lateral deviation	Temporal	Mandible

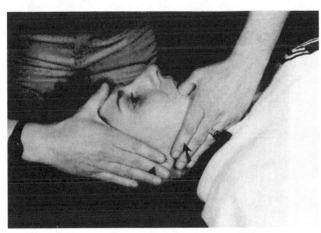

▲ **Figure 8.55** Medial-lateral glide of the mandible.

Fixed Segment. Examiner's one hand holds subject's head (temporal bone), with the distal interphalangeal joints of the fingers just superior to the joint space.

Moving Segment. Examiner's other hand is placed along the mandible with the thenar eminence immediately inferior to the joint space.

Summary of Joint Play of the Temporomandibular Joint

Table 8-1 provides a summary of TMJ play.

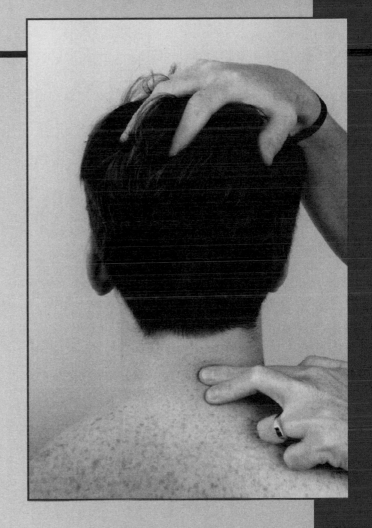

Cervical Spine

The vertebrae serve many important functions. They protect the spinal cord and assist in breathing and swallowing. They provide a base of support for the head and internal organs and indirect attachments for the limbs. They allow mobility for the trunk. The articulations for each vertebra are numerous. The bodies articulate with each other, and the articulations are cushioned by intervertebral disks. The vertebral arches articulate through the superior and inferior articulating facets. The facet joints are plane synovial joints and have three degrees of freedom of motion. The articulation with the intervertebral disks permits minimal motion and is referred to as a symphysis type of amphiarthrodial joint.

The atlanto-occipital joint has two degrees of freedom of motion—flexion and extension and lateral bending. The atlantoaxial articulation produces the primary motion of rotation. The direction of motion permitted in the remaining vertebrae depends on the direction of the facets (except for the sacrum, the segments of which are fused). The sacrum articulates with the ilium, and the sacroiliac joint is capable of a limited amount of flexion and extension. The vertebrae are reinforced by intersegmental and intrasegmental ligaments and muscles.

GONIOMETRY

Cervical Vertebrae

CERVICAL FLEXION

Flexion in the sagittal plane occurs between all cervical vertebrae, the occipital bone, and the upper five to seven thoracic vertebrae (T5–T7). The majority of the movement occurs between the superior and inferior facet joints followed by movement between the intervertebral disks.

Motion

- Preferred: From 0 to 45 degrees of neck flexion in the sagittal plane.
- Alternate: When using a measuring tape, 0 in.

Position. Subject sits with the trunk well supported and the neck in the anatomical position. The hands are placed in the lap, and the shoulder joints are relaxed.

Goniometric Alignment (Fig. 9-1)

Axis. Placed over the external auditory meatus.

Stationary Arm. Placed parallel to the floor.

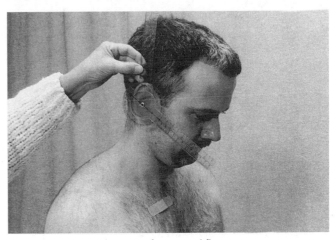
▲ **Figure 9.1** End position for cervical flexion.

Moving Arm. Placed along a line parallel to the inferior border of the nose.

Alternates

1. A bubble or gravity-activated goniometer is fixed to the head over the ear with the base parallel to the top of the ear. The goniometer is set at 0 degrees (Fig. 9-2).
2. The number of inches from the point of the chin to the midpoint of the sternal notch is measured with a tape; the subject's mouth remains closed (Figs. 9-3 and 9-4).
3. The distance in inches from the external occipital protuberance and the spinous process of C7 is measured.

Stabilization. The trunk is stabilized.

Precautions

- Prevent trunk flexion.
- Prevent neck rotation and lateral flexion.

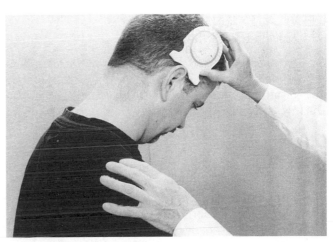
▲ **Figure 9.2** Alternate end position for cervical flexion using a gravity-activated goniometer.

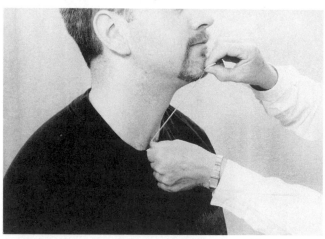

▲ **Figure 9.3** Alternate starting position for cervical flexion using a measuring tape.

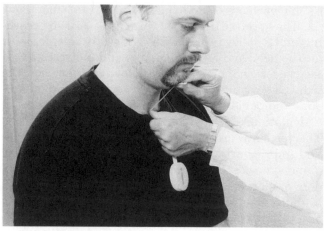

▲ **Figure 9.4** Alternate end position for cervical flexion using a measuring tape.

OCCIPITAL FLEXION

It is difficult for a subject to flex only the occiput without cervical vertebra motion.

Motion. From 0 to 10 or 15 degrees in the sagittal plane. The motion is one of nodding as in tucking the chin without cervical vertebral motions.

Position. Subject sits or is supine with the trunk well supported and the neck in the anatomical position.

Goniometric Alignment. Same as for cervical flexion.

Stabilization. The natural lordosis remains within the cervical vertebra.

Precautions

- Prevent cervical flexion.
- Stabilize the trunk.

CERVICAL EXTENSION AND HYPEREXTENSION

The extension motion is the return from neck flexion. Hyperextension increases the anterior convexity of the cervical vertebrae. The motion occurs in the sagittal plane between the articulating facets of all the cervical vertebrae and at the atlanto-occipital joint.

Motion. From 45 to 0 degrees for extension and 0 to 45 degrees for hyperextension of the cervical vertebrae. When using a measuring tape, the distance is approximately 7 to 10 in from complete flexion into hyperextension of the cervical vertebrae.

Position and goniometric alignment are the same as for cervical flexion (Figs. 9-5 and 9-6).

Alternates

1. The bubble or gravity-activated goniometer is fixed to the head with the base over the top of the ear. The goniometer is set at zero (Fig. 9-7).

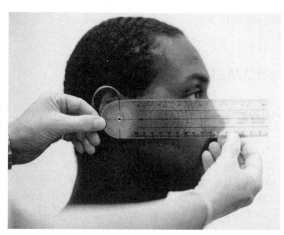

▲ **Figure 9.5** Starting position for cervical extension and hyperextension.

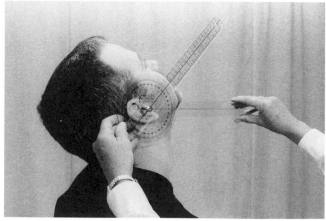

▲ **Figure 9.6** End position for cervical extension and hyperextension.

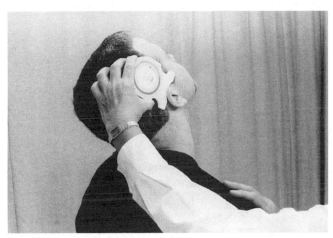

▲ **Figure 9.7** Alternate end position for cervical extension and hyperextension using a gravity-activated angle finder.

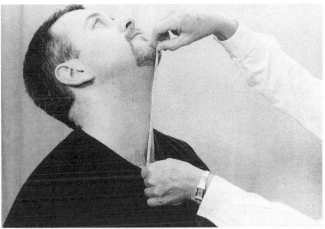

▲ **Figure 9.8** Alternate end position for cervical extension and hyperextension using a measuring tape anteriorly.

2. The tape measure is used to determine the distance in inches between the tip of the chin and the sternal notch (Fig. 9-8).
3. The tape measure is placed from the external occipital protuberance to the spinous process of C7. The difference between the starting and ending positions is the range of motion (Figs. 9-9 and 9-10).

Stabilization. The trunk and shoulder girdle are stabilized.

Precautions

• Prevent trunk flexion.
• Prevent neck lateral flexion and rotation.

OCCIPITAL EXTENSION

Extension of the occiput on the cervical vertebra may be a difficult motion for the subject to perform. This motion occurs in the sagittal plane around an axis through the mastoid processes.

Motion. From 0 to 25 degrees. The subject extends the head by tilting the chin upward.

Position. Subject sits with the trunk well supported, and the natural cervical lordotic curve is maintained.

Goniometric Alignment. The same as for cervical extension.

Stabilization. The cervical vertebra is motionless.

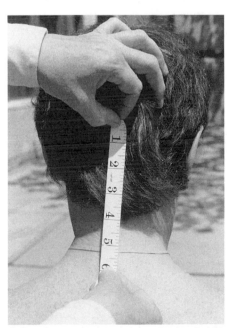

▲ **Figure 9.9** Alternate starting position for cervical extension and hyperextension using a measuring tape.

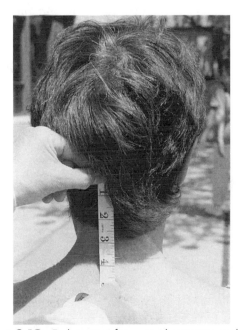

▲ **Figure 9.10** End position for cervical extension and hyperextension using a measuring tape.

Precautions

- Prevent cervical vertebral extension.
- Stabilize the trunk.

CERVICAL ROTATION

Rotation of the cervical vertebrae occurs in the transverse plane. The greatest amount of rotation occurs between the first (atlas) and the second (axis) cervical vertebrae, at the atlantoaxial joint. Rotation does occur between the articulating facets of each of the cervical vertebrae and the intervertebral disks. Cervical vertebral rotation is accompanied by lateral flexion to the same side as the rotation.

Motion. From 0 to 60 to 75 degrees of cervical rotation in each direction. The distance is approximately 5 in to each side, as measured by tape.

Position. Subject sits with the trunk supported and the neck in the anatomical position. The subject's hands are resting in the lap, and the shoulder joints are relaxed.

Goniometric Alignment (Fig. 9-11)

Axis. Placed over the center of the top of the head.

Stationary Arm. Placed in line with the acromion process of the side being measured.

Moving Arm. Placed in line with the tip of the nose.

Alternate. Place the measuring tape on the midline of the chin and the acromion process. Measure the difference between the starting and ending positions. The difference in the measurement is the amount of range of motion (Fig. 9-12).

Stabilization. The trunk and shoulder girdle are stabilized.

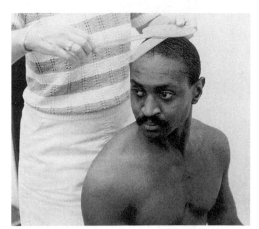

▲ **Figure 9.11** End position for cervical rotation.

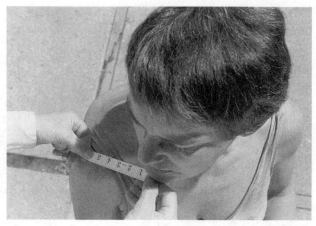

▲ **Figure 9.12** Alternate end position for cervical rotation using a tape measure.

Precautions

- Prevent the trunk from rotating.
- Keep the neck in the transverse plane.
- Prevent scapular elevation.

CERVICAL LATERAL FLEXION

The motion of lateral flexion occurs in the frontal plane. The lateral flexion motion is more or less equally distributed among all the joints of the cervical vertebrae. It is accompanied by rotation of the vertebrae to the same side because of the stretch of the soft-tissue structures.

Motion. From 0 to 45 to 60 degrees of cervical joint lateral flexion. Using a measuring tape, the distance between the starting and ending positions is approximately 5 in to each side.

Position. Subject sits with the trunk supported and the neck in the anatomical position. The hands lie in the lap, and the shoulder girdle joints are relaxed.

Goniometric Alignment (Fig. 9-13)

Axis. Placed over the spinous process of C7.

Stationary Arm. Placed along the thoracic spinous processes.

Moving Arm. Placed over the external occipital protuberance of the occipital bone.

Alternates

1. The lower edge of a bubble goniometer is centered over the external occipital protuberance (Fig. 9-14).

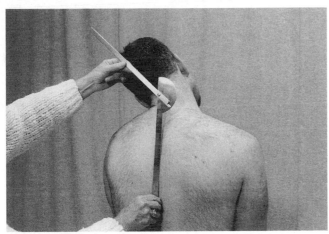

▲ **Figure 9.13** End position for cervical lateral flexion.

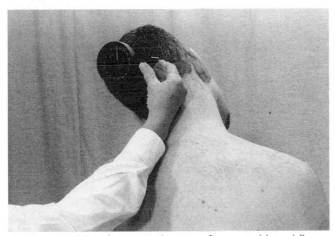

▲ **Figure 9.14** Alternate end position for cervical lateral flexion using a gravity-activated angle finder.

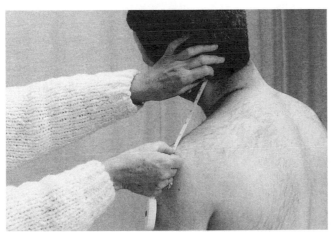

▲ **Figure 9.15** Alternate end position for cervical lateral flexion using a tape measure.

2. A tape measure is used to measure the distance between the mastoid process of the temporal bone and the acromion process of the scapula. An average amount of lateral flexion motion is approximately 5 in (Fig. 9-15).

Stabilization. The upper trunk and shoulder girdle are stabilized.

Precautions

- Prevent shoulder elevation on the test side.
- Prevent upper trunk lateral flexion to the test side.

MUSCLE LENGTH TESTING

Cervical Lateral Flexion (Sidebending)

Limitations of neck and trunk motions may occur as a result of bony impingements or of muscles that are too tight for a desired motion. Muscles are considered multijoint and contract in the three planes of movement because they cross the individual cervical vertebra. Cervical lateral flexion is accompanied by rotation to the same side. The muscles showing a decrease in length that are assessed are the levator scapulae, anterior, middle, and posterior scalene, sternocleidomastoid, upper trapezius, splenius capitis, and cervicis.

LEVATOR SCAPULAE MUSCLE

Position. The subject is in a sitting position with the shoulder joint abducted so that the scapula is in an upwardly rotated position. The head and neck are in the anatomical position.

Movement. The examiner laterally flexes the head to the opposite side of the abducted shoulder, maintaining the upward rotation of the scapula.

Measurement. Use any of the methods that are indicated for lateral flexion in the goniometry section (Fig. 9-16).

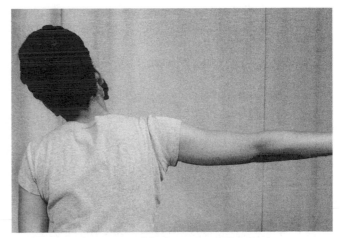

▲ **Figure 9.16** Testing of the levator scapulae muscle.

Considerations

- The levator scapulae muscle may show limitations in length during rotation of the neck with the scapulae rotated upwardly.
- The other neck lateral flexor muscles do not attach to the medial side of the scapula; therefore, shoulder position would not be a factor.

ANTERIOR, MIDDLE, AND POSTERIOR SCALENE; STERNOCLEIDOMASTOID; UPPER TRAPEZIUS; AND SPLENIUS CAPITIS AND CERVICIS MUSCLES

Position. The subject is in a sitting position with the shoulder girdle in the anatomical position.

Movement. The examiner flexes the head laterally to one side while the shoulder girdle is stabilized on the opposite side (Fig. 9-17).

Measurement. The same techniques are used as for goniometry.

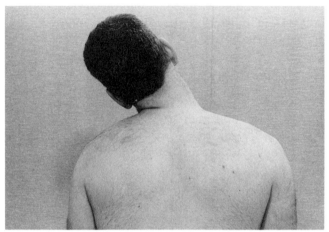

▲ **Figure 9.17** Muscle length testing of right lateral flexor muscle for the cervical region.

Considerations

- The trunk must remain upright and not allowed to flex laterally.
- The shoulder girdle must not elevate on either side during the movement.
- It is difficult to isolate selectively a single muscle of the neck; however, the sternocleidomastoid and upper portions of the trapezius muscles may be assessed as neck rotators.

Cervical Rotators

The rotators of the neck and head also laterally flex. Follow the assessment procedure as outlined previously.

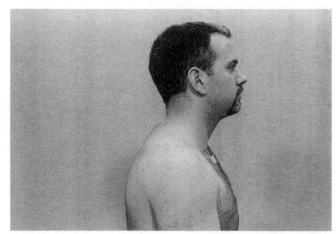

▲ **Figure 9.18** Subject demonstrates a forward head.

CERVICAL FLEXORS

The neck flexor muscles produce motion in the sagittal plane. When the subject's mastoid process lies anterior to the axis of motion, the sternocleidomastoid muscle acts as a cervical flexor; if it does not, the sternocleidomastoid muscle is a cervical extensor. Other anterior cervical muscles that may exhibit tightness are the longus coli, longus capitis, and suprahyoid and infrahyoid muscles. The muscle length assessment cannot be isolated from goniometric measurements (Fig. 9-18). Excessive extension in the cervical vertebra is an increase in the normal anterior curve and results from tilting the head backward, which leads to increased length of the anterior flexor muscles (Fig. 9-19).

Cervical Extensors

The cervical extensor muscles lie posterior to the axis and produce motion in the sagittal plane. The extensor muscles that lie superficial to deep are the

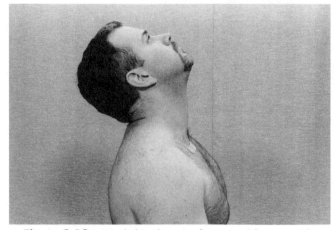

▲ **Figure 9.19** Muscle length testing for cervical flexor muscles.

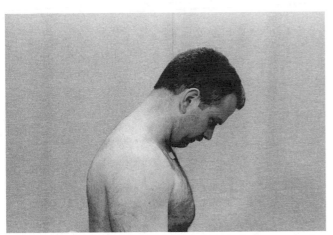

▲ **Figure 9.20** Muscle length testing of cervical extensor muscles.

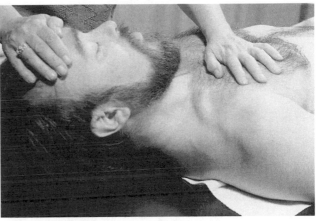

▲ **Figure 9.22** Testing the sternocleidomastoid muscle in the AG supine position.

upper portions of the trapezius, splenius capitis and splenius cervicis, iliocostalis cervicis, longissimus cervicis and capitis, spinalis cervicis and capitis, semispinalis cervicis and capitis, multifidis, rotators longus and brevis, and the suboccipital muscles. The length of these muscles is examined during occipital and cervical flexion. The length of the extensor muscles cannot be isolated from goniometry measurements (Fig. 9-20). Forward head posture is demonstrated with tightness of the cervical extensor muscles (see Fig. 9-18).

MANUAL MUSCLE TESTING

STERNOCLEIDOMASTOID MUSCLES

The sternocleidomastoid muscles produce the basic motion of flexion of the neck in the sagittal plane through a test range of 45 degrees or just beyond the straightening of the lordosis. Usually both sides are tested simultaneously, but they may be tested unilaterally by having the subject rotate to the opposite side.

Palpation. Superficially on the anterolateral aspect of the neck (Fig. 9-21).

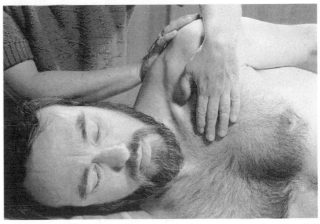

▲ **Figure 9.23** Testing the sternocleidomastoid muscle in the GM sidelying position.

Position

Against gravity (AG): Subject lies supine (Fig. 9-22).

Gravity minimized (GM): Subject is in sidelying position with the head supported on a surface that allows easy motion (Fig. 9-23).

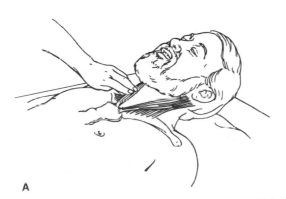

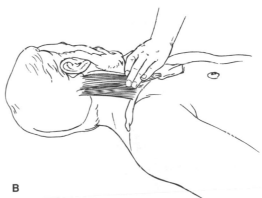

▲ **Figure 9.21** **(A)** Palpation for the sternocleidomastoid muscle in neck flexion. **(B)** Palpation for the sternocleidomastoid muscle during neck flexion with rotation to the opposite side.

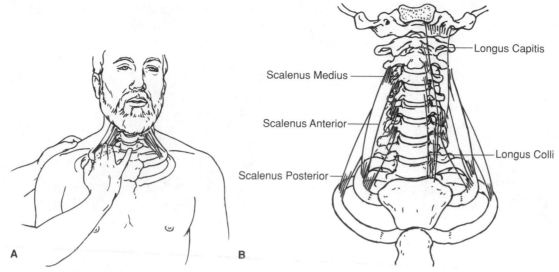

▲ **Figure 9.24** (**A**) Palpation for the anterior, middle, and posterior scalene muscles. (**B**) Location of the scalene muscles.

Movement. Flexion of the neck in the sagittal plane.

Resistance. Applied to the anterior forehead into extension.

Stabilization. The thorax is stabilized.

Substitutions

- Palpate each muscle to be sure that both sternocleidomastoid muscles are functioning.
- Rectus capitis anterior and the rectus capitis lateralis muscles are accessory neck flexors.
- Suprahyoid, infrahyoid, and platysma are also accessory muscles for the motion of neck flexion.
- Scalene muscles and the longus colli and capitis flex the neck.

ANTERIOR, MIDDLE, AND POSTERIOR SCALENE MUSCLES; LONGUS COLLI MUSCLE; LONGUS CAPITIS MUSCLE

The scalene muscles flex the neck when both sides contract simultaneously. Unilaterally, the muscles flex laterally and rotate the neck to the same side. The longus colli and capitis muscles produce neck flexion in the sagittal plane. The starting position is with the neck in extension.

Palpation

Scalene Muscles. Place the fingertips above the clavicle in the triangle formed by the sternocleidomastoid and trapezius muscles. Have the subject force inspiration (Fig. 9-24).

Longus Colli and Longus Capitis. The longus colli and longus capitis muscles are too deep to palpate.

Position

AG: Subject lies supine.
GM: Subject is in sidelying position with the head supported on a surface that allows easy motion.

Movement. Flexion of the neck in the sagittal plane.

Resistance. Applied to the anterior forehead into extension.

Stabilization. The thorax is stabilized.

Substitutions

- Sternocleidomastoid muscle is a neck flexor.
- Rectus capitis anterior, rectus capitis lateralis, suprahyoid and infrahyoid, and platysma muscles also flex the neck.

▼ Attachments of Sternocleidomastoid (Sternal and Clavicular) Muscles			
Muscle	**Proximal**	**Distal**	**Innervation**
Sternocleidomastoid (sternal) (clavicular)	Superior aspect of manubrium sterni medial third of clavicle	Mastoid process	Spinal accessory CN IX

▼ Attachments of Scalene, Longus Colli, and Longus Capitis Muscles

Muscle	Proximal	Distal	Innervation
Scalenus Anterior	Anterior tubercles of C3-6	Superior crest of first rib	Ventral primary rami of cervical spinal nerves
Middle Posterior	Posterior tubercles of C2-7 Posterior tubercles of C5-7	Superior crest of first rib Outer surface of second rib	
Longus colli	Anterior tubercles of C3-5, anterior surface of C5-7, T1-3	Tubercle of the atlas, anterior tubercles of C5 and C6, anterior surface of C2-4	Ventral primary rami of cervical spinal nerves
Longus capitis	Anterior tubercles of C3-6	Inferior occipital bone, basilar portion	Ventral primary rami of cervical spinal nerves

SPLENIUS CAPITIS AND CERVICIS MUSCLES

The splenius capitis and cervicis muscles produce the motion of extension of the neck through a range of 90 degrees, or 10 in from a starting position of 45 degrees of flexion. Usually both sides are tested simultaneously, although they may be tested separately.

Palpation. The splenius capitis and cervicis muscles lie deep to the upper trapezius muscles. Place the fingertips under the lateral border of the upper trapezius muscle. The fibers are directed toward the mastoid process (Fig. 9-25).

Position

AG: Subject lies prone with a pillow under the thorax or with the head over the edge of the treatment table (Fig. 9-26).

GM: Subject is in sidelying position with the head supported on a low-friction surface (Fig. 9-27).

Movement. Extension of the head and neck.

Resistance. Applied to the occiput in a downward and forward direction.

Stabilization. Upper posterior thorax is stabilized.

Substitutions

- Deviations to the left or right indicate that one side is stronger than the other.
- Upper trapezius, erector spinae, and intertransversarii muscles extend the neck.

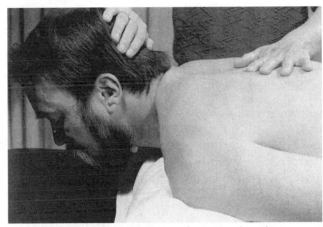

▲ **Figure 9.26** AG prone position for testing the splenius capitis and cervicis muscles.

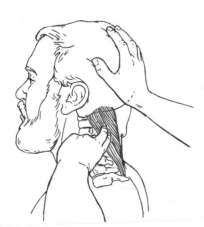

▲ **Figure 9.25** Palpation for the splenius capitis and cervicis muscles.

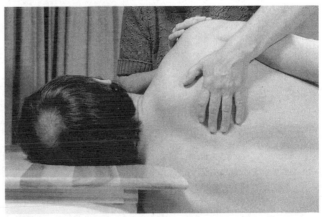

▲ **Figure 9.27** GM sidelying position for testing the splenius capitis and cervicis muscles.

▼ Attachments of Splenius Capitis and Cervicis Muscles			
Muscles	**Proximal**	**Distal**	**Innervation**
Splenius capitis	Inferior ligamentum nuchae, spinous process of C7 and T1-4 vertebrae	Mastoid process, occipital bone, and lateral third of superior nuchal line	Cervical spinal nerve and ventral primary rami of the cervical spinal nerves
Splenius cervicis	Spinous processes of T3-6 vertebrae	Posterior tubercles of C1-3	Cervical spinal nerve and ventral primary rami of the cervical spinal nerves

CLINICAL ASSESSMENT

In addition to examination of the cervical spine itself, the examiner should clear associated areas for dysfunction, including the shoulder girdle, thoracic region (including the thoracic outlet), and temporomandibular joint.

Observation and Screening

Evaluation of sitting and standing posture and identification of postural abnormalities are important in individuals complaining of cervical spine symptoms. Postural abnormalities resulting in muscular imbalances and increased ligamentous stress commonly produce pain in the cervical and upper trunk areas. Refer to Chapter 4 for detailed information on postural assessment.

Using anterior and posterior observation, the examiner can detect deviations of the head away from the midline, occurring secondary to torticollis, cervical spine pain, Klippel-Feil syndrome, or hysteria. Torticollis, resulting from shortening or spasm of the sternocleidomastoid muscle, is manifested in the subject sidebending the neck toward the affected side and rotating the chin toward the uninvolved side. Cervical pain usually results in sidebending and rotation away from the painful side, with the face directed upward. Conversely, subjects with hysteria typically sidebend and rotate toward the painful side, with the face directed downward. An anterior view of the subject allows the examiner to identify certain mandibular asymmetries. It should be noted that asymmetry between shoulder heights, seen in posterior observation, is commonly associated with upper limb dominance with the dominant shoulder being lower.

Lateral observation permits the identification of postural abnormalities, including a forward head; increased or decreased cervical, thoracic, and lumbar curves; and round shoulders. Additionally, protrusion or retrusion of the mandible can be appreciated from this view.

Palpation

The following structures and landmarks should be palpated or observed during cervical spine evaluation (Fig. 9-28). Areas of pain, tenderness, muscle guarding, atrophy, swelling, or congestion should be noted:

1. Spinous processes of C2 through T3*
2. Transverse processes of C1

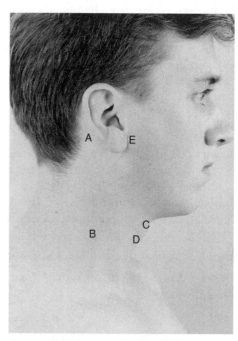

A = Mastoid Process   C = Hyoid Bone
B = Sternocleido-   D = Thyroid Cartilage
     mastoid Muscle   E = TMJ

▲ **Figure 9.28** Surface anatomy of cervical region.

---

* Note: The spinous process of C2 is the first palpable spinous process and is found just inferior to the external occipital protuberance. Forward and backward bending of the cervical spine may make it easier for the examiner to locate this landmark (Fig. 9-29). To differentiate between C6, C7, and T1 spinous processes, locate the first prominent spinous process at the cervicothoracic junction. Palpate the spinous process of the superior vertebra and the interspinous space. Bend the head and neck backward while continuing palpation (Fig 9-30). If the superior spinous process seems to "disappear" in the backward bent position, the C6-7 interspace has been identified. If both spinous processes remain palpable, the C7 to T1 interspace has been identified.

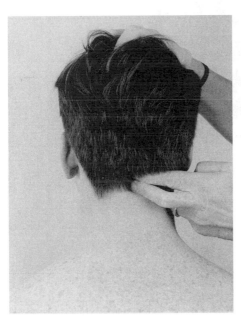

▲ **Figure 9.29** Palpation of spinous processes of the second and third cervical vertebrae.

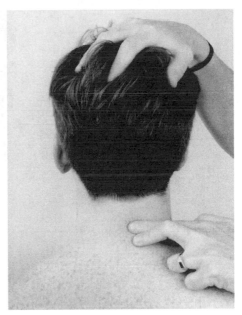

▲ **Figure 9.30** Palpation of spinous processes of the sixth and seventh cervical vertebrae.

3. Mastoid process
4. Angles of the mandible
5. External occipital protuberance
6. Articular pillars
7. Zygapophyseal joints (facet articulations)
8. Carotid (Chassaignac's) tubercle of C6
9. First rib, anterior and posterior attachments
10. Hyoid bone
11. Thyroid cartilage
12. Sternal notch
13. Sternoclavicular articulations
14. Boundaries of anterior and posterior triangles
15. Carotid arteries
16. Trunks of the brachial plexus
17. Scapula
   Superior angle
   Medial (vertebral) border

   Spine
   Acromion process
18. Muscles and their attachment sites
   Trapezius
   Sternocleidomastoid
   Levator scapulae
   Scalenes
   Rhomboids
   Posterior suboccipital muscles

Gross Active and Passive Movements

The motions to be assessed for the active and passive range include the following:

1. Forward bend (Fig. 9-31)
2. Backward bend (Fig. 9-32)

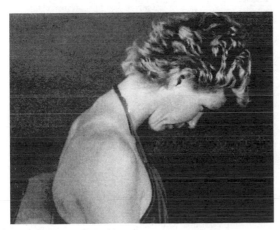

▲ **Figure 9.31** Forward bend.

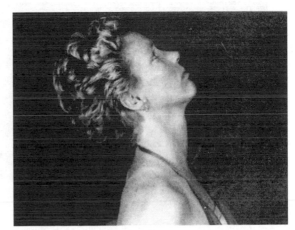

▲ **Figure 9.32** Backward bend.

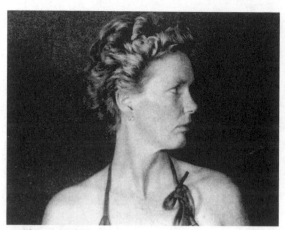
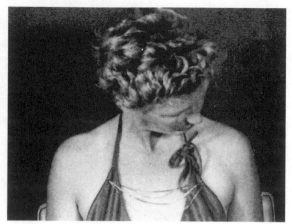

▲ **Figure 9.33** **(A)** Rotation in neutral position. **(B)** Rotation in forward bent position.

3. Right and left rotation in neutral and forward bent positions (Fig. 9-33)
4. Right and left sidebending with rotation to the same and opposite sides (Fig. 9-34). (Note: In true sidebending, the head naturally rotates to the same side. If the subject artificially keeps the head facing forward during sidebending, as is commonly done, rotation in the opposite direction must occur at the atlantoaxial articulation.)

End feel is assessed by gentle overpressure at the end of painless range. Sustained positioning assesses for the onset of latent paresthesia.

Contractile Testing

Contractile testing of the cervical spine should include the following:

1. Forward bending
2. Backward bending
3. Right and left sidebending
4. Right and left rotation

SPECIAL CLINICAL TESTS

VERTEBRAL ARTERY INSUFFICIENCY TESTS

The following four tests all assess vertebrobasilar artery insufficiency. Tests should be performed bilaterally, starting with the side on which no symptoms are expected. A test is terminated immediately with the onset of signs or symptoms, which typically abate when the head is returned to the neutral position. These symptoms include faintness, dizziness, nystagmus, and personality changes. It is suggested that no thrust manipulations be performed if there is a positive result. Also, the vertebral artery should be retested after each manual therapy procedure, because an increase in cervical range of motion may produce a positive result in the new range.

Vertebral Artery Test (Quadrant Test)

Method. Subject lies supine with a pillow beneath the upper and middle thoracic spine. The head is supported by the therapist in a neutral position. The head is brought into sidebending with

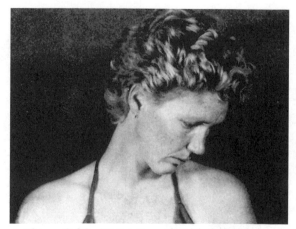
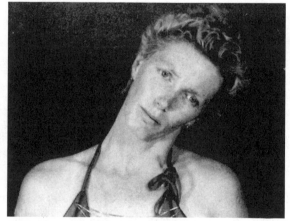

▲ **Figure 9.34** **(A)** Rotation with sidebend to the same side. **(B)** Rotation with sidebend to the opposite side.

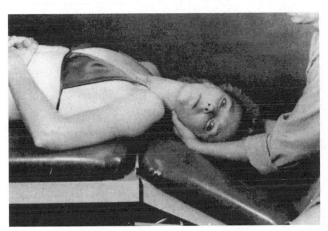

▲ **Figure 9.35** Quadrant test.

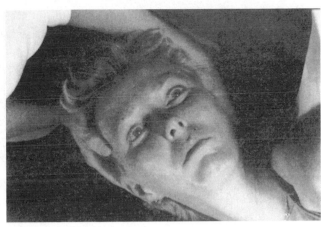

▲ **Figure 9.37** Maigne's test.

rotation to the same side, and the subject is observed for 8 to 12 seconds for signs or symptoms. If there are none, the head is moved into backward bending and again observed for signs or symptoms (Fig. 9-35). The test is terminated immediately if signs or symptoms develop.

Backward Bending Test

Method. With subject and examiner positioned as in the quadrant test, the subject's head is brought into full backward bending, without sidebending or rotation. The subject is observed for signs or symptoms for 8 to 12 seconds (Fig. 9-36).

Maigne's Test

Method. With the subject supine, the examiner brings the head into a position of full backward bending and rotation or into the setup position for the intended manipulation. The subject holds the position for as long as 30 seconds, while the examiner observes and questions the subject for signs and symptoms (Fig. 9-37).

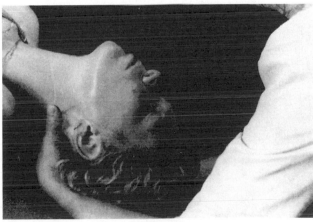

▲ **Figure 9.36** Backward bending test.

Results. The results of these tests are positive if the subject experiences or demonstrates signs of vertigo, nystagmus, slurred speech, tinnitus, nausea, vomiting, syncope, or visual disturbance. The subject's eyes should be open, and the subject should be speaking to be properly assessed. Again, the test is terminated immediately if symptoms are observed.

Hautant's Test

Indication. Hautant's test is for vertebrobasilar artery insufficiency.

Method. Subject is seated with the arms outstretched and forearms supinated (Fig. 9-38A). Subject is instructed to close the eyes and bring the head into full backward bending and rotation (see Fig. 9-38B).

Results. Observe the subject for signs and symptoms. A positive test result is indicated if one hand sinks and pronates on the side of compromise.

Additional Notes on Vertebral Artery. Inner ear involvement can produce signs and symptoms like those of a positive vertebral artery test. For this reason, the subject may also be tested sitting or standing and should rotate the trunk while maintaining the head orientation. If this rotation of the cervical spine also causes signs and symptoms, the vertebral artery is still suspected of compromise. If negative, an inner ear problem is a potential source of symptoms.

ALAR LIGAMENT TEST

Indication. The alar ligament test reveals rupture of the alar ligament or fracture of the odontoid process of C2.

Method. Subject lies supine. The therapist supports the head beneath the occipital region while palpating the C2 spinous process. A gentle force is

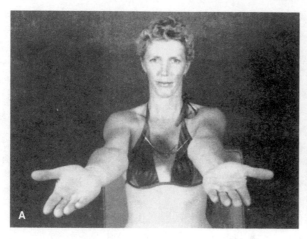

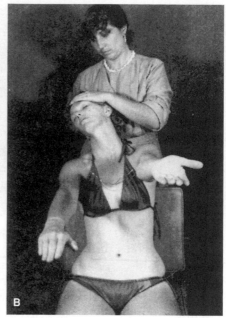

▲ **Figure 9.38** (**A**) Hautant's test. (**B**) Positive Hautant's test result.

given to produce suboccipital sidebending of the atlanto-occipital articulation, first to one side, then to the other (Fig. 9-39). The spinous process is palpated during this movement to assess concurrent C2 rotation (the spinous process of C2 is palpated rotating in the opposite direction).

Results. The C2 rotation to the same side must be immediate. If there is a lag or no concurrent movement, the result is positive. This is a potentially life-threatening situation.

COMPRESSION TEST (SPURLING TEST)

Indication. The compression test may be used in the assessment of disk protrusion or intervertebral foramen compromise, ligamentous lesions, and irritation of facet joint capsules.

Method. The subject is seated, with the head and neck in a neutral position. The examiner, with fingers interlocked and placed on top of the subject's head, provides gentle downward force (Fig. 9-40). Take care not to cause forward, backward, or sideways bending of the cervical spine. Variations on this test include the addition of sidebending, rotation, and backward bending of the cervical spine. Compression force directed through the cervical spine in a position of rotation is referred to as Jackson's test. The compression force in the maximum cervical compression test is performed with the cervical spine rotated and sidebent to the same side.

Results. In the presence of a disk protrusion or compromised intervertebral foramen, compression of the spine tends to increase symptoms, while decreasing symptoms in ligamentous lesions or irrita-

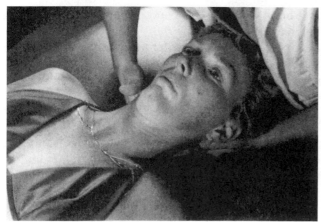

▲ **Figure 9.39** Alar ligament test.

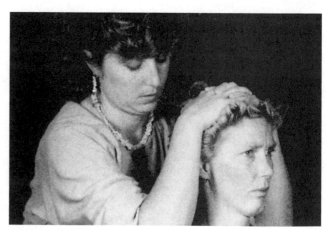

▲ **Figure 9.40** Compression test.

tion of facet joint capsules. Compression tests described previously, which involve rotation and sidebending, will refer symptoms toward the side of sidebending and rotation.

DISTRACTION TEST

Indication. The distraction test may be used in the assessment of disk protrusion or intervertebral foramen compromise, ligamentous lesions, and irritation of facet joint capsules.

Method. The subject may be positioned either supine or seated.

The examiner contacts the mastoid processes with the base of the palms. A gentle, even force lifts the weight of the subject's head straight upward (Fig. 9-41). An alternate hand placement is to place the thumb and fingers of one hand over each mastoid process and the opposite hand beneath the chin. Care must be taken to ensure that the distraction force is produced through the mastoid processes and not through the mandible. Excessive force through the mandible may produce TMJ dysfunction or increase already existing TMJ symptomatology in subjects with upper limb radicular symptoms.

Results. In the presence of a disk protrusion or compromised intervertebral foramen, distraction of the spine tends to relieve symptoms, while increasing symptoms in ligamentous lesions or irritation of facet joint capsules.

SHOULDER DEPRESSION TEST

Indication. This test may be performed in suspected cases of nerve root or nerve compression, foraminal compromise, dural adhesions, or facet joint capsule irritation.

Method. The subject is positioned either supine or seated. The examiner depresses the shoulder of the side being tested while simultaneously sidebending the neck away from that side.

Results. Reproduction of symptoms or exacerbation of already existing symptoms on the side being stretched indicates a positive test.

UPPER LIMB TENSION TEST

This test should be conducted in subjects with upper limb radicular symptoms that could be referred from the cervical spine nerve roots, brachial plexus, or thoracic outlet. See Chapter 5 for a discussion of this test.

THORACIC OUTLET TESTS

The battery of thoracic outlet tests should be incorporated as part of a cervical region evaluation in subjects with upper limb radicular symptoms of unknown etiology.

JOINT PLAY: PASSIVE INTERVERTEBRAL MOVEMENT

PALPATION OF PASSIVE INTERVERTEBRAL MOVEMENT DURING ASSESSMENT OF GROSS RANGE OF MOTION

Segmental movement is assessed at the interspinous space. Forward and backward bending movements (Figs. 9-42 and 9-43) are palpated by contacting the spinous processes with opposite sides of one digit and guiding the head through these motions. The spinous processes will be felt to approach each other in backward bending and to separate in forward bending. To assess sidebending and rotation movements, the

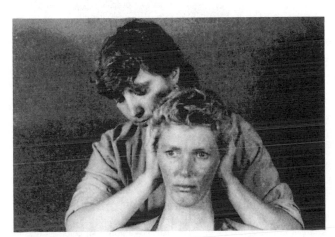

▲ **Figure 9.41** Distraction test.

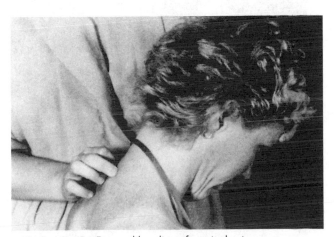

▲ **Figure 9.42** Forward bending of cervical spine.

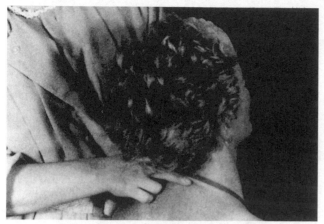

▲ **Figure 9.43** Backward bending of cervical spine.

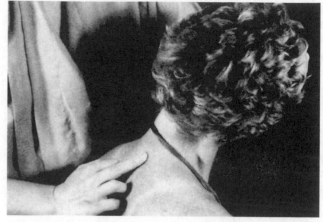

▲ **Figure 9.44** Sidebending of cervical spine.

spine should first be bent forward to the level of testing for localization. Sidebend (Fig. 9-44) and rotation (Fig. 9-45) are assessed with contact on the lateral aspect of the spinous processes and the interspinous space. The contact will be on the side toward which the upper spinous process is expected to move. (For example, right rotation of C5 on C6 will cause the spinous process of C5 to move to the left. The examiner, therefore, palpates on the left.)

Suboccipital Forward Bending

Method. Subject lies supine. The examiner stabilizes the axis with a contact over the articular pillars (Fig. 9-46A). With the opposite palm on the fore-

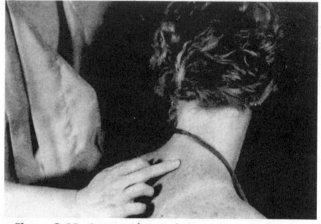

▲ **Figure 9.45** Rotation of cervical spine.

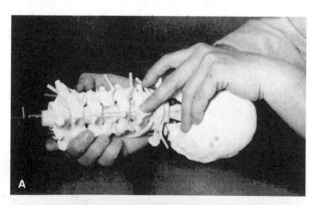

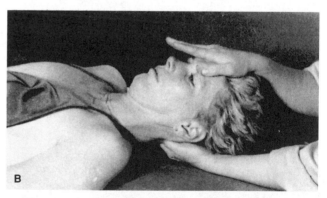

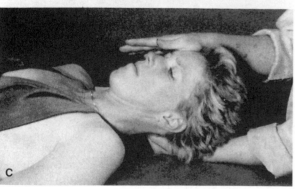

▲ **Figure 9.46** (**A**) Hand contact for suboccipital forward bending. (**B**) Central pressure producing bilateral movement. (**C**) Lateral pressure testing unilateral movement.

head, the examiner attempts to bend the head forward as if the subject were nodding. Centrally applied pressure produces bilateral movement (see Fig. 9-46*B*), while more lateral pressure tends to localize testing to the same side (see Fig. 9-46*C*).

Results. Suboccipital forward bending assesses backward glide of the atlantooccipital articulation and forward glide of the atlantoaxial joint.

Suboccipital Backward Bending

Method. The subject lies supine. The examiner supports the head under the occiput with the second digits at the level of the atlas. The examiner can now use these digits as a fulcrum to bend the head backward at the suboccipital level. The examiner can assess one or both sides.

Results. Suboccipital backward bending assesses forward glide of the occipital condyles on the atlas and backward glide and tilt of the atlas on the axis.

Suboccipital Sidebending

Method. Subject lies supine. The examiner supports the head at the occiput, with the second digit metacarpophalangeal joint of each hand lying just distal to the mastoid process but not contacting the transverse process of C1. Gentle sidebending is produced by the hands acting as a force couple, localizing movement to the occipitoatloid level, which causes rotation of the axis to the same side by way of the alar ligaments.

Results. Suboccipital sidebending assesses lateral glide of the atlanto-occipital joint in the opposite direction, forward glide of the same side of the atlantoaxial joint, and backward glide of the atlantoaxial joint to the opposite side.

Suboccipital Rotation

The subject must pass the vertebral artery test before this test is performed.

Method. With the subject supine, the neck is brought into very slight forward bending and is then passively bent and rotated to one side. This action will cause facet locking on the side of the bend or rotation. The head is then rotated toward the opposite side, with the apposed facets blocking forward gliding movement of the lower segment facet (Fig. 9-47). The test movement is then repeated in the opposite direction.

Results. Suboccipital rotation assesses backward glide of the facets on the side toward which the head is rotated and forward glide of the facets on the side of bending.

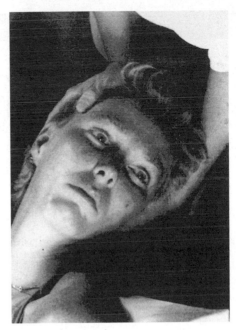
▲ **Figure 9.47** Suboccipital rotation.

Forward and Backward Glide: C2, C3 to T3, T4

Method

- Unilateral: The pad of the thumb is placed over the articular pillar of one side. Force is applied in a direction parallel to the joint plane to assess for end feel or provocation of symptoms (Fig. 9-48).
- Bilateral: Contact to bilateral articular pillars of the same vertebra is made with the pad of the thumb and the metacarpophalangeal joint of the second digit of the same hand. Force is applied parallel to the joint plane (Fig. 9-49).

Results. The forward and backward glide test assesses forward glide of the inferior motion segment and backward glide of the superior segment.

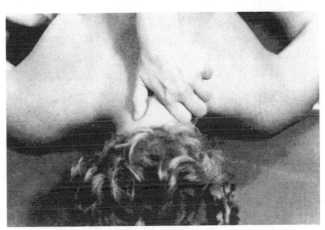
▲ **Figure 9.48** Hand contact for forward and backward glide.

TABLE 9.1	**Summary of Cervical Spine Joint Play**		
GLIDE	RESTRICTION	FIXED BONE	MOVING BONE
Atlanto-occipital Joint			
Anterior	Backward bend	Atlas	Occiput
Backward	Forward bend	Atlas	Occiput
Frontal plane	Sidebend, same direction	Atlas	Occiput
Rotation	General hypomobility	Atlas	Occiput
Atlantoaxial Joint			
Forward	Forward bend, atlantoaxial rotation in opposite direction Atlanto-occipital sidebend in opposite direction	Axis	Atlas
Backward	Backward bend, atlantoaxial rotation in same atlanto-occipital direction; sidebend in same direction	Axis	Atlas
Frontal	General hypomobility	Axis	Atlas
C2, C3–T3, T4 Joints			
Forward	Forward bend, sidebend in opposite direction, rotation in opposite direction	Inferior vertebra	Superior vertebra
Backward	Backward bend; sidebend in same direction, rotation in opposite direction	Inferior vertebra	Superior vertebra
Side	General hypomobility	Inferior vertebra	Superior vertebra

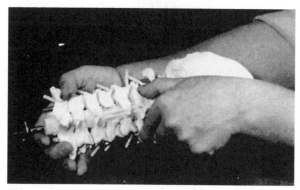

▲ **Figure 9.49** Forward and backward glide.

Midcervical Side Glide

Method. Subject lies supine with the neck in a neutral position. The examiner places the metacarpophalangeal joint of the second digit on the articular pillar. Using the opposite hand to support the neck, the examiner applies lateral force along the transverse plane. This force tends to "gap" the facet of the opposite side at the same level as a test of joint play.

Summary of Joint Play of the Cervical Spine

As a standard of reference, vertebral movement or position is always described by the superior vertebra with respect to the inferior vertebra, independent of which vertebra actually moves (i.e., cephalad-caudal versus caudal-cephalad sequence). Table 9-1 provides a summary of joint play of the cervical spine.

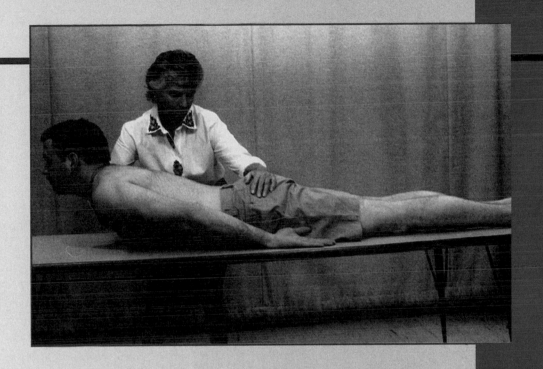

10

Thoracolumbar Spine

GONIOMETRY

Thoracic and Lumbar Vertebrae

THORACIC AND LUMBAR FLEXION

The motion of thoracic and lumbar vertebral flexion occurs in the sagittal plane. The greatest amount of motion occurs in the lumbar region, because the articular facets are positioned in the sagittal plane. The motion occurs also between the articular facets and the intervertebral disks. The disks compress anteriorly and distract posteriorly.

Motion. There is approximately a 4-in difference between the starting and ending positions. The range of motion in the lumbar region amounts to a straightening of the lordotic curve, with little or no reversal of the lumbar lordosis.

Position

- Preferred: Subject sits with the knee joints flexed.
- Alternate: Subject stands with the trunk erect.

Measuring Tape

Starting. The tape is placed proximally on the spinous process of C7 and distally to S1.

Ending. Following flexion of the vertebrae, using the same bony landmarks, calculate the difference in distance between the starting and ending positions (Fig. 10-1).

Stabilization. The pelvis and hip joints are stabilized.

Precautions

- Prevent increased hip joint flexion.
- Prevent anterior tilt of the pelvis.
- Allow for cervical vertebral flexion.

THORACIC AND LUMBAR EXTENSION AND HYPEREXTENSION

The motion of vertebral extension occurs in the sagittal plane. The majority occurs between the lumbar articular facets, because they are oriented in the sagittal plane. Extension also occurs between the intervertebral disks, which are compressed posteriorly and distracted anteriorly. The motion in the lumbar regions increases the normal lordosis and in the thoracic region, decreases the normal kyphosis, or posterior convexity.

Motion. The extension motion is the distance between the starting and ending points when using a measuring tape. The difference is approximately 2 in of thoracolumbar extension.

Position, measuring, and stabilization are the same as for thoracic and lumbar flexion (Fig. 10-2).

Precautions

- Prevent an increase in hip joint extension.
- Prevent posterior pelvic tilt.
- Prevent trunk rotation.

THORACIC AND LUMBAR LATERAL FLEXION

The thoracolumbar motion of lateral flexion occurs in the frontal plane and is accompanied by thoracic and lumbar rotation to the opposite side. The most lateral flexion occurs between the thoracic articular facets and less between the intervertebral disks. The disks are compressed on the test side and distracted on the other side.

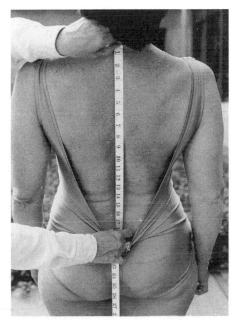

▲ **Figure 10.2** End position for thoracic and lumbar extension and hyperextension.

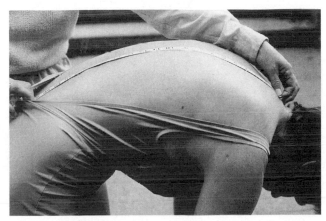

▲ **Figure 10.1** End position for thoracic and lumbar flexion.

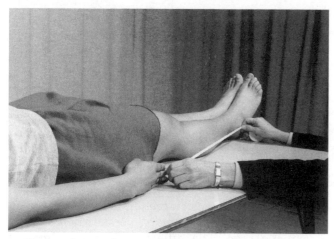

▲ **Figure 10.3** End supine position for lateral trunk flexion.

Motion. Subject bends to one side, rotating as little as possible. The motion is determined by the difference between the starting and ending positions. Because of such variances in body proportions as arm and trunk length, the amount of motion is determined by comparing the sides.

Position

- Preferred: Subject lies supine with the medial malleoli touching (Fig. 10-3).
- Alternate: Subject stands erect with the feet flat on the floor, approximately 2 in apart (Fig. 10-4).

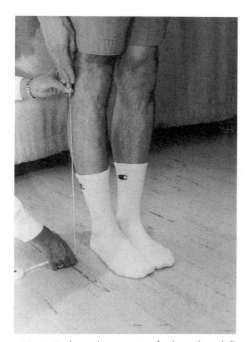

▲ **Figure 10.4** End standing position for lateral trunk flexion.

Measuring Tape

Starting

- Preferred: Place one end of a measuring tape on the tip of the middle finger and the other on the tip of the lateral malleolus.
- Alternate: Place one end of a measuring tape on the tip of the middle finger and the other on the floor on a point directly beneath the middle finger.

Ending. Measure the difference in inches following the lateral flexion motion.

Stabilization. The pelvis is stabilized.

Precautions

- Avoid trunk flexion, extension, and rotation.
- Prevent lateral tilting of the pelvis.

THORACIC AND LUMBAR ROTATION

The rotation motion occurs in the transverse plane between the articular facets and the intervertebral disks. The lumbar vertebrae exhibit little or no rotation, the most occurring in the thoracic region. The motion of thoracolumbar vertebral rotation is accompanied by lateral flexion to the opposite side.

Motion. Objective measurements usually are not taken. The motion of thoracolumbar rotation is observed, and the amount of motion is compared to that on the opposite side.

Position. Subject sits erect with the feet flat on the floor in a chair without a back support or facing the back of the chair (Fig. 10-5).

Measurements. No actual measurements are taken. The motion on each side is observed.

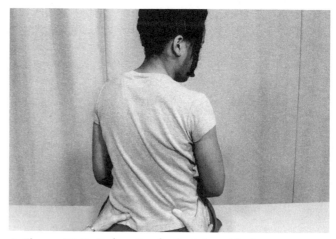

▲ **Figure 10.5** End position for thoracic and lumbar rotation.

Stabilization. The pelvis is stabilized.

Precautions

- Prevent pelvic rotation.
- Avoid trunk flexion and extension and lateral flexion.

MUSCLE LENGTH TESTING

Thoracic Flexors

When the abdominal muscles are too short, the thoracic vertebrae increase their normal curve. An excess of thoracic flexion is called kyphosis. Tightness in the rectus abdominus muscle leads to a depressed sternal angle.

RECTUS ABDOMINUS, INTERNAL AND EXTERNAL ABDOMINAL OBLIQUE, TRANSVERSIS ABDOMINUS, AND PYRAMIDALIS (IF PRESENT) MUSCLES

Position. The subject is in a prone position with the upper limbs at the side of the trunk.

Movement. The examiner assists the subject in extension (hyperextension) of the trunk while the lower limbs are held firmly on the surface of the treatment table.

Measurement. Same as for goniometry (Fig. 10-6).

Considerations

- The anterior superior iliac spines remain flat on the table.
- Extension of the thoracic vertebrae is considered as the ability to straighten out the vertebrae. If the motion is excessive, the thoracic vertebrae will show a slight anterior curve.

Thoracic Extensors

The intrinsic thoracic muscles seldom show any tightness and may show an increase in length, resulting in kyphosis. The assessment of these muscles is the same as goniometer measurements for the thoracic vertebrae.

Lumbar Extensors

The intrinsic lumbar extensor muscles are thick and powerful. The motion of extension is to increase the normal anterior convexity of the lumbar vertebra and flexion is to decrease the curve. Excessive flexion of the low back beyond the straight position is referred to as hyperflexion or hypermobility. The extension range of motion is quite variable among individuals (Fig. 10-7).

ERECTOR SPINAE (LUMBORUM), TRANSVERSARIOSPINALES (LUMBAR), AND QUADRATUS LUMBORUM MUSCLES (WITH HAMSTRING MUSCLES)

Position. The subject is in a long sitting position with the lower limbs supported and ankle joints in anatomical position.

Movement. The examiner helps the subject forward flex with knees extended, reaching toward the toes.

Measurement. The ruler is used to measure the distance between the fingertips of the subject and

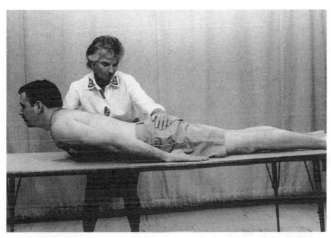

▲ **Figure 10.6** Muscle length testing of the abdominal muscles.

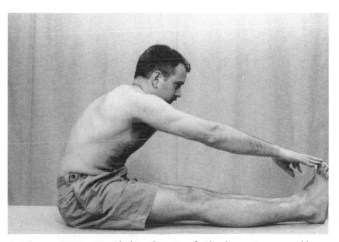

▲ **Figure 10.7** Muscle length testing for lumbar extensor and hamstring muscles.

the toes. Excessive motion would be measured by the distance the finger tips went beyond the toes. This measurement only indicates a change in forward bending, no standard has been established because of variability among individuals.

Considerations

- Normal length of the hamstring muscles permits the pelvis to flex forward so that the angle between the table and the sacrum is approximately 80 degrees according to Kendall.
- Normal lumbar flexion allows the low back to flatten.
- The long sitting position will not isolate limited range of motion from the hamstring muscles, low back muscles, gastrocnemius, or excessive length of the thoracic extensors.

ERECTOR SPINAE (LUMBORUM), TRANSVERSARIOSPINALES (LUMBAR), AND QUADRATUS LUMBORUM MUSCLES (WITHOUT HAMSTRING MUSCLES)

Position. The subject is short sitting with the knees flexed over the edge of the treatment table.

Movement. The examiner flexes the subject's low back without motion occurring in the pelvis.

Measurement. A ruler or a gravity-activated tool is used following the guidelines as in goniometry (Fig. 10-8).

Considerations

- Trunk flexion occurs without an anterior tilt of the pelvis.

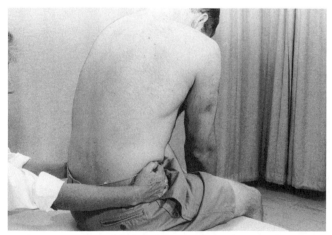

▲ **Figure 10.8** Muscle length testing of the thoracic spine extensors.

- If a subject has excessive low back muscle length, then guard the subject during forward flexion.

MANUAL MUSCLE TESTING

UPPER RECTUS ABDOMINIS MUSCLE

The upper portion of the rectus abdominis muscle is tested for flexion of the upper trunk in the sagittal plane, through a range such that the inferior angles of the scapulae clear the table. The subject should curl up slowly.

Palpation. Palpate the rectus abdominis on both sides of the midline between the umbilicus and the xiphoid process (Fig. 10-9).

Position. Subject lies supine.

Movement

- For 0 to P or 0 to 2 grades: Depression of the lower portion of the thorax (Figs. 10-10 and 10-11).

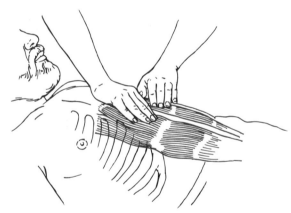

▲ **Figure 10.9** Palpation for the upper rectus abdominis muscle.

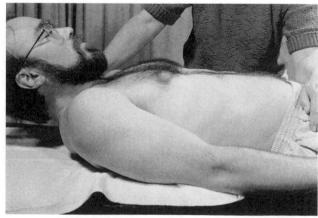

▲ **Figure 10.10** Appearance of "poor minus" performance of the rectus abdominis muscle.

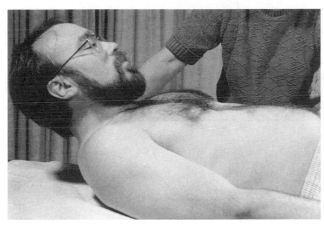

▲ **Figure 10.11** Appearance of "poor" performance of the rectus abdominis muscle.

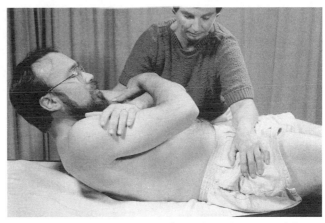

▲ **Figure 10.14** Appearance of "good" performance of the rectus abdominis muscle.

- For P+ to N or 2+ to 5 grades: Partial sit-up (Figs. 10-12 to 10-16).

Resistance. No external resistance is given; resistance is determined by position of the upper limbs.

Stabilization. Pelvis and lower limbs are stabilized.

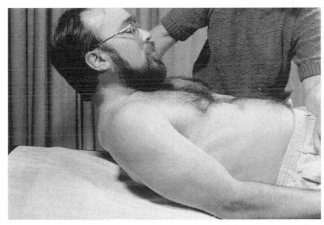

▲ **Figure 10.12** Appearance of "poor plus" performance of the rectus abdominis muscle.

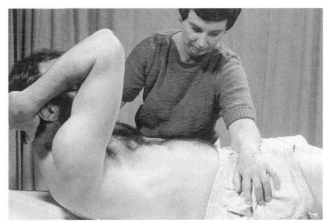

▲ **Figure 10.15** Appearance of "good plus" performance of the rectus abdominis muscle.

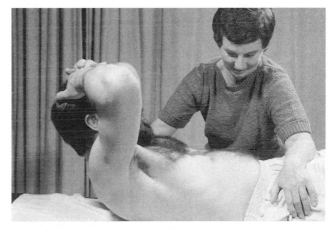

▲ **Figure 10.16** Appearance of "normal" performance of the rectus abdominis muscle.

Grades

0: No contraction palpated

T or 1: Contraction without depression of the thorax

P−: Contraction with partial depression of the thorax

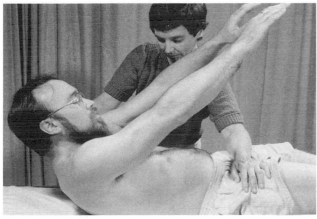

▲ **Figure 10.13** Appearance of "fair plus" performance of the rectus abdominis muscle.

▼ Attachments of Rectus Abdominis Muscle

Muscle	Proximal	Distal	Innervation
Rectus abdominis, upper	Pubic crest and symphysis	Costal cartilages of fifth to seventh ribs and xiphoid process	Ventral primary rami T5–10
Lower			T10–L1

P or 2: Contraction with full depression of the thorax

P+: Upper limbs at side of trunk; trunk begins motion against gravity.

F–: Upper limbs at side of trunk; spines of scapulae clear the table.

F or 3: Upper limbs at side of trunk; inferior angles of the scapulae clear the table.

F+: Upper limbs held straight in front of subject; inferior angles of scapulae clear the table.

G or 4: Upper limbs across chest; inferior angles of scapulae clear the table.

G+: Hands placed behind the head with elbows pointing forward; inferior angles clear the table.

N or 5: Hands on top of head with the shoulder horizontally abducted; inferior angles clear the table.

Substitutions

- Subject may jerk up using momentum; the sit-up should be performed slowly.
- For grades of P+ to F or 2+ to 3, subject may push up with the upper limbs.
- For grades of T to P or 1 to 2, the subject may breathe deeply, causing depression of the lower portion of the thorax.
- The internal and external abdominal obliques of each side contracting together can produce trunk flexion in the sagittal plane.
- Deviation of the umbilicus to one side indicates greater strength of that side.

LOWER RECTUS ABDOMINIS MUSCLE

The lower portion of the rectus abdominis muscle is tested during the motion of flexion of the lower trunk until the sacrum clears the treatment table.

Palpation. Palpate the rectus abdominis on both sides of the midline between the umbilicus and the symphysis pubis (Fig. 10-17).

Position. The subject lies supine, with the hips and knees flexed and the feet flat on the table; the upper limbs are crossed over the chest (Figs. 10-18 and 10-19).

Movement. Posterior pelvic tilt: The sacrum is lifted from the table.

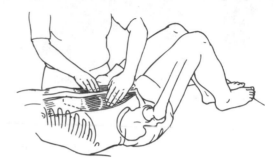

▲ **Figure 10.17** Palpation for the lower rectus abdominis muscle.

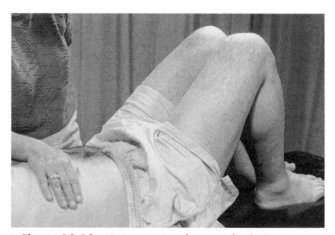

▲ **Figure 10.18** "Poor minus" performance for the lower portion of the rectus abdominis.

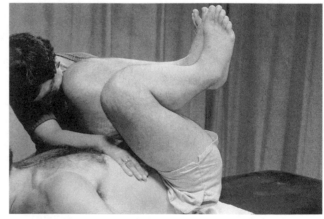

▲ **Figure 10.19** "Fair" performance for the lower portion of the rectus abdominis.

Resistance. No external resistance is applied. Weight of the lower limbs and the number of repetitions provide the resistance.

Stabilization. No stabilization is necessary.

Grades

0: No contraction
T or 1: Contraction felt but no movement
P−: Partial pelvic tilt
P or 2: Complete pelvic tilt
P+: Initiates lifting of sacrum
F−: Lifts sacrum through half the range
F or 3: Lifts sacrum through full range one time
F+: Lifts sacrum through full range two to three times
G or 4: Lifts sacrum through full range four to six times
G+: Lifts sacrum through full range seven to nine times
N or 5: Lifts sacrum through full range 10 times
P+ to N or 2+ to 5: Subject brings knees to chest, then lifts sacrum off the table.

Substitutions

• For grades of P− and P or 2, subject may breathe deeply, causing the abdomen to depress, thus giving the appearance of posterior pelvic tilt.
• For grades of P+ to N or 2+ to 5, subject may push with the upper limbs or jerk up. Be sure subject comes up slowly and keeps the upper limbs relaxed.
• The umbilicus may deviate toward the strong side.

Attachments. See attachments for upper rectus abdominis muscle.

EXTERNAL AND INTERNAL ABDOMINAL OBLIQUE MUSCLES

The external and internal abdominal oblique muscles are tested against gravity (AG) during trunk flexion and rotation or a diagonal sit-up. In the gravity-minimized (GM) position, the motion is rotation only. The end point of the test range is when both scapulae clear the table. Both rotation and flexion occur at the same time, and the trunk must roll up evenly without extension in the lumbar area. The movement takes place at the same speed over the full range, without a jerk at the beginning of motion. The external abdominal oblique muscle contracts when the subject rotates to the opposite side, and the internal abdominal oblique muscle contracts when the subject rotates to the same side. If the

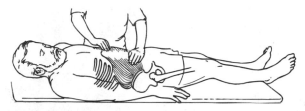

▲ **Figure 10.20** Palpation for the external and internal oblique abdominal muscles.

trunk is rotating toward the left, the right external abdominal oblique and the left internal abdominal oblique contract to perform the diagonal sit-up.

Palpation

External Abdominal Oblique. Palpate below the ribs and costal cartilages of the lowest ribs in the midclavicular line.

Internal Abdominal Oblique. Palpate immediately medial to the anterior superior iliac spine in the midclavicular line (Fig. 10-20).

Position

AG: Subject lies supine with the lower limbs extended (Figs. 10-21 to 10-24).
GM: Subject sits with the upper limbs at the sides of the trunk. If the subject is unable to sit, an alternate position is used: subject lies supine with the hips and knees flexed, feet flat on the table. In this position, however, the subject may depress the lower thorax and elevate the pelvis when performing the rotation.

Movement. Subject attempts to perform a diagonal sit-up.

Resistance. No external resistance is applied; it is determined by the position of the upper limbs.

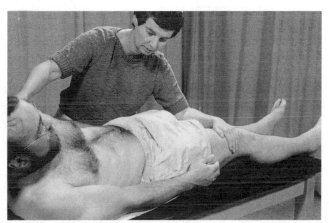

▲ **Figure 10.21** "Poor plus" performance for the external and internal oblique abdominal muscles.

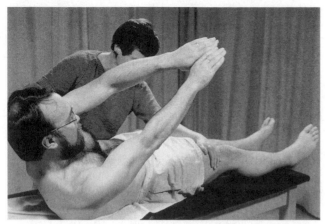

▲ **Figure 10.22** "Fair plus" performance for the external and internal oblique abdominal muscles.

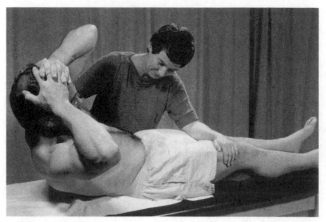

▲ **Figure 10.24** "Normal" performance for the external and internal oblique abdominal muscles.

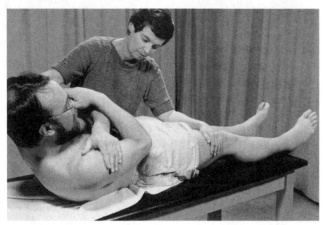

▲ **Figure 10.23** "Good" performance for the external and internal oblique abdominal muscles.

F−: Elevation of half of the opposite scapula, upper limbs relaxed

F or 3: Upper limbs relaxed; inferior angle of the opposite scapula clears table.

F+: Upper limbs straight in front of subject; opposite scapula clears the table, and part of the scapula on the side toward which the person is reaching comes off the table.

G or 4: Upper limbs across chest; opposite scapula clears the table and part of the scapula on the side toward which the person is reaching comes off the table.

G+: Upper limbs behind the neck with the elbows directed forward; both scapulae clear the table.

N or 5: Upper limbs on top of head with the shoulders abducted; both scapulae clear the table.

Stabilization. Pelvis and lower limbs are stabilized.

Grades

0: No contraction palpated

T or 1: Contraction felt, but no rotation

P−: Partial rotation

P or 2: Full rotation

P+: Beginning elevation of the opposite scapula, upper limbs relaxed

Substitutions

• In the GM position, the deep rotators of the back may rotate the trunk.
• In the AG position, subject may jerk up. Motion should be performed slowly and evenly.
• Rectus abdominis and the short rotators of the back assist in the motion of trunk flexion with rotation.

▼ Attachments of External and Internal Abdominal Oblique Muscles

Muscle	Proximal	Distal	Innervation
External abdominal oblique	Lateral surface of caudal eight pairs of ribs	Linea alba, inguinal ligament, anterior superior iliac spine, pubic tubercle, and anterior half of iliac crest	Ventral primary rami of T5–L1
Internal abdominal oblique	Inguinal ligament, iliac crest, and thoracolumbar fascia	Pubic crest, linea alba, and 10th–12th ribs	Ventral primary rami of T7–L1

ERECTOR SPINAE, TRANSVERSISPINALIS, INTERSPINALES, THORACIC, AND LUMBAR INTERTRANSVERSARII MUSCLES

The intrinsic back muscles are tested in the motion of cervical, thoracic, and lumbar vertebral extension from a starting position of slight flexion. The motion is tested through a range of minimal extension.

Palpation. Palpate the erector spinae on either side of the midline in the thoracic and lumbar vertebral region (Figs. 10-25 and 10-26).

Position

AG: For the thoracic muscles, subject lies prone with pillows under the abdomen and the upper limbs resting on the buttocks (Fig. 10-27). For the lumbar muscles, subject lies prone with pillows under the hips and the hands resting on the buttocks (Fig. 10-28).

GM: For the thoracic muscles, subject sits backward in a chair with the back slightly rounded and relaxed and the hands on the back of the chair (Fig. 10-29). For the lumbar muscles, subject sits with the

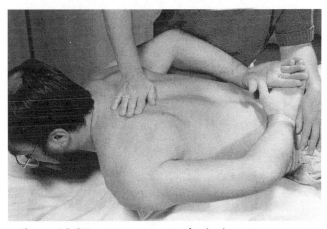

▲ **Figure 10.27** AG prone position for the thoracic erector spinae muscles.

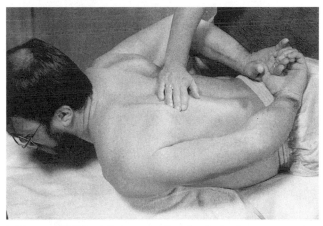

▲ **Figure 10.28** AG prone position for the lumbar erector spinae muscles.

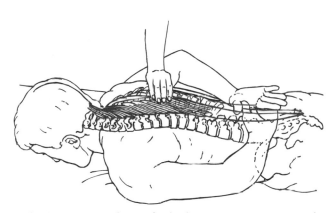

▲ **Figure 10.25** Palpation for the thoracic erector spinae muscles.

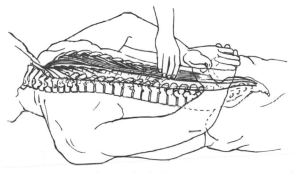

▲ **Figure 10.26** Palpation for the lumbar erector spinae muscles.

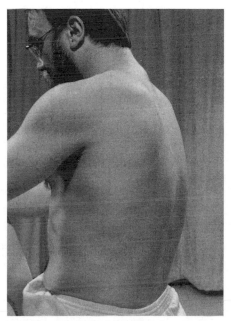

▲ **Figure 10.29** GM sitting position for the thoracic erector spinae muscles.

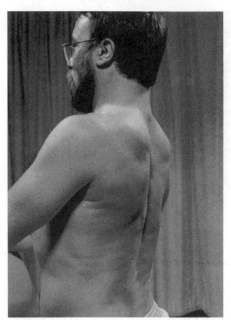

▲ **Figure 10.30** GM sitting position for the lumbar erector spinae muscles.

lower back arched, increased lumbar lordosis, and the pelvis tilted anteriorly (Fig. 10-30). Alternatively, subject lies supine, and the back is arched in the thoracic and lumbar regions.

Movement. Subject extends the upper and lower portions of the trunk.

Resistance. Applied to the upper portion of the thoracic spine for the thoracic portion and to the lower portion of the thoracic spine for the lumbar portion.

Stabilization

Thoracic. Pelvis and lumbar vertebrae are stabilized.

Lumbar. Pelvis and hips are stabilized.

Substitutions

- Observe the motion of intrinsic extensors in adjacent areas in the specific test area.
- The subject may push off from the table with an anterior thrust of the shoulders. Keep scapulae adducted.
- To ensure contraction of the trunk extensors, have the subject relax the shoulders at the completion of the test range.
- Observe lumbar vertebrae motion during hip extension.

▼ Attachments of Intrinsic Back Muscles

Muscle	Proximal	Distal	Innervation
Cervical Spine Suboccipital muscles	Atlas and axis	Transverse processes of atlas and occipital bone	Dorsal primary rami of the cervical spinal nerves
Iliocostalis cervicis	Third to sixth rib angles	Posterior tubercles of C4-6	Dorsal primary rami of the cervical spinal nerves
Longissimus cervicis	Transverse processes of T1-4 or T5	Posterior tubercles of C2-6	Dorsal primary rami of the cervical spinal nerves
Longissimus capitis	Transverse processes of T1-4 or T5 and C4 or 5-7	Mastoid process	Dorsal primary rami of the cervical spinal nerves
Spinalis cervicis	Ligamentum nuchae, spinous process of C7	Spinous processes of axis and C3 and C4	Dorsal primary rami of the cervical spinal nerves
Spinalis capitis	Transverse processes of upper thoracic and lower cervical vertebrae	Occipital bone between superior and inferior nuchal lines	Dorsal primary rami of the cervical spinal nerves
Semispinalis cervicis	Transverse processes of T1-6	Spinous processes of C2-5	Dorsal primary rami of the cervical spinal nerves
Semispinalis capitis	Transverse processes of T1-6 and C4-7	Between superior and inferior nuchal lines	Dorsal primary rami of the cervical spinal nerves
Multifidi	Transverse processes of cervical vertebrae	Cervical vertebra's spinous process of each two vertebrae immediately superior	Dorsal primary rami of the cervical spinal nerves

continued on page 251

▼ Attachments of Intrinsic Back Muscles *(Continued)*

Muscle	Proximal	Distal	Innervation
Rotatores	Transverse process of cervical vertebrae	Lamina of immediately superior cervical vertebra	Dorsal primary rami of the cervical spinal nerves
Interspinalis	Between spinous processes six pairs of cervical vertebrae		Dorsal primary rami of the cervical spinal nerves
Intertransversarii	Between transverse processes six pairs of cervical vertebrae		Posterior: dorsal and ventral primary rami Anterior: ventral primary rami of spinal nerves
Thoracic Spine Iliocostalis thoracis	Angles of the lower six ribs	Angle of upper six ribs and transverse process of C7	Dorsal primary rami of the thoracic spinal nerves
Longissimus thoracis	Lumbar transverse processes Thoracolumbar fascia	Transverse processes of all thoracic vertebrae and lower nine pairs of ribs between the angle and tubercle	Dorsal primary rami of the thoracic spinal nerves
Semispinalis thoracis	Transverse processes of thoracic vertebrae	Spinous process of C6 and C7 and T1-4	Dorsal primary rami of the thoracic spinal nerves
Multifidi	Transverse processes of thoracic vertebrae	Spinous process of two to four immediately superior vertebrae	Dorsal primary rami of the thoracic spinal nerves
Rotatores	Transverse processes of thoracic vertebrae	Lamina of vertebra immediately superior	Dorsal primary rami of the thoracic spinal nerves
Intertransversarii	11 pairs between thoracic transverse processes		Dorsal primary rami of the thoracic spinal nerves
Interspinales	Two to three pairs between 1st and 2nd and 11th and 12th spinous processes		Dorsal primary rami of the thoracic spinal nerves
Lumbar Spine Iliocostalis lumborum	Spinous processes of lumbar vertebrae and T11 and T12 Posterior iliac crest and supraspinous ligament Crest of the sacrum	Inferior border of the angles of the lower six or seven ribs	Dorsal primary rami of the lumbar spinal nerves
Multifidis	Sacrum Posterior superior iliac spine Sacroiliac ligaments Transverse processes of lumbar vertebrae	Spinous process of two to four immediately superior vertebrae	Dorsal primary rami of the lumbar spinal nerves
Rotatores	Transverse processes of lumbar vertebrae	Lamina of immediately superior vertebra	Dorsal primary rami of the lumbar spinal nerves
Interspinalis	Four pairs between lumbar spinous processes		Dorsal primary rami of the lumbar spinal nerves
Intertransversarii	Four pairs between lumbar transverse processes	Dorsal and ventral primary rami of lumbar spinal nerves	Dorsal primary rami of the lumbar spinal nerves

QUADRATUS LUMBORUM MUSCLE

The quadratus lumborum muscle is tested in the motion of hip hiking, moving the pelvis in the coronal plane unilaterally. The iliac crest approximates the 12th rib. The test range is 25 to 30 degrees, or 3 in.

Palpation. Palpate the quadratus lumborum with subject either supine or standing. The lateral trunk flexors must be relaxed so that the examiner can place the fingers deep under the erector spinae muscles. The subject should bend the trunk laterally, then relax. The fingers are placed over the posterior iliac crest and below the 12th rib directed toward the vertebrae (Fig. 10-31).

Position

AG: Subject stands on a block or stool holding onto the examiner lightly to maintain balance, with the test leg hanging free (Fig. 10-32).

GM: Subject is either supine or prone, with test leg abducted 15 degrees and the pelvis laterally tilted (Fig. 10-33).

Movement. Subject hikes the hip by elevating the pelvis on the test side.

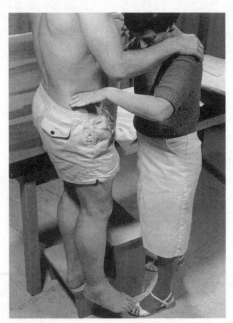

▲ **Figure 10.32** Testing the quadratus lumborum muscle in the AG standing position.

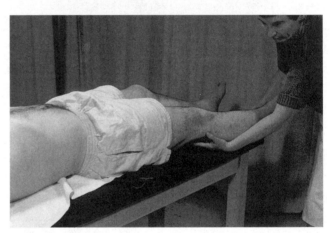

▲ **Figure 10.33** Testing the quadratus lumborum muscle in the GM supine position.

Resistance. Applied to the iliac crest in the direction of lateral tilt of the pelvis.

Stabilization. Trunk is stabilized on the opposite side.

Substitution

- Flexion of the trunk to the opposite side may give the appearance of hip hiking.

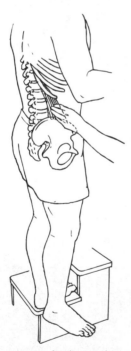

▲ **Figure 10.31** Palpation for the quadratus lumborum muscle.

▼ Attachments of Quadratus Lumborum Muscle			
Muscle	**Proximal**	**Distal**	**Innervation**
Quadratus lumborum	Iliolumbar ligaments Iliac crest Transverse processes of lower lumbar vertebrae	Inferior border of 12th rib Transverse processes of L1-4	Ventral primary rami of L1-3

CLINICAL ASSESSMENT

Observation and Screening

Associated areas to be cleared for dysfunction include the cervical spine, shoulder girdle (especially for scapulothoracic dysfunction), lumbosacral spine, sacroiliac joints, and lower limbs using the lower quarter screening examination. A complete postural examination should be conducted with particular attention given to the thoracolumbar and pelvic regions.

From a lateral view, any deviations from the normal thoracic kyphotic curvature and lumbar lordotic curvature should be noted. An increase in the thoracic kyphosis is commonly accompanied by rounded shoulders and a forward head. An excessive lumbar lordosis is typically seen with an anterior pelvic tilt and the potential for hip flexor tightness. A diminished or flattened lumbar lordotic curve tends to be associated with a posterior pelvic tilt and possible hamstring tightness. Abdominal tone should also be assessed from a lateral perspective.

Anterior observation allows for examination of symmetry of ASIS heights and iliac crest heights. Posterior observation permits evaluation of scoliosis, lateral shifts, and symmetry of iliac crest and PSIS heights between right and left sides. Scoliosis, which can either be classified as structural or functional, is identified by a lateral curvature of the spine within the thoracolumbar area. These lateral curves can be composed of a single primary or OCO curve or an OSO curve that possesses a larger primary curve and a smaller secondary compensatory curve. Regardless of the type of curve evident, the scoliosis is classified according to the convex side of the curve. For example, an OSO curve with the convex side of the thoracic curve to the right and the convex side of the lumbar curve to the left would be called a right thoracic, left lumbar scoliosis. Determination as to whether the scoliosis is structural or functional can clinically be made by marking the spinous processes of the thoracolumbar spine with a skin marker in an upright position, followed by observing the spinal alignment with the subject in full trunk flexion. In cases of structural scoliosis, the curve(s) will remain in both positions of erect standing and trunk flexion. A subject with a functional scoliosis will exhibit the curve(s) in erect standing, but on trunk flexion, the curve(s) will straighten.

The presence of a lateral shift, seen in subjects with lumbar derangements, is indicated by the shoulders being offset laterally relative to the pelvis. The shift is classified according to the direction that the shoulders are offset. For example, a left lateral shift would be present when the shoulders are offset to the left relative to the pelvis (Fig. 10-34).

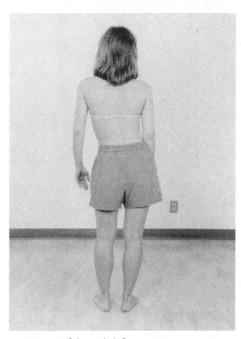

▲ **Figure 10.34** Left lateral shift.

A posterior view also allows for identification of sciatic scoliosis secondary to a lumbar derangement. When the disk lies lateral to the nerve root, the subject will usually sidebend away from the involved side. However, the subject will typically sidebend toward the involved side when the disk is situated medial to the nerve root.

Palpation and Surface Anatomy

Palpation during evaluation of the thoracolumbar spine should include the following (Fig. 10-35):

1. Spinous processes
2. Transverse processes
3. Ribs (including costochondral and costovertebral attachments, rib margin, and intercostal spaces; special attention should be paid to the first rib and its relationship to the clavicle anteriorly.)
4. Sternum (including manubrium, body, xiphoid process, and the sternal angle)
5. Sternoclavicular joint
6. Scapula
7. Cervicothoracic junction
8. Paravertebral muscles
9. 12th rib
10. ASIS
11. PSIS
12. Iliac crests
13. Lumbosacral junction
14. Gluteal folds
15. Greater trochanters

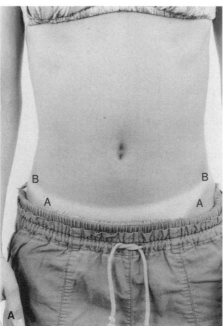

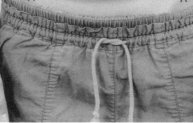

▲ **Figure 10.35** Surface anatomy of the thoracolumbar region. (**A**) Anterior view. (**B**) Posterior view.

A = ASIS   B = Iliac Crests

A = Iliac Crests   C = Lumbar Spinous
B = PSIS   Process

Gross Active Movements

The movements to be assessed for range and quality of movement include the following:

1. Forward bending (Fig. 10-36)
2. Backward bending (Fig. 10-37)
3. Sidebending (Fig. 10-38)
4. Rotation (Fig. 10-39)

Note: In the thoracic spine, sidebending and rotation occur in opposite directions. In the erect posi-

tion in the lumbar spine, sidebending and rotation occur in opposite directions. In forward bend of the lumbar spine, sidebending and rotation occur in the the same direction.

Rotation of the spine is best observed by evaluating the sidebending component. The rules of sidebending and rotation change; the midthoracic levels are transitional. The lower segments follow the rule of opposite sidebending and rotation as in the lumbar spine in the erect position. The upper segments follow the rule of same sidebending and rotation as in the cervical spine.

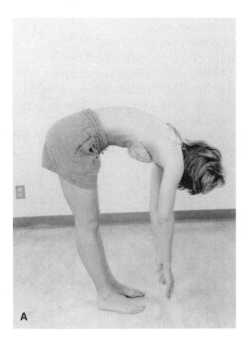

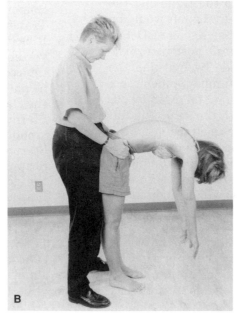

▲ **Figure 10.36** (**A**) Unrestricted forward bending of the thoracolumbar spine. (**B**) Restricted movement of the pelvis during forward bending of the thoracolumbar spine.

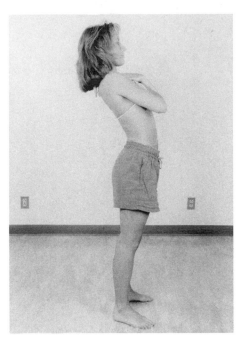

▲ **Figure 10.37** Backward bending of the thoracolumbar spine.

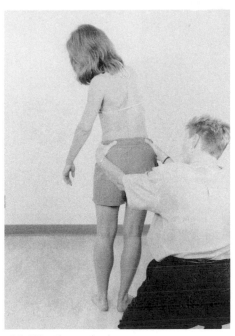

▲ **Figure 10.39** Thoracolumbar rotation.

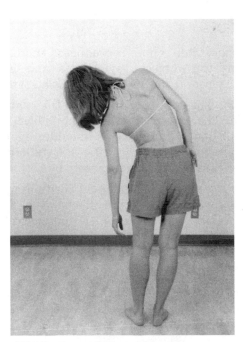

▲ **Figure 10.38** Thoracolumbar sidebending.

REPEATED FORWARD AND BACKWARD BENDING: STANDING AND LYING (MCKENZIE'S REPEATED MOVEMENT TESTING)

Indication. Repeated bending is performed to differentiate between derangement of the disk and mechanical dysfunction of other spinal structures.

Method. For all of the following tests, the effect of the first movement on the subject's pain is noted.

The effect is noted again after the repeated movements have been performed. Movements should be repeated as many as 10 times unless the subject reports reproduction or increased intensity or radiation of pain into the lower limb. The subject's range of motion during the repeated motions should also be observed.

Standing Forward Bending. The subject stands with the feet about 12 in apart and is asked to run the hands down the front of the legs, as if to touch the toes, as far as can be tolerated and then to return to the upright position (Fig. 10-40).

Standing Backward Bending. The subject stands with the feet 12 in apart and the hands placed in the small of the back. The subject bends backward over the hands, then returns to the upright position (Fig. 10-41). (Note: If the subject is in a lateral shift position related to the symptoms, the examiner should attempt to correct this postural fault with a side glide technique before repeated testing of backward bending.)

Supine Forward Bending. The subject is supine, grasping both knees with the hands. The subject bends forward, pulling the knees to the chest (Fig. 10-42). Knee flexion eliminates compression of the spine by the body weight and tension on the nerve root.

Prone Backward Bending. The subject lies prone with the hands positioned as if to do a push-up. The subject is asked to straighten the upper limbs and raise the trunk, keeping the pelvis and lower limbs

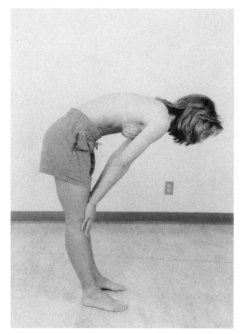

▲ **Figure 10.40**   Repeated forward bending.

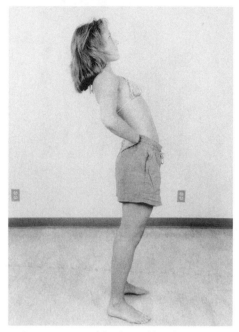

▲ **Figure 10.41**   Repeated backward bending.

in contact with the table and then to return to the starting position (Fig. 10-43). In this position, body weight compression is diminished and muscular activity of the trunk muscles eliminated.

Results. The results of these tests are considered to indicate disk derangement, joint or soft-tissue dysfunction, or a postural syndrome. No pain during testing indicates that pain experienced at other times by the subject is due to a postural syndrome in which time and positioning are key factors. Pain felt at the extremes of motion that does not progressively worsen with repetition and is relieved with return from the end position is indicative of joint or soft-tissue dysfunction. Disk derangement is indicated by progressive worsening of symptoms, especially with repeated movements, with increasingly intense pain or peripheralization of pain.

SIDE GLIDE

Indication. Side glide reproduces, increases, or decreases the subject's symptoms and indicates whether a lateral shift is relevant to the symptoms.

Method. The subject stands with the examiner at one side. The examiner grasps the subject's pelvis with both hands and places a shoulder against the subject's lower thorax (Fig. 10-44). Equal and opposite forces are applied transversely by both hands.

Results. End feel and sustained positioning (10–15 seconds) are assessed for the effects on the subject's symptoms (increase or decrease and centralization or peripheralization of pain).

CONTRACTILE TESTING

Contractile testing should include all the motions assessed during gross active movement.

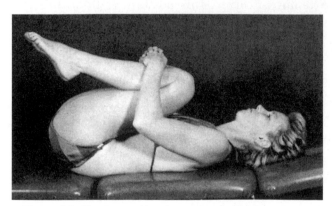

▲ **Figure 10.42**   Forward bend in supine position.

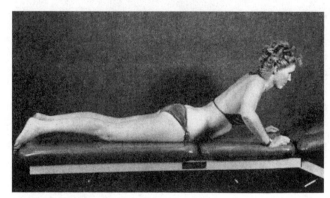

▲ **Figure 10.43**   Backward bend in prone position.

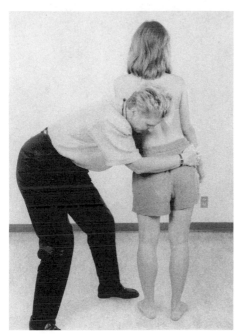

▲ **Figure 10.44** Side glide.

SPECIAL CLINICAL TESTS

POSITIONAL FAULTS

Indication. Testing for positional faults enables the examiner to locate a possible spinal dysfunction. A finding of misalignment of the spinous processes must be correlated with the actual detection of mobility dysfunction at the same vertebral level to be considered valid.

Method. The examiner pinches the spinous processes of two adjacent vertebrae between the thumb and forefinger of each hand and evaluates them for alignment along the length of the spine (Fig. 10-45A). The examiner then evaluates the distance between successive vertebrae (see Fig. 10-45B).

Results. Each spinous process should be aligned between adjacent vertebrae, and the interspinous distances should be similar, though it gradually changes, being narrower at both the upper and lower thoracic levels and greatest in the midthoracic region. A misaligned spinous process or an abnormal intervertebral space indicates either a potential motion segment dysfunction or a bony abnormality. If the segment moves normally with passive intervertebral movement testing, it is considered normal. If mobility is abnormal at the level of the positional fault, treatment is indicated. For example, a vertebra in an apparently forward bent position indicates restriction of forward glide of the superior motion segment or restriction of backward glide of the inferior one; this can be unilateral or bilateral. Therefore, only with motion testing can a more definitive assessment of the actual dysfunction be concluded.

SKIN ROLLING

Indication. Skin rolling is used to assess soft-tissue mobility and to locate trigger points, areas of congestion, and temperature discrepancies.

Method. The examiner lifts an area of skin between the thumb and forefinger of each hand. The skin is "rolled" forward along the length and in the direction desired (Fig. 10-46).

Results. Ease, looseness, and lack of tenderness of the skin, although variable from person to person, are normal. Areas that feel tethered, congested, hot, or cold or that are tender are usually sites of involvement that require treatment.

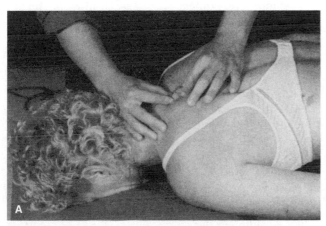
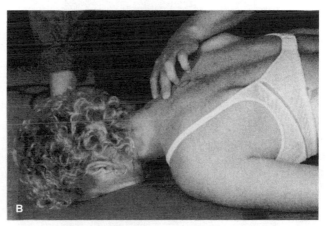

▲ **Figure 10.45** Testing for positional faults. **(A)** Palpation for rotational positional faults. **(B)** Palpation for forward and backward positional faults.

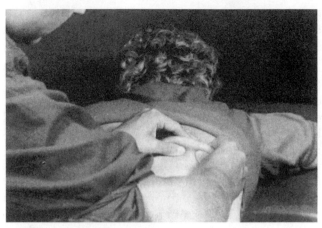

▲ **Figure 10.46** Skin rolling.

COMPRESSION AND DISTRACTION TESTS

Indication. Compression and distraction tests are used to assess the presence of a space-occupying lesion (i.e., disk) in the lumbar spine that may be compressing the spinal nerve roots.

Method

- Compression: The examiner stands behind the seated subject. Placing the hands on the subject's shoulders, the examiner provides a moderate and even downward force through the trunk, taking care not to cause forward, backward, or sidebending of the trunk (Fig. 10-47).
- Distraction: The subject sits with upper limbs crossed. The examiner stands behind the subject and reaches around the thorax, grasping

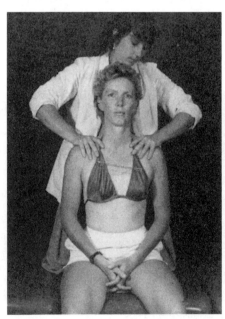

▲ **Figure 10.47** Compression test.

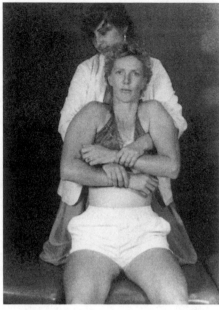

▲ **Figure 10.48** Distraction test.

the subject's forearms. By straightening up or leaning back, the examiner can distract the spine along its vertical axis (Fig. 10-48). If the subject has shoulder pathology, the examiner may put less strain on that area by holding around the thorax and distracting through the trunk.

Results. In the presence of a space-occupying lesion, increased compression tends to exacerbate symptoms, while distraction tends to alleviate them.

STORK STANDING TEST (ONE-LEG STANDING EXTENSION TEST)

Indication. This test may be used in the overall assessment of a stress fracture involving the pars interarticularis.

Method. The subject stands with most of the body weight borne through one lower limb while the other limb is used primarily for balance. The subject then actively backward bends the trunk (Fig. 10-49). The test is repeated while weight bearing on the opposite limb.

Results. A positive test results when pain is reproduced in the low back.

SEGMENTAL INSTABILITY TEST

This test may assist in the determination of lumbar spine instability.[17]

Method. The subject is positioned prone with the lower limbs off the table and the toes resting on the

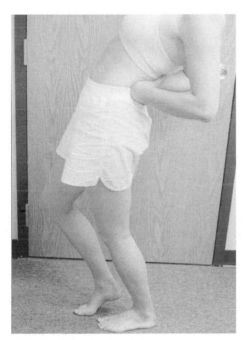

▲ Figure 10.49 Stork standing test.

floor. The examiner applies pressure segmentally over the lumbar spine while the subject remains relaxed (Fig. 10-50A). The subject is then instructed to lift the legs off the floor by contracting the hip and spinal extensors. While in this position, the examiner again applies pressure segmentally over the lumbar spine (see Fig. 10-50B).

Results. A positive test results in low back pain reproduced with pressure applied to the lumbar spine with the subject relaxed but no pain with pressure

applied during muscular contraction. This lack of pain is attributable to the area of instability being protected and masked by the muscular contraction.

PHEASANT TEST

Indication. This test may assist the examiner in the detection of an unstable lumbar spinal segment.

Method. The subject is positioned prone while the examiner fully flexes both knees with one hand and then carefully applies a hyperextension pressure to the lumbar spine with the other hand.

Results. Pain reproduced in the back or legs during the applied lumbar pressure indicates a positive test.

QUADRANT TEST

Indication. The quadrant test is beneficial in the evaluation of intervertebral foramina narrowing.

Method. The examiner stands behind the subject, who is also standing. As the subject moves into backward bending, the examiner places a hand on the subject's shoulder to guide the movement. Simultaneously, the subject also moves into rotation and sidebending toward the painful side (Fig. 10-51). The test is completed when the combined range of motion is complete or the subject experiences reproduction of symptoms.

Results. Limited range of motion by provocation of symptoms represents a positive test.

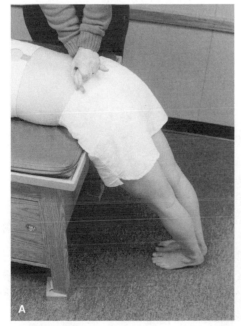
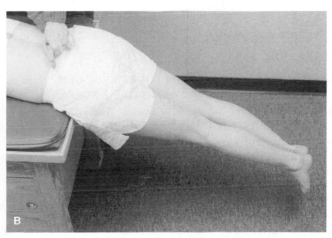

▲ Figure 10.50 **(A & B)** Segmental instability tests.

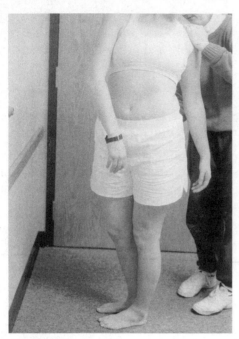

▲ **Figure 10.51** Quadrant test.

TESTS FOR DURAL SIGNS BY INCREASED TENSION ON SPINAL NERVE ROOTS

The following tests were designed and interpreted as tests of involvement or irritability of the lumbar spinal nerve roots by assessing reproduction of symptoms when the nerve roots are tensed. The examiner must remember that the spinal nerve roots are not the only structures provoked by these tests. In addition to the spinal nerve root, vertebral facets, and sacroiliac and hip joint structures, the hamstrings and fascial elements are also put under stress. The examiner must be aware that one of these other structures may be the source of symptoms or influence them. These elements must be properly assessed before it is possible to conclude which structure is at fault.

Straight Leg Raise Test (Laseque's Test)[2,5,8-10,16,18]

Method. The subject lies supine with the nontest limb positioned in extension and resting on the table. The examiner passively raises the test lower limb, keeping the hip slightly adducted and internally rotated and the knee fully extended (Fig. 10-52).

The angle of the hip, measured between the elevated lower limb and the table, is recorded.

Results. Reproduction of symptoms in the back or along the distribution of the sciatic nerve indicates a positive test.

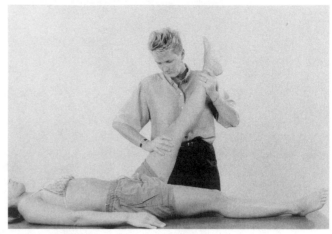

▲ **Figure 10.52** Straight leg test (Laseque test).

The sciatic nerve is on full stretch at approximately 70 degrees of hip flexion; therefore, a positive test for sciatic nerve involvement will occur prior to that amount of hip flexion.

Braggard's Test[5,10,16]

Method. The subject lies supine as positioned above. The examiner raises the involved lower limb to the point just short of where symptoms begin. The ankle of the limb is then passively dorsiflexed (Fig. 10-53).

Results. The result is positive if symptoms are reproduced in the lower back or the involved extremity. A variation of this test would be to raise the involved limb to the point of symptom reproduction and then slightly lower the limb to a point of no symptoms. The examiner then passively dorsiflexes the ankle, which should again reproduce the symptoms.

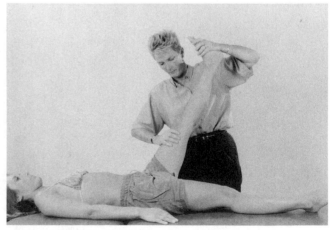

▲ **Figure 10.53** Braggard's test.

Lermitte's Test (Crossed Extension Straight Leg Raise)

Method. The subject lies supine as previously described while the examiner passively performs a straight leg raise of the uninvolved lower limb.

Results. The result is positive if pain is reproduced in the back or in the involved limb. A positive test is usually representative of some space-occupying lesion, such as a disk herniation.

Brudzinski's Test[3,12]

Method. The subject lies supine with both hands behind the neck. The examiner assists the subject in flexing the head, neck, and upper back (Fig. 10-54).

Results. A positive result is indicated by pain in the low back, pelvic girdle, or lower limb.

Soto-Hall Test[5,10,16]

Method. The subject lies supine. The examiner raises the involved lower limb, keeping it straight, to a point just short of the onset of pain. The subject's head and neck are then passively flexed (Fig. 10-55).

Results. Test results are positive if symptoms are reproduced.

Slump Test[13]

Method. The subject is seated with the upper limbs clasped at the hands behind the back. The subject is asked to "slump" forward at the trunk. The examiner, using one arm, next applies an overpressure through the shoulders to the slumped trunk. The examiner then directs the subject to forward bend the neck, after which the examiner again applies an overpressure. With this overpressure

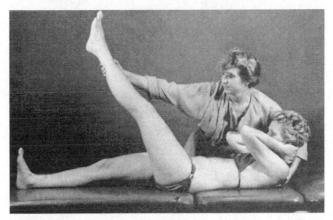

▲ **Figure 10.55** Soto-Hall test.

being maintained by the examiner at the head, neck, and trunk, the subject then extends the knee; the ankle is dorsiflexed by the examiner (Fig. 10-56*A*). Finally, the subject's head and neck are released and allowed to return to a neutral position (see Fig. 10-56*B*).

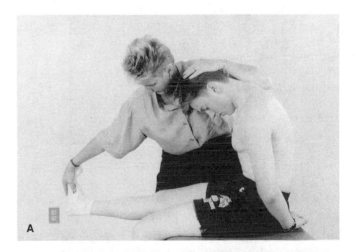

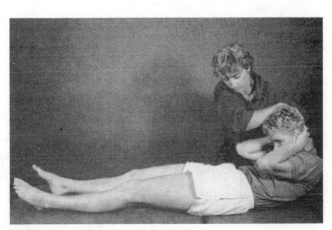

▲ **Figure 10.54** Brudzinski's test.

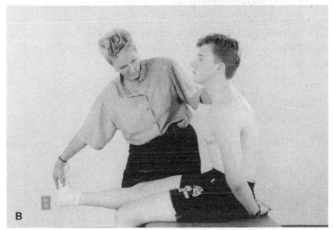

▲ **Figure 10.56** (**A** & **B**) Slump test.

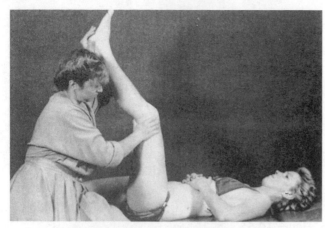

▲ **Figure 10.57** Cram's test.

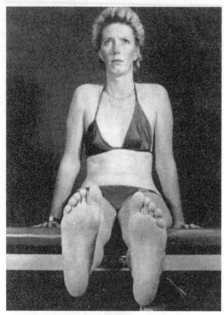

▲ **Figure 10.58** Brechterew's test.

Results. Symptoms should progressively increase with each added component of the test, as the dura is progressively stretched from above and below. Once the head and neck are released, there should be a noticeable decrease in the intensity of the symptoms.

Cram's Test (Bowstring Test, Popliteal Pressure Test)[6]

Method. The subject lies supine. The examiner raises the involved straight leg to the point of onset of pain, then slightly flexes the knee until the pain is alleviated. The knee position is maintained; the hip is flexed further to a point just short of the onset of pain. The examiner then presses on the posterior tibial nerve where it passes through the popliteal fossa (Fig. 10-57).

Results. Test results are positive if symptoms are reproduced.

Brechterew's Test

Method. The subject is seated and asked to extend both knees simultaneously (Fig. 10-58).

Results. Test results are positive if symptoms are reproduced in the involved limb.

FEMORAL NERVE STRETCH[7]

Indication. Femoral nerve stretch is used to determine whether there is any irritation of the femoral nerve or root.

Method. The subject is prone. The examiner flexes the subject's knee while supporting the thigh just proximal to the knee (Fig. 10-59). The examiner stabilizes the pelvis while extending the hip to provide a further stretch of the femoral nerve.

Results. Pain reproduced or exacerbated in the subject's back or throughout the femoral nerve distribution indicates a positive result for femoral nerve or nerve root irritation.

TESTS TO EVALUATE MALINGERING

Flip Sign

Indication. The flip sign is used to assist in determining whether the subject may be inventing symptoms.

Method. If the subject has a positive straight leg raise test when supine but the examiner suspects malingering, the subject is requested to assume a short sitting position with the legs dangling over the side of the table. Under the guise of examining for an unrelated problem (e.g., to check the knee or

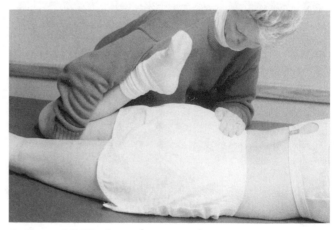

▲ **Figure 10.59** Femoral nerve stretch.

foot), the examiner extends the knee now set up in a variant of the straight leg raise position.

Results. Reproduction of stretch of an irritated nerve root should occur in both the supine and sitting positions for this test. The subject who is malingering may fail to report symptoms in the variant position. The examiner should then be alerted to observe the subject carefully in the seated position as the subject with true symptoms may lean the trunk backward or grimace rather than verbalize the complaints.

Hoover's Test[1,11]

Indication. Hoover's test is used to help determine whether the subject may be malingering or withholding effort.

Method. With the subject supine, the examiner places one hand under each heel and asks the subject to raise one lower limb. The examiner should feel an increase in pressure under the opposite heel as the subject tries to gain leverage with the effort (Fig. 10-60). The test is repeated with the opposite limb.

Results. If no increased pressure is felt from the opposite limb, the subject is probably not putting forth full effort, and the test is positive.

Burn's Test

Method. The subject is asked to kneel on a chair and bend forward to touch fingers to the floor (Fig. 10-61).

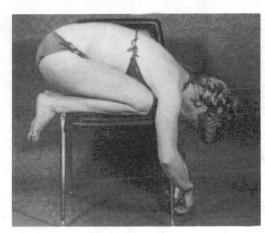

▲ **Figure 10.61** Burn's test.

Results. The subject who is unable to perform the task or overbalances the chair is likely to be malingering.

TESTS TO INCREASE INTRATHECAL PRESSURE

The following three tests assess the effect of increased intrathecal pressure. A positive result suggests either intrathecal or extrathecal pathology (e.g., disk protrusion, tumor), including the meninges themselves.

Valsalva's Maneuver[15]

Method. The subject is asked to hold a breath and then bear down, as if to have a bowel movement.

Results. Test results are positive if the subject reports reproduction or exacerbation of spinal pain or radiation into the limb.

Milgram's Test

Method. The subject lies supine. The examiner asks the subject to lift both lower limbs simultaneously 2 to 4 in off the table while holding the position for 30 seconds (Fig. 10-62A).

Results. Test results are positive if the subject is unable to hold the limbs elevated for 30 seconds or experiences reproduction of pain in the spine or radiation into the limb (see Fig. 10-62B).

Naphziger's Test

Method. The subject lies supine. The examiner gently compresses the internal jugular veins bilaterally for approximately 10 seconds, then asks the subject to cough.

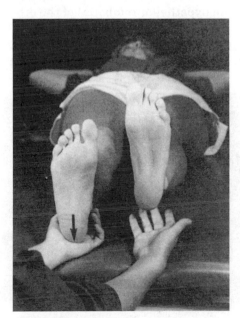

▲ **Figure 10.60** Hoover's test.

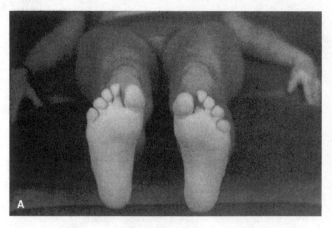

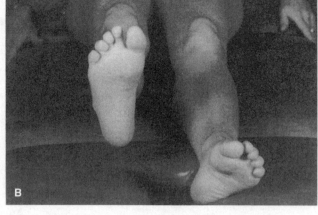

▲ **Figure 10.62** (**A**) Milgram's test. (**B**) Positive Milgram's test result.

Results. Pain experienced in the low back during coughing indicates a positive test. This results from compression of the spinal theca and a subsequent increase in intrathecal pressure.

JOINT PLAY

Passive Intervertebral Movement Testing of the Thoracic Spine

PALPATION OF PASSIVE INTERVERTEBRAL MOVEMENT DURING GROSS RANGE OF MOTION

Segmental movement is assessed at the interspinous space as in cervical spine evaluation for the upper thoracic levels. The examiner can support and guide movement of the midthoracic and lower thoracic levels by controlling the shoulders and thorax (Fig. 10-63). The spinous process is palpated during forward and backward bending, sidebending, and rotation. Assessment of sidebending and rotation is facilitated by forward bending to the level of testing.

The examiner decides whether the end feel is normal, hypermobile, or hypomobile and observes for provocation of symptoms.

Spring Test

Method. The examiner places the pisiform of the cephalad hand on the spinous process of each vertebra, producing a gentle springing force in a direction perpendicular to the contour of the spine (Fig. 10-64).

Results. The spring test assesses forward bending of the superior motion segment and backward bending of the inferior segment.

Posterior and Anterior Glide

Method. The examiner touches the transverse processes of a vertebra with the pads of the second and third digits of the caudal hand (Fig. 10-65*A*) and presses the hypothenar eminence of the other (mobilizing) hand over these two digits (see Fig. 10-65*B*). Gentle force is applied in the posterocaudal–anterocephalic direction to follow the plane of the joint.

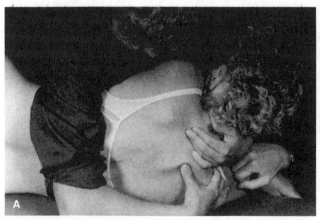

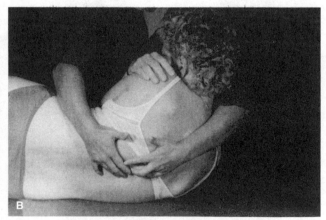

▲ **Figure 10.63** Assessment of segmental movement at the (**A**) midthoracic and (**B**) lower thoracic levels.

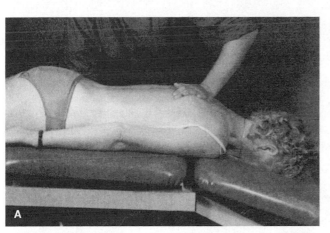
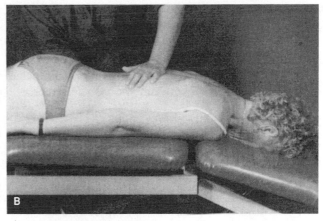

▲ **Figure 10.64** Spring testing of the (**A**) midthoracic and (**B**) lower thoracic levels.

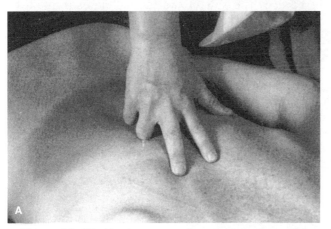
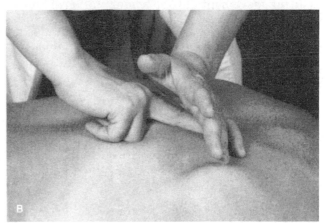

▲ **Figure 10.65** Hand positioning for posterior–anterior glide.

Results. This method assesses forward bending of the inferior motion segment and backward bending of the superior segment.

Rotatory Glide

Method. Contact is made as for posterior and anterior glide, except that the dummy hand touches two adjacent vertebrae, for example, the left transverse process of T6 and the right transverse process of T7. (The reverse setup will also be tested.) The hypothenar eminence of the mobilizing hand produces a posterior and anterior force.

Results. This method tests right rotation of T6 on T7 by producing forward glide of the left T6-7 articulation and backward glide of the right T6-7 articulation. This test is fairly well localized to single motion segments.

Rib (Costovertebral) Mobility

Method. The subject lies in a prone position. The examiner uses the thumb web space along the length of the rib, including the costovertebral angle (Fig. 10-66). The examiner assesses mobility in the posterior and anterior (following the obliquity of the rib), cranial-caudal, and caudal-cranial directions.

Results. The examiner identifies areas of normal mobility, hypermobility, and hypomobility of the costovertebral articulations.

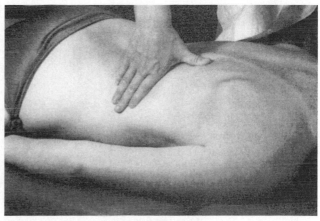

▲ **Figure 10.66** Costovertebral mobility.

Passive Intervertebral Movement Testing of the Lumbar Spine

All movements are described as the motion of the superior segment in relation to the inferior one.

Forward Bend

Method. The subject is in the sidelying position. The examiner brings the uppermost limb or both limbs into hip and knee flexion (Fig. 10-67). The hip must typically be flexed at least 90 degrees before lumbar movement is recruited. While using the cephalad hand to palpate the interspinous space, the examiner brings the hip into further flexion, thereby recruiting movement at each segmental level for assessment of mobility.

Results. This test assesses the superior glide of the facets.

Sidebending

Method 1. The subject is in the sidelying position, with hips and knees flexed 90 degrees. The examiner uses the craniad hand to palpate at the interspinous level on the side of sidebending. The caudad hand contacts the ischial tuberosity of the upper innominate (pelvis) and rocks the pelvis superiorly (Fig. 10-68A). The result is sidebending of the lumbar spine in the direction of the upper side. The spine is bent forward to each segmental level to localize testing. The examiner then contacts the iliac crest and pushes inferiorly to rock the pelvis and produce lumbar sidebending to the opposite direction (see Fig. 10-68B). The examiner palpates the other side.

Method 2. The subject is in the sidelying position with the hips and knees flexed 90 degrees. The subject is moved toward the edge of the table, guarded by the examiner, so that the lower limbs may be lowered over the side of the table. The examiner, supporting at the ankles, raises the subject's limbs to rock the pelvis, in turn causing ("upward") sidebending of the lumbar spine (Fig. 10-69). The examiner palpates each segment at the interspinous space on the side toward which the subject is bent. The opposite sidebend is tested by lowering the limbs below the level of the table to rock the pelvis in the opposite direction. The palpating finger moves to the lower side in the direction of sidebending.

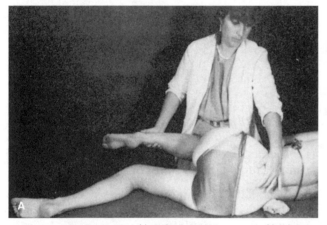
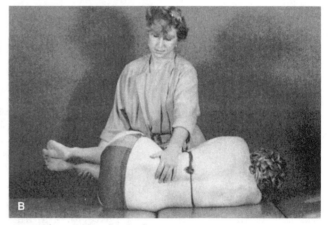

▲ **Figure 10.67** Forward bending. **(A)** Assessment of lumbar intersegmental forward bending by flexion of uppermost limb. **(B)** Assessment of lumbar intersegmental mobility by flexion of both lower limbs.

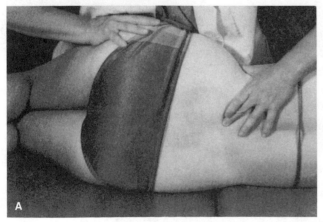
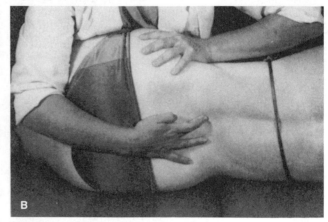

▲ **Figure 10.68** Sidebending. **(A)** Lumbar sidebending to the left. **(B)** Lumbar sidebending to the right.

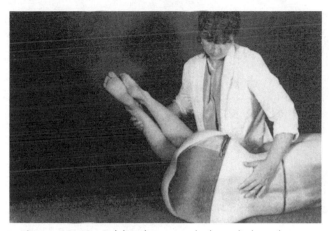

▲ **Figure 10.69** Sidebending using the lower limbs as leverage.

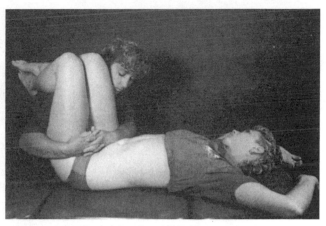

▲ **Figure 10.70** Sidebending of L5–S1.

Results. Sidebending evaluates inferior and medial glide of the ipsilateral side and superior and lateral glide of the contralateral facet joints.

Sidebending of L5 to S1

Method. The subject lies supine. The examiner "slings" the subject's knees over the examiner's shoulders so that the hips and knees are flexed 90 degrees. The examiner locks the fingers together and with the forearm, contacts the top of the subject's thighs as far proximally as possible (Fig. 10-70). Caudal distraction is produced to the side away from the examiner.

Results. Sidebending of L5 to S1 assesses inferior glide of the sacrum on the L5 inferior facet of that side.

Rotation

Method 1. The subject lies prone as the examiner flexes the knees to 90 degrees to use as a lever. The spine is palpated at the interspinous space on the side toward which the limbs are rotated or the side opposite the direction of rotation. Even though rotation is being imparted from inferior to superior, the standard reference position of the superior vertebra in relation to the inferior vertebra is maintained (Fig. 10-71*A*). The examiner moves the limbs in the opposite direction to produce the opposite rotation, changing the palpation to the appropriate side.

Method 2. The subject lies prone. The examiner rotates the lumbar spine by lifting the ASIS of one side (see Fig. 10-71*B*). The spine rotates toward the side opposite the side lifted. The examiner palpates at the interspinous level on the side opposite the direction of rotation. The examiner then lifts the opposite ASIS.

Method 3. The subject is in a sidelying position facing the examiner. The examiner localizes the segment by having the subject bend forward to the level being tested. The examiner rotates the thorax to the segment being tested. Palpation will be on the lower side of the interspinous space.

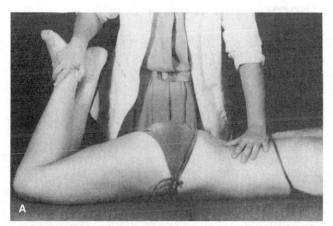

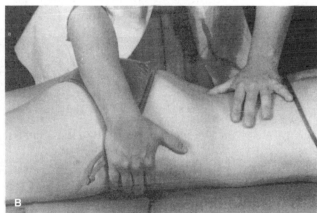

▲ **Figure 10.71** Rotation: **(A)** Method 1, using lower limbs for leverage; **(B)** Method 2, using pelvis as leverage.

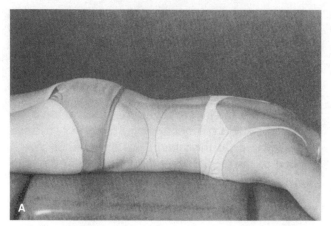
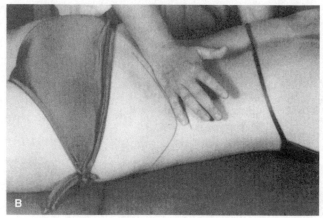

▲ **Figure 10.72** **(A)** Identification of 12th rib and iliac crest. **(B)** Spring test for rotation of vertebrae.

Results. Rotation evaluates lateral and superior glide of the ipsilateral facet joints and medial and inferior glide of the contralateral facet joints.

Posterior–Anterior Spring Test

Method. The subject lies prone. The examiner presses the pisiform to the spinous process to spring the vertebra in a posterior-anterior direction. The forearm of the examiner is perpendicular to the contour of the subject's back.

Results. The posterior-anterior spring test evaluates general hypomobility of the superior and inferior motion segments.

Rotation

Method. The subject lies prone. The examiner palpates the 12th rib and the iliac crest (Fig. 10-72A). Pressing the pisiform over the level of the transverse process, the examiner applies downward force on one side to produce rotation of that vertebra (note that two motion segments are involved) to the oppo-

TABLE 10.1	**Summary of Thoracic Spine Joint Play**
GLIDE	RESTRICTION
Forward	Forward bend, sidebend to the opposite side, rotation to the opposite side
Backward	Backward bend, sidebend to the same side, rotation to the same side
Rotation	Rotation to the same side, backward glide of the same side, and forward glide of the opposite side facets
Spring test	General hypomobility of the costo-vertebral facet joints

TABLE 10.2	**Summary of Lumbar Spine Joint Play**
GLIDE	RESTRICTION
Forward	Forward bend, sidebend to the opposite side, rotation to the same side
Backward	Backward bend, sidebend to the same side, rotation to the opposite side
Rotation	Rotation to the same side, sidebending to the opposite side

site side (see Fig. 10-72B). L2, L3, and L4 can be tested in this fashion. The examiner will have to angle the testing hand to follow the oblique angles of the 12th rib and the iliac crest to make proper contact.

Results. The rotation spring test evaluates general mobility of the ipsilateral facet joints of the superior and inferior motion segments.

Summary of Joint Play of the Thoracic and Lumbar Spine

Tables 10-1 and 10-2 provide a summary of thoracic and lumbar joint play.

REFERENCES

1. Arieff AJ, Tigay EI, Kurtz JI, Larmon WA: The Hoover sign: An objective sign of pain and/or weakness in the back or lower extremities. Arch Neurol 5:673, 1961
2. Brieg A, Troup JDG: Biomechanical considerations in straight-leg raising test: Cadaveric and clinical studies of the effects of medial hip rotation. Spine 4:242, 1979
3. Brody IA, Williams RH: The signs of Kernig and Brudzinski. Arch Neurol 21:215, 1969
4. Brudzinski J: A new sign of the lower extremities in meningitis of children (neck sign). Arch Neurol 21:217, 1969

5. Charnley J: Orthopedic signs in the diagnosis of disc protrusion with special reference to the straight-leg-raising test. Lancet 1:156, 1951

6. Cram RH: A sign of sciatic nerve root pressure. J Bone Joint Surg 35B:192, 1953

7. Dyck P: The femoral nerve traction test with lumbar disc protrusion. Surg Neurol 6:163, 1976

8. Edgar MA, Park WM: Induced pain patterns on passive straight-leg-raising in lower lumbar disc protrusion. J Bone Joint Surg 56B:658, 1974

9. Fahrni WH: Observations on straight-leg-raising with special reference to nerve root adhesions. Can J Surg 9:44, 1966

10. Goddard BS, Reid JD: Movements induced by straight-leg-raising in the lumbo-sacral roots, nerves and plexus and in the intrapelvic section of the sciatic nerve. J Neurol Neurosurg Psychiatry 28:12, 1965

11. Hoover CF: A new sign for the detection of malingering and functional paresis of the lower extremities. JAMA 51:746, 1908

12. Kendall FP, McCreary EK, Provance P: Muscles, Testing, and Function, 4th ed. Baltimore, Williams & Wilkins, 1993.

13. Kernig W: Concerning a little noted sign of meningitis. Arch Neurol 21:216, 1969

14. Maitland GD: The slump test: Examination and treatment. Aust J Physiother 31:215, 1985

15. Scham SM, Taylor TKF: Tension signs in lumbar disc prolapse. Clin Orthop 75:195, 1971

16. Urban LM: The straight-leg-raising test: A review. J Orthop Sports Phys Ther 2:117, 1981

17. Wadworth CT, DeFabio RF, Johnson D: The spine. In Manual Examination and Treatment of the Spine and Extremities. Baltimore, Williams & Wilkins, 1988

18. Wilkins RH, Brody IA: Laseque's sign. Arch Neurol 21:219, 1969

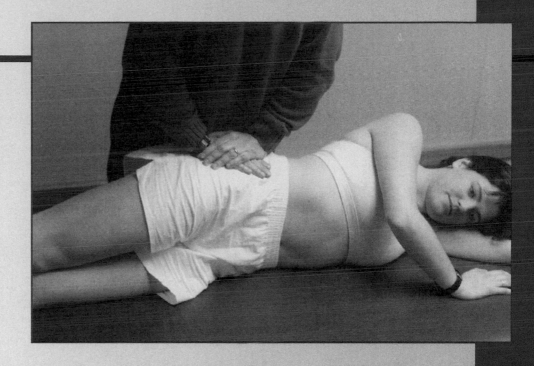

Sacroiliac Joint

CLINICAL ASSESSMENT

Observation and Screening

As stated in a previous chapter, because of the biomechanical relationship of the lumbosacral spine, sacroiliac (SI) joints, hips, and lower limbs, patients with symptom complaints involving these areas may require specific examinations of all regions.

Gross observation should include a careful and detailed postural evaluation of the patient's entire body, concentrating on trunk and lower limb alignments. Refer to Chapter 4 for information on postural examination. Inspection and palpation of pelvic landmarks help to determine the presence of SI malalignment or leg-length discrepancy. Malalignment may also be indicated by other clinical signs and symptoms.

A wealth of information can be gained by noting the symmetry of the anterior superior iliac spines (ASIS) and posterior superior iliac spines (PSIS) from one side of the patient to the other. Nutation, defined as forward bending of the sacrum relative to the ilium, results in a relative posterior torsion of the joint on the ipsilateral side. This postural deviation will cause the ASIS to lie higher and the PSIS to lie lower on the involved side compared with those same landmarks on the uninvolved side. Nutation results in the pelvic brim becoming smaller in diameter and the pelvic outlet becoming larger. Conversely, counternutation, or a backward bending of the sacrum on the ilium, creates a relative anterior torsion of the joint on the same side. As a result, examination of the bony landmarks reveals the ASIS to be lower and the PSIS to be higher on the involved side compared with the normal uninvolved side. Counternutation results in the pelvic brim becoming larger in diameter and the pelvic outlet smaller.

Cephalic and caudal shearing injuries to the SI joint result in both the ASIS and PSIS landmarks on one side being higher or lower compared with those same landmarks on the opposite side. In the case of a cephalic shear injury in which the ilium on the affected side is displaced inferior relative to the sacrum, the ASIS and PSIS will both lie lower than on the uninvolved side. On the other hand, a caudal shear with the ilium positioned superior relative to the sacrum causes the ASIS and PSIS landmarks to sit higher than on the uninvolved side.

Abnormalities of the SI joint not only affect the ASIS and PSIS landmarks, but also the symmetry of the pubic symphysis. In a torsional injury of the SI joint, palpable asymmetry between the right and left components of the pubic symphysis may be felt on the anterior and superior surfaces. In a shearing injury, palpable asymmetry may be appreciated on the superior surface of the pubic symphysis but not necessarily on its anterior surface.

Finally, SI dysfunction may result in apparent leg-length discrepancies. In SI torsional injuries, true leg length is unaffected while apparent leg-length differences exist. Typically, a posterior torsion of the joint produces an apparently shorter leg length, whereas an anterior torsion creates an apparently longer limb length. A cephalic shear injury may produce an apparent lengthening of the limb secondary to the inferior displacement of the affected ilium. Conversely, a caudal shear may result in an apparent shortening of the limb on the involved side.

Palpation and Surface Anatomy

The following structures and landmarks should be palpated or observed during SI joint evaluation:

1. ASIS
2. PSIS
3. Iliac crests
4. Pubic tubercle
5. Posterior sulci
6. S2 tubercle
7. Sacrotuberous ligament
8. Greater trochanters
9. Muscles

Although many of the following muscles are primarily considered to be hip muscles, their attachments on the innominate bone make them susceptible to aberrant stresses and strains when there is mechanical dysfunction of the SI joint. Special attention should be paid to such things as the innominate attachments and locating trigger points and areas of congestion. The following muscles should be examined:

1. Piriformis
2. Tensor fasciae latae
3. Gluteus maximus
4. Hamstrings
5. Rectus femori
6. Sartorius
7. All adductor group muscles
8. Iliotibial band

SPECIAL CLINICAL TESTS

The following tests permit the examiner to assess the SI joint for hypermobility or hypomobility by evaluating end feel or observing relationships of bony landmarks. Most are additionally provocation tests of joint irritability to test for reproduction of symptoms, especially those localized to the SI joint.

Supine-Sit Test

Indication. The supine-sit test evaluates SI torsion by comparing functional leg lengths. Because of the eccentric position of the acetabulum, a functional leg-length discrepancy due to SI torsion will become apparent by rotating the pelvis from the supine to the sitting position.

Method. The subject lies supine. The examiner holds both ankles and gives a slight even traction force to make sure the subject is lying straight. The lower limbs are then placed on the table. With the thumbs placed just distal to the medial malleoli of the ankles, the examiner compares leg lengths (Fig. 11-1*A* and *B*). The subject is then asked to rise into the straight leg sitting position, and leg lengths are again compared (see Fig. 11-1*C* and *D*). The examiner must note whether the relationships remain the same or change with the change of position.

Results. A change in length between the two positions is a positive indication of SI torsion. No change in relationship suggests no torsion. Posterior torsion is identified when the shorter limb in the supine position becomes the longer limb in the sitting position. Anterior torsion is ascertained when the longer

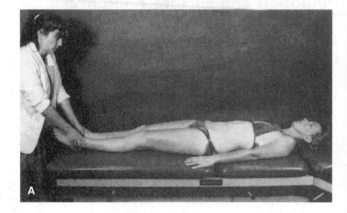

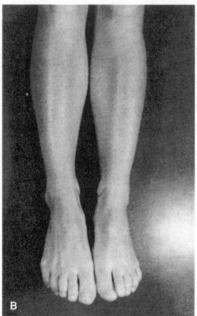

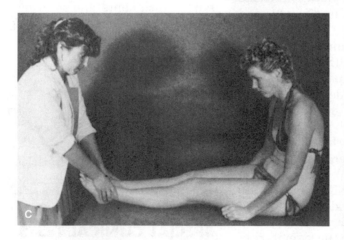

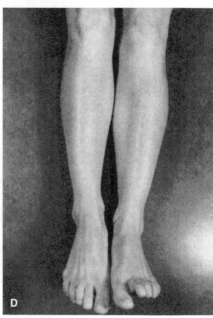

▲ **Figure 11.1** (**A**) Initial position of supine-to-sit test. (**B**) Symmetrical level of medial malleoli. (**C**) Final position for supine-to-sit test. (**D**) Asymmetrical position of medial malleoli.

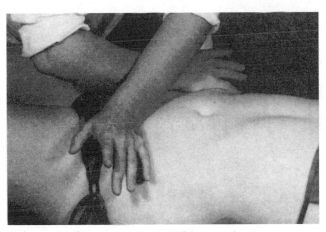

▲ **Figure 11.2** Anterior gapping of the sacroiliac joint.

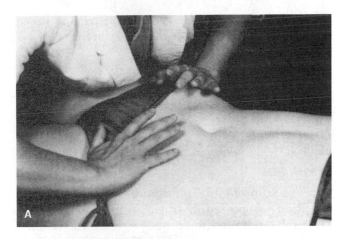

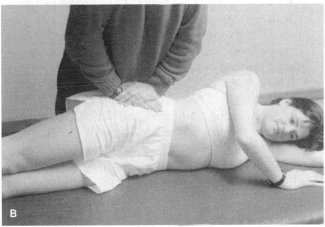

▲ **Figure 11.3** **(A)** Posterior gapping of the sacroiliac joint. **(B)** Alternate position for posterior gapping test.

limb supine becomes the shorter limb sitting. Posterior torsional dysfunctions are more commonly found than anterior torsional problems.

Anterior Gapping Test
(Transverse Anterior Stress Test)

Indication. Anterior gapping implicates the SI articulation as a source of symptoms, specifically the anterior SI ligaments.

Method. The subject lies supine (a pillow can be placed beneath the knees to decrease lumbar lordosis). The examiner crosses the upper limbs to contact the subject's right ASIS with the right hand and the subject's left ASIS with the left hand. A force directed laterally and posteriorly through each ASIS is given as though to separate them (Fig. 11-2). This force causes tension on the anterior structures of the SI joint while compressing the posterior structures. Pressure can be constant or oscillating.

Results. The result is positive if motion reproduces localized unilateral SI pain.

POSTERIOR GAPPING TEST
(TRANSVERSE POSTERIOR STRESS TEST)

Indication. Posterior gapping implicates the posterior SI ligaments as a source of symptoms. This test is the complement to the anterior gapping test.

Method. The subject lies supine. The examiner contacts the lateral aspect of the ASIS bilaterally. Force is directed medially and anteriorly as if to approximate the ASIS, producing tension on the posterior SI ligaments while compressing the anterior structures (Fig. 11-3A). The force can be constant or oscillating. An alternate position is to place the subject sidelying with the examiner standing behind the subject. Both of the examiner's hands are placed on the lateral aspect of the uppermost ilium and a force is directed through the subject's pelvis toward the table (see Fig. 11-3B).

Results. The result is positive if pain is reproduced, localized to an SI joint.

Posterior-Anterior Spring Test
(Sacral Apex Pressure Test)

Indication. The posterior-anterior spring test implicates the SI joint as a source of pain.

Method. The subject lies prone. The innominate is stabilized by contact of the ASIS with the table (contact can be improved by placing a rolled towel beneath the ASIS bilaterally) and the hypothenar eminence of the caudal hand of the examiner contacts the PSIS on the side to be tested. The cranial hand of the examiner contacts the apex of the sacrum and produces a short posterior-anterior stress to "spring" the joint. The examiner should spring test several levels of the sacrum, working toward the base.

Results. Test results are positive if pain is reproduced, especially if it is localized to the SI joint.

Torsion

Indication. Torsion testing assesses for provocation of torsional dysfunction of the SI joint.

Method

Posterior Torsion

1. The subject sits. The examiner, standing behind, supports the subject at the shoulders and leans the subject back against the trunk while stepping backward. The examiner then rotates the subject to one side while contacting the ASIS of the opposite side, blocking it from movement, thereby producing posterior torsion on that side (Fig. 11-4).
2. The subject is lying on the side opposite that to be tested. The examiner contacts the ASIS with the cephalad hand and the posterior aspect of the ischial tuberosity with the other. The hands are used as a force couple to produce a posterior rotation torque to the innominate along the anterolateral-posteromedial plane of the joint.

Anterior Torsion. Hand position is changed from that for posterior torsion so that the caudal hand now contacts the ischial tuberosity for the anterior-inferior aspect, and the cephalad hand contacts the forearm along the iliac crest. Following the plane of the joint, a force couple produces an anterior rotatory torque to the innominate (Fig. 11-5). Forces can be constant or oscillating.

Results. Test results are positive if symptoms are provoked, especially if they are localized to the SI joint.

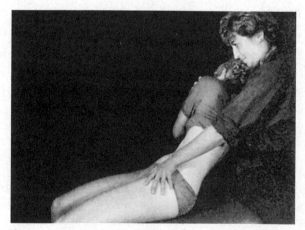

▲ **Figure 11.4** Posterior torsion test of the sacroiliac joint.

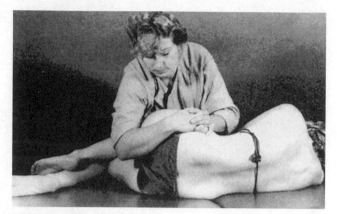

▲ **Figure 11.5** Anterior torsion test of the sacroiliac joint.

Piedallu's Sign

Indication. Piedallu's sign indicates restriction of SI joint mobility.

Method. The subject is sitting on a firm surface. The examiner locates and compares the levels of the left and right PSIS to each other and then compares each PSIS to the level of the S2 tubercle (Fig. 11-6A). The subject is asked to bend forward, flexing the hips and trunk. The positional relationships of the landmarks are again compared (see Fig. 11-6B).

Results. Frequently, SI dysfunction is indicated by the PSIS of the restricted side being inferior to that on the uninvolved side. Test results are positive if, with a finding of uneven PSISs, the relationship of PSIS to S2 reverses with forward bending. This result occurs due to the hypomobile SI joint moving prematurely during the forward bending of the subject.

Sacroiliac Rocking Test (Sacrotuberous Ligament Stress Test)

Indication. This test can be used to identify irritation of the sacrotuberous ligament.

Method. With the subject positioned supine, the examiner passively and maximally flexes the test hip and knee. The examiner maintains the flexed limb position while simultaneously adducting the hip in the direction of the opposite shoulder.

Results. Pain in the area of the SI joint is a positive test.

Gillet's Test (Sacral Fixation Test)

Indication. Gillet's test evaluates the SI joint for restricted mobility.

Method. The subject stands. The examiner stands behind the subject and locates and compares the po-

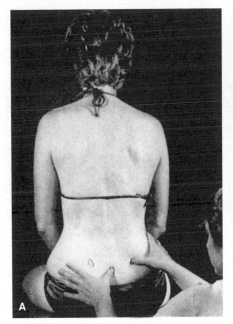
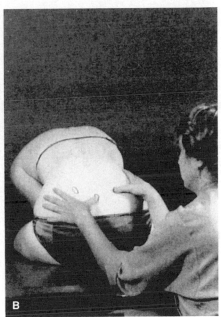

▲ **Figure 11.6** Piedallu's sign. (**A**) Comparison of the PSIS levels and the S2 tubercle in sitting. (**B**) Comparison of the PSIS levels and the S2 tubercle in the forward bent position.

sition of one PSIS relative to the S2 tubercle (Fig. 11-7*A*). The subject is then asked to raise the knee of the side being palpated (as in marching). The examiner again compares the positional relationship of the landmarks (see Fig. 11-7*B*). The ischial tuberosity and the S2 tubercle should also be compared.

Results. With normal SI mobility, the PSIS on the limb being flexed would move caudally and the ischial tuberosity would move laterally with respect to the S2 tubercle. Test results are positive if the PSIS or the tuberosity is restricted in the cephalad direction.

Gaenslin's Test (Passive Hip Extension)

Indication. Gaenslin's test implicates the SI joint as a source of symptoms.

Method. The subject is supine, holding knees to chest. The examiner helps the subject move the lower trunk to the edge of the table, so that the nearside innominate bone has fully cleared the table and the (padded) edge of the table supports the sacrum (Fig. 11-8*A*). The lower limb of the unsupported side is then lowered over the side of the table (see Fig. 11-8*B*).

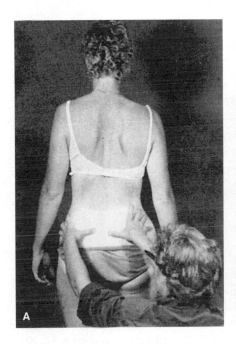
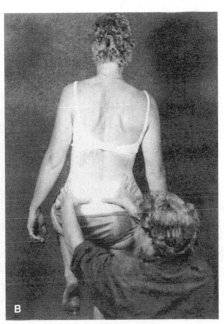

▲ **Figure 11.7** Test for sacroiliac restriction standing.

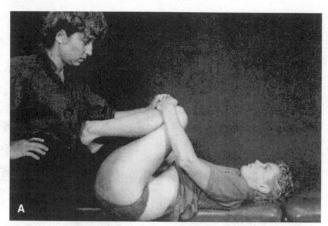
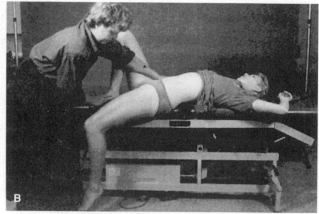

▲ **Figure 11.8** **(A)** Gaenslin's test. **(B)** Lower limb of unsupported side is lowered over the side of the table.

Results. Test results are positive if pain is reproduced, particularly if it is localized to the SI joint.

Yeoman's Test

Indication. Yeoman's test is designed to assess pathology of the anterior SI ligaments.

Method. As the subject lies prone, the examiner passively flexes the knee to 90 degrees and then extends the hip.

Results. Pain in the area of the SI joint may indicate a positive test, but the examiner must be aware of other tissues being stressed with this maneuver that have the potential to elicit pain.

Flamingo Test

Indication. This test can be used in the identification of SI or pubic symphysis dysfunction.

Method. The standing subject is directed to lift one leg off the ground, creating a unilateral weight-bearing situation.

Results. Pain in the area of the SI joint on the side of the weight-bearing limb or in the pubic symphysis indicates a positive test for that particular structure.

SHEAR TESTS

Indication. The shear tests implicate the SI joint as a source of symptoms, assessing the joint in the caudad and cephalad directions.

Method

Caudal Shear. The subject lies prone. The examiner contacts the base of the sacrum with the cephalad hand and stabilizes the innominate bone at the ischial tuberosity. With the forearms parallel to the table, a shear force is applied to move the sacrum on the innominate in the caudad direction (Fig. 11-9).

Cephalad Shear. The caudad hand contacts the apex of the sacrum, while the cephalad hand stabilizes the innominate along the iliac crest. A shear force is given to move the sacrum on the innominate in the cephalad direction (Fig. 11-10).

Results. Results are positive if symptoms are reproduced, particularly if they are localized to the SI joint.

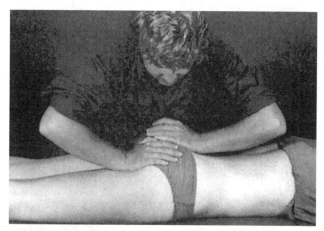

▲ **Figure 11.9** Caudal shear of the sacrum on the ilium.

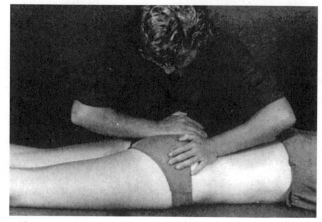

▲ **Figure 11.10** Cephalad shear of the sacrum on the ilium.

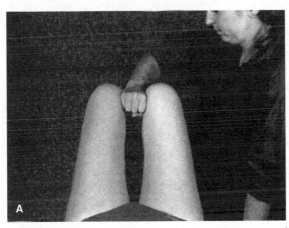 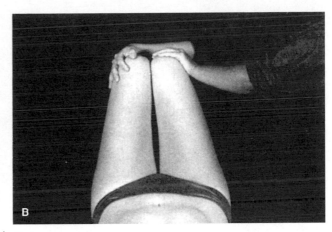

▲ **Figure 11.11** (**A**) Isometric adduction. (**B**) Isometric abduction.

ISOMETRIC ADDUCTION AND ABDUCTION

Indication. Isometric adduction and abduction implicate the SI joint as a source of symptoms by stressing the joint with resisted muscle contraction.

Method. The subject lies supine with the hips and knees flexed, feet flat on the table. The examiner isometrically resists bilateral adduction and then abduction contractions (Fig. 11-11).

Results. Test results are positive if pain is reproduced and localized to the SI joint.

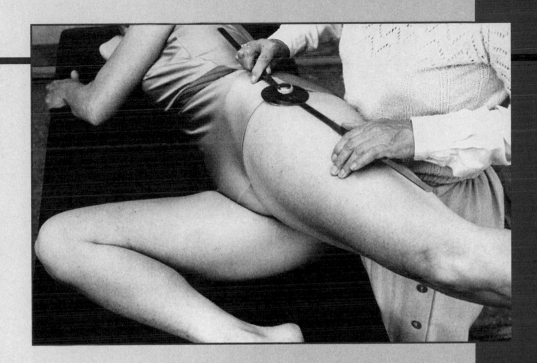

12

Hip

The hip joint is a synovial ball-and-socket type of joint with the head of the femur articulating with the acetabulum. It has greater congruency than any other joint in the body. The hip joint transmits a great force between the trunk and the floor; in addition, it plays a major role in ambulation. The articular arrangement is designed for stability but does permit limited mobility. The hip joint has three degrees of freedom of motion. The true axis of motion goes through the center of the femoral head. Clinically, the axis is at the level of the greater trochanter.

GONIOMETRY

HIP FLEXION

Hip flexion occurs in the sagittal plane between the head of the femur and the acetabulum of the os coxa. As the hip moves into flexion, the head of the femur glides in a posterior and inferior direction. Hip flexion motion is accompanied by secondary movements, such as posterior pelvic tilt and lumbar vertebral flexion. The subject is stabilized so that the secondary motions do not affect hip joint flexion and are not included in the measurement.

Motion. From 0 to 115 to 125 degrees into a position of hip flexion with knee flexion.

Position

- Preferred: Subject lies supine with the opposite lower limb flat on the table top (Fig. 12-1).
- Alternate: Subject is in sidelying position on the opposite side (Fig. 12-2).

Goniometric Alignment

Axis. Placed on the lateral aspect of the hip approximately a fingerbreadth anterior and superior to the greater trochanter of the femur.

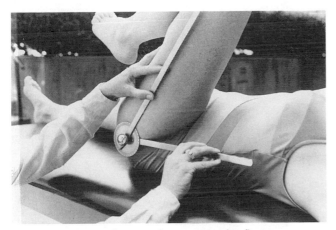

▲ **Figure 12.1** End position for measuring hip flexion.

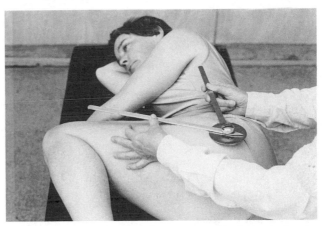

▲ **Figure 12.2** End position for measuring hip flexion in the alternate sidelying position.

Stationary Arm. Placed parallel to the long axis of the trunk, in line with the greater trochanter of the femur.

Moving Arm. Placed along the lateral midline of the femur toward the lateral epicondyle.

Stabilization. The pelvis is stabilized.

Precautions

- Allow the knee to flex to prevent a stretch on the hamstring muscles.
- Keep the opposite lower limb flat on the table to control posterior pelvic tilt.
- Avoid lumbosacral motion.

HIP EXTENSION AND HYPEREXTENSION

Extension and hyperextension motion occurs in the sagittal plane as the return from hip flexion. The test position for hip joint hyperextension is lying on the side opposite the hip joint being measured. As the femur extends and hyperextends, the head glides in an anterior and inferior direction in the acetabulum of the os coxa. The extension-hyperextension motion at the hip is usually accompanied by anterior pelvic tilt and increased lumbar lordosis. The subject is stabilized, and the secondary motions are not included in the measurement.

Hyperextension of the hip joint is rare as a true motion. Careful analysis of the motion will show that it is an extension of the lumbar vertebrae with forward tilt of the pelvis.

Motion. From 115 to 125 degrees to 0 degrees of hip extension and 0 to 10 to 15 degrees of hip hyperextension. In the prone test position, the subject must keep the anterior superior iliac spines (ASIS) flat on the table to ensure that the motion is occurring at the hip joint and not at the lumbar vertebrae.

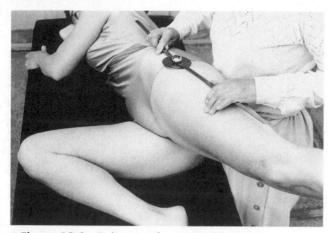

▲ **Figure 12.3** End position for measuring hip extension.

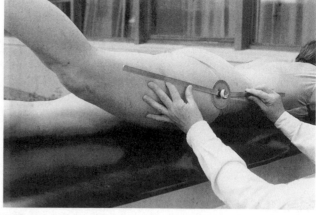

▲ **Figure 12.4** End position for measuring hip hyperextension in the alternate prone position.

Position

- **Preferred:**
  1. Subject is in sidelying position on the opposite side with the nontest hip flexed to 90 degrees to prevent anterior rotation of the pelvis (Fig. 12-3).
  2. Subject lies prone with the hip and knee joints in the anatomical position (Fig. 12-4).
- **Alternate:** Subject lies supine with both lower limbs in the anatomical position.

Goniometric Alignment. Same as for hip flexion.

Stabilization. The pelvis and lumbar vertebrae are stabilized.

Precautions

- Avoid lumbar extension.
- Keep the knee joint extended to prevent stretch on the rectus femoris muscle.
- Avoid anterior pelvic tilt.

HIP ABDUCTION

In the anatomical position, hip abduction motion occurs in the frontal plane. The motion of hip joint abduction occurs between the head of the femur gliding in an inferior direction in the acetabulum of the pelvis. Hip joint abduction is usually accompanied by contralateral pelvic tilt, which is not included in the measurement.

Motion. From 0 to 45 degrees of hip abduction.

Position. Subject lies supine with the lower limb to be tested in the anatomical position (Figs. 12-5 and 12-6).

Goniometric Alignment

Axis. Placed on the anterior surface of the hip joint in line with the greater trochanter of the femur.

Stationary Arm. Placed parallel to and below the ASIS at the level of the hip joint.

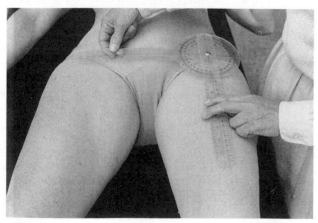

▲ **Figure 12.5** Starting position for measuring hip abduction.

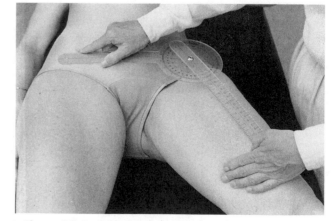

▲ **Figure 12.6** End position for measuring hip abduction.

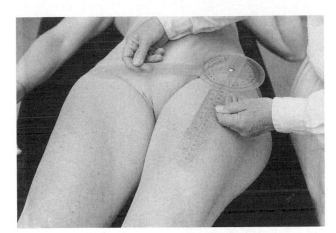

▲ **Figure 12.7** End position for measuring hip adduction.

Moving Arm. Placed on the anterior surface of the thigh parallel to the anterior midline of the femur, toward the midline of the patella.

Stabilization. The pelvis is stabilized.

Precautions

• Prevent lateral rotation at the hip joint.
• Prevent lateral tilt of the pelvis (hip hiking).

HIP ADDUCTION

In the test position, adduction of the hip joint occurs in the frontal plane. The head of the femur glides in a superior direction in the acetabulum. The adduction motion of the hip is usually accompanied by ipsilateral tilt of the pelvis, which is not included in the measurement.

Motion. From 0 to 20 to 30 degrees of hip joint adduction.

Position. Subject lies supine with the hip and knee joints in the anatomical position. The opposite lower limb is abducted to allow full range of motion on the test side (Fig. 12-7).

Goniometric alignment and stabilization are the same as for hip abduction.

Precautions

• Prevent medial rotation of the hip joint.
• Prevent ipsilateral tilt of the pelvis.

HIP MEDIAL ROTATION

In the test position, hip medial rotation motion occurs in the transverse plane. The motion of medial rotation is produced between the head of the femur

and the acetabulum. The head of the femur glides in a posterior direction in the acetabulum during medial rotation of the joint. In the alternate test position, the hip is flexed and not in the anatomical position. Greater range of motion occurs with the hip joint flexed because it is in the open-packed position.

Motion. From 0 to 30 to 45 degrees of hip joint medial rotation. The total range of motion varies depending on whether the hip joint is flexed or extended.

Position

• Preferred: Subject lies supine with the hip joint in the anatomical position and the knee flexed to 90 degrees over the edge of the table. The opposite hip and knee are flexed, and the foot lies flat on the table (Figs. 12-8 and 12-9).
• Alternate:
  1. Subject sits with the knee flexed over the edge of the table. The femur is parallel with the table top, and the hip joint is flexed 90 degrees.
  2. Subject lies prone with the hip joint in the anatomical position and the knee joint flexed 90 degrees (Figs. 12-10 and 12-11).
  3. Subject lies supine with the knee joints flexed 90 degrees and the stationary arm of the goniometer perpendicular to the floor (Fig. 12-12).

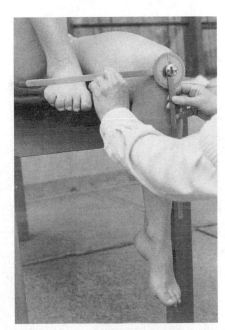

▲ **Figure 12.8** Starting position for measuring hip medial rotation.

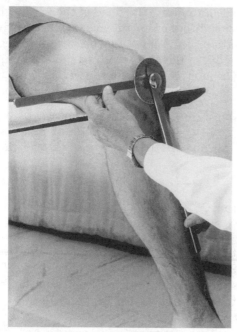

▲ **Figure 12.9** End position for measuring hip medial rotation.

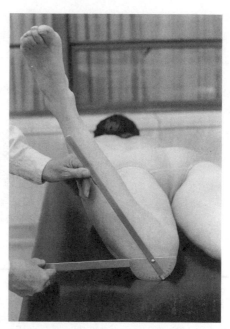

▲ **Figure 12.11** End position for measuring hip medial rotation in the alternate prone position.

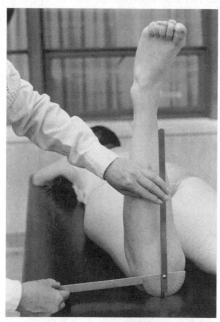

▲ **Figure 12.10** Starting position for measuring hip medial rotation in the alternate prone position.

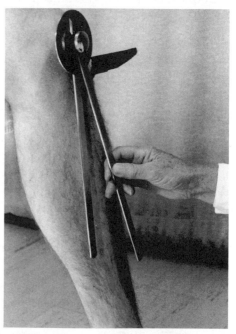

▲ **Figure 12.12** End position for measuring hip medial rotation in the alternate supine position using the effect of gravity on the stationary arm of the goniometer.

Goniometric Alignment

Axis. Placed over the anterior midpatella to project through the shaft of the femur to the femoral head.

Stationary Arm

- Preferred: Placed parallel to the table top.
- Alternate: Placed perpendicular to the floor or parallel to the midline of the tibia.

Moving Arm. Placed along the crest of the tibia to a point midway between the malleoli.

Stabilization. Stabilize the distal end of the thigh.

Precautions

- Avoid rotation and lateral tilting of the pelvis toward the same side.
- Prevent the pelvis from lifting off the table.

- In the sitting position, prevent contralateral trunk flexion.
- Prevent adduction at the hip joint.

HIP LATERAL ROTATION

In the anatomical position, lateral rotation of the hip occurs in the transverse plane. As the motion of hip lateral rotation occurs, the head of the femur glides in an anterior direction in the acetabulum. In the preferred test position, the hip joint is in the anatomical position. Less range of motion in lateral rotation occurs because the hip joint is in a closed-packed position.

Motion. From 0 to 30 to 45 degrees of hip joint lateral rotation. In the preferred test position, the hip joint is in the anatomical position.

Position

- Preferred: Subject is supine, with the knee flexed to 90 degrees over the edge of the table. The nontest hip and knee joint are flexed, and the foot is flat on the table (Fig. 12-13).
- Alternate:
  1. Subject sits with the hip and knee joints flexed to 90 degrees.
  2. Subject lies prone with the test knee joint flexed to 90 degrees (Fig. 12-14).
  3. Subject lies supine with the stationary arm of the goniometer perpendicular to the floor (Fig. 12-15).

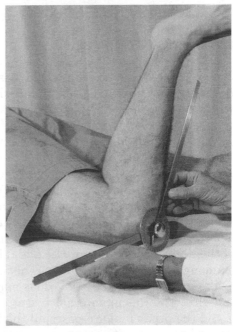

▲ **Figure 12.14** End position for measuring hip lateral rotation in the alternate prone position.

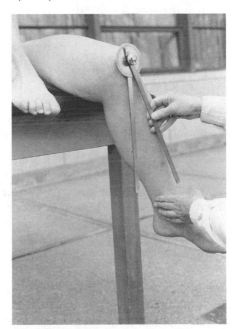

▲ **Figure 12.15** End position for measuring hip rotation in the alternate supine position, using the effects of gravity on the stationary arm of the goniometer.

Goniometric alignment and stabilization are the same as for hip medial rotation.

Precautions

- Avoid rotation of the pelvis toward the opposite side.
- Prevent hip joint adduction or flexion.
- Avoid contralateral tilt of the pelvis.
- Prevent ipsilateral trunk flexion or rotation.

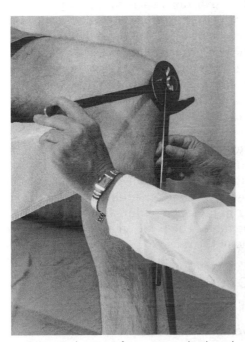

▲ **Figure 12.13** End position for measuring hip lateral rotation.

MUSCLE LENGTH ASSESSMENT

Hip Joint Flexor Muscles

The hip flexor muscles lie anterior to the axis of motion in the sagittal plane. The group of muscles that cross the hip joint includes the iliacus, psoas major, sartorius, rectus femoris, tensor fascia lata, pectineus, adductor longus, and gracilis. The identified muscles are two-joint or multijoint muscles, except for the pectineus and adductor longus muscles. Each crosses the hip proximally and the knee distally. As a group, the muscles tend to contract during an erect standing posture because the gravity line lies slightly posterior to the hip joint. A decrease in length of the anterior hip joint muscles is relatively common among sedentary individuals. The iliopsoas muscle is the muscle formed by the psoas major and iliacus muscles. The iliacus muscle crosses only the hip joint and the psoas major crosses all the lumbar vertebrae and joins the iliacus muscle prior to its exit from the pelvic cavity to its distal attachment on the lesser trochanter of the femur.

ILIOPSOAS (ILIACUS AND PSOAS MAJOR), ADDUCTOR LONGUS, AND PECTINEUS MUSCLES

Position. The subject is supine, with the pelvis in a neutral position and the knee joints over the edge of the table (Thomas test).

Movement. The examiner flexes both knees toward the chest, allowing the back to flatten on the treatment table. The other thigh is lowered toward the table. The knee joint is allowed to be relaxed. If the thigh is not flat on the treatment table, the iliopsoas, adductor longus, and pectineus muscles have a decrease in length.

Excessive hip joint mobility would be assessed with the test hip joint off the end of the treatment table. The low back remains flat on the surface of the table, and the opposite knee is held toward the chest.

Measurement. Align the goniometer using the bony landmarks for measuring hip flexion. The difference from the table and the position of the hip is the amount of hip flexor muscle shortening. The range of motion should be recorded in degrees lacking in complete hip joint extension. Excessive motion is evident if the test hip joint is positioned off the edge of the treatment table and the hip joint continues into hyperextension while the opposite knee is held toward the chest and the low back remains flat on the table (Fig. 12-16).

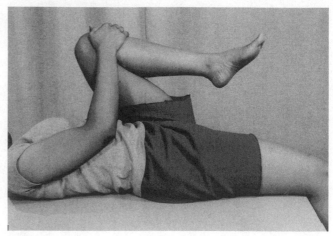

▲ **Figure 12.16** Muscle length testing of hip flexor muscles (Thomas test).

Considerations

- The iliopsoas muscle attaching to the lumbar vertebra and the lesser trochanter of the femur may have a tendency to pull the lumbar vertebrae into hyperextension (lordosis) unless the low back is kept flat on the table.
- If the hip joint is extended and the knee joint is allowed to extend, this indicates that the one-joint hip flexors are normal in length and the two-joint rectus femoris and tensor fascia lata muscles are probably shortened. An indication of tightness of the two-joint rectus femoris muscle is demonstrated when the test leg's knee joint extends while the test hip joint is extended completely.
- The sartorius muscle may be tight if the hip joint is extended accompanied by lateral rotation.
- The tensor fascia lata muscle shows limitation in length if the hip joint is extended accompanied by medial rotation.
- The pectineus or adductor longus may be too short if the hip joint tends to drift into adduction during extension.
- Excessive low back flexibility may not produce a true length test of the hip flexor muscles. The buttock (sacrum) must remain flat on the treatment table with the lumbar vertebrae remaining in flexion, avoiding lifting of the buttock off the table. The position maintains the proximal end of the muscle in its elongated state.

SARTORIUS MUSCLE

Position. Same as previous test.

Movement. Same as previous test. The examiner supports the knee joint in extension and holds the

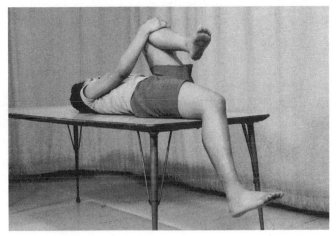

▲ **Figure 12.17** Muscle length testing of the sartorius muscle.

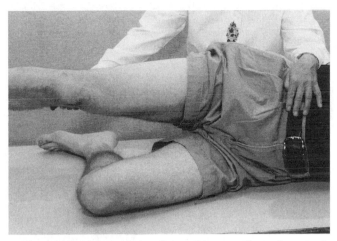

▲ **Figure 12.18** Muscle length test of the tensor fascia lata muscle (Ober test).

hip joint in neutral rotation/abduction-adduction. If lateral rotation occurs at the hip on the test side with the hip joint in extension, then the sartorius is probably shortened.

Measurement. Same as previous test. An increase in flexion indicates shortness in the sartorius muscle with the hip joint in neutral rotation (Fig. 12-17).

Considerations

- With the knee joint in extension, the rectus femoris muscle may also be too tight.
- If medial rotation at the hip joint occurs, the tensor fascia lata muscle may be too tight.
- If the hip joint does not completely extend, the knee joint remains extended, and rotation does not occur at the hip, then the iliopsoas may be the only muscle showing too little length.
- The Thomas test should be performed to eliminate the effect of one-joint flexor muscles.

TENSOR FASCIA LATA (ACCOMPANYING ILIOTIBIAL BAND; OBER TEST)

Position. The subject is sidelying. The nontest leg is supported on the treatment table slightly flexed at the hip and knee joints for stability, to decrease lumbar lordosis, and to prevent an anterior pelvic tilt.

Movement. The test knee joint is flexed to 90 degrees or completely extended (modified Ober*). The examiner abducts and hyperextends the hip joint. Rotation at the hip does not occur. In this position, the hip joint is allowed to adduct toward the table.

Measurement. If the hip joint remains abducted and does not come to the horizontal, the distance from the treatment table to the medial border of the knee may be measured with a ruler. If the hip adducts to the surface of the table, shortening of the tensor fascia lata muscle and accompanying iliotibial band has not occurred (Fig. 12-18).

Considerations. If the examiner allows the hip joint to rotate medially or flex, then the test length for the tensor fascia lata muscle will not be accurate, allowing slack in the muscle.

RECTUS FEMORIS MUSCLE

Position. The subject is supine, with the test knee joint flexed over the edge of the treatment table. The nontest hip joint is flexed to flatten the low back area.

Movement. The examiner completely extends the hip joint to the surface of the treatment table. If the knee joint extends, then the two-joint rectus femoris muscle is too short.

Measurement. Measure with a goniometer the degrees of knee joint flexion. Start the measure from a position of 80 degrees of flexion to the end position. The number of degrees from 80 degrees indicates the amount of shortness in the muscle (Fig. 12-19).

Considerations

- If the hip joint can be completely extended only if the knee joint is allowed to extend, then the one-joint hip flexors have a normal length and the rectus femoris is tight.
- The above action may indicate that the tensor fascia lata muscle may also be tight.

---

* The modified Ober test, knee joint extended, was developed by Kendall to lessen the strain placed on the knee joint.

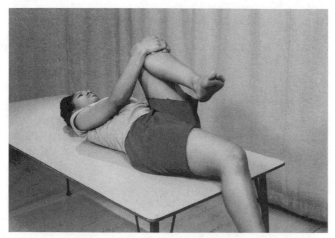

▲ **Figure 12.19** Muscle length test for the rectus femoris muscle.

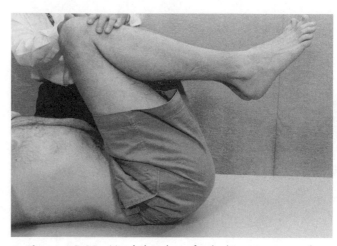

▲ **Figure 12.20** Muscle length test for the hip extensor muscle.

Hip Extensor Muscles

The extensor muscles of the hip joint lie posterior to the axis in the sagittal plane. The hip joint extensor muscles more commonly involved in limitations are the one-joint gluteus maximus and the two-joint hamstrings (short head of the biceps femoris only crosses the knee joint). The action of the hamstring muscles at the knee joint is dependent on the position of the hip joint. When they are stretched by hip flexion, their efficiency as knee flexors increases.

GLUTEUS MAXIMUS MUSCLE

Position. The subject is supine with the knee joints flexed and the pelvis in neutral with regard to anterior and posterior pelvic tilt. A short sitting position may also be used as long as the pelvis and low back remain in a neutral position.

Movement. The examiner flexes the thigh toward the pelvis without an accompanying posterior pelvic tilt. The sacrum remains flat on the treatment table.

Measurement. Hip flexion is measured with a goniometer when the sacrum begins to lift off the table. The total number of degrees of hip flexion is subtracted from the normal range of motion at the hip, and the difference is the amount of gluteus maximus limitation. Any excessive motion will be limited by the abdomen on the anterior thigh (Fig. 12-20).

Considerations

- Low back (lumbar) hypermobility into flexion may produce motion that appears to be at the hip joint. The sacrum must remain flat on the table.
- To eliminate the effect of the hamstring muscles, the knee joint remains flexed.

HAMSTRINGS: BICEPS FEMORIS LONG HEAD, SEMIMEMBRANOSUS, AND SEMITENDINOSUS MUSCLES (STRAIGHT LEG RAISE TEST)

Position. The subject is supine with the knee joint extended and the low back and sacrum flat on the surface of the treatment table. The nontest leg is held down on the table.

Movement. The examiner flexes the test hip joint, holding the knee joint in extension with the ankle joint relaxed (Fig. 12-21).

Measurement. The degree of hip joint flexion is measured with a goniometer. The normal adult range of motion is 70 to 80 degrees. Less than that range indicates that the hamstring or gluteus maximus muscle is too tight. Excessive hamstring length is indicated if hip flexion is greater than 80 degrees of flexion.

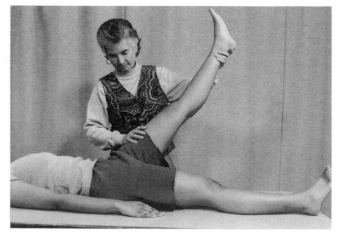

▲ **Figure 12.21** Muscle length test for the hamstrings (straight leg raise).

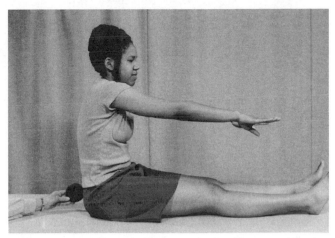

▲ **Figure 12.22** Muscle length test for hamstring muscles (alternate).

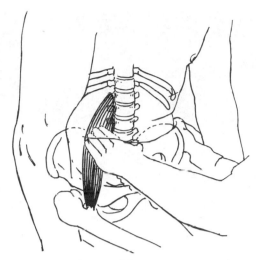

▲ **Figure 12.23** Palpation of the psoas major muscle.

Considerations

- If the hip flexors are tight, then a roll or pillow may be placed under the nontest leg to allow the low back to be flat on the table.
- A posterior pelvic tilt would provide an increase in hamstring muscle length. The pelvis must remain neutral in the sagittal plane.
- An anterior pelvic tilt or a hyperextended low back will give the appearance of the hamstring muscles being too short.

HAMSTRINGS (ALTERNATE TEST)

A study was performed by Cornbleet and Woolsey using a sit and reach test.

Position. The subject is in a long sitting position with the lower limbs supported.

Movement. The examiner asks the subject to reach forward actively to reach the toes.

Measurement. An inclinometer is used over the sacrum to measure the hip joint angle for a mean value of 81 degrees (Fig. 12-22).

MANUAL MUSCLE TESTING

PSOAS MAJOR AND ILIACUS MUSCLES

The psoas major and the iliacus muscles have a common insertion and are called the iliopsoas muscle. The combined muscle produces the motion of hip flexion in the sagittal plane through a test range of 30 degrees from a starting position of 90 degrees of flexion. During the movement, the pelvis remains fixed in a posterior pelvic tilt.

Palpation

Psoas Major. With the subject seated and bent forward to relax the abdominal muscles, place fingers deep into the abdomen below the ribs and above the iliac crest, gently pushing toward the posterior abdominal wall (Fig. 12-23).

Iliacus. It is difficult to palpate the iliac muscle, which lies on the iliac fossa.

Position

Against gravity (AG): Subject sits with the knees flexed and the pelvis in posterior tilt. Hands should be holding on to the edge of the table (Fig. 12-24).

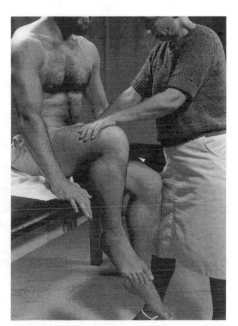

▲ **Figure 12.24** Testing the iliopsoas muscle in the AG position.

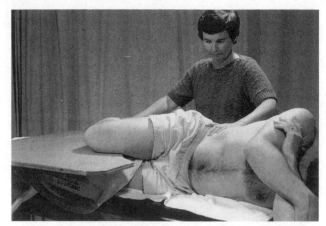

▲ **Figure 12.25** Testing the iliopsoas muscle in the GM position.

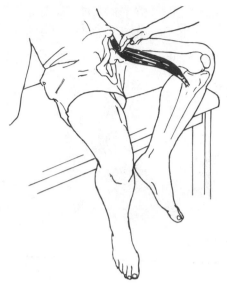

▲ **Figure 12.26** Palpation of the sartorius muscle.

Gravity minimized (GM): Subject is in sidelying position with the lower limb supported on a powder board; the hip is in neutral rotation, and the knee is flexed 90 degrees (Fig. 12-25).

Movement. Flexion of hip in the sagittal plane.

Resistance. Applied to the proximal knee on the anterior surface of the thigh.

Stabilization. The opposite side of the pelvis is stabilized.

Substitutions

• The hip abducts and laterally rotates as the sartorius flexes.
• The hip abducts and medially rotates as the tensor fasciae latae flexes.
• Rectus femoris is an accessory muscle to hip flexion.

SARTORIUS MUSCLE

The sartorius muscle performs hip flexion accompanied by abduction and lateral rotation. It is a two-joint muscle that crosses the knee joint and assists in flexing it.

Palpation. Palpate below and slightly medial to the anterior superior iliac spine (Fig. 12-26).

Position

AG: Subject sits with the pelvis in posterior pelvic tilt and both knees flexed to 90 degrees off the edge of the table (Fig. 12-27).
GM: Subject lies supine with the heel of the test limb on the opposite ankle; the nontest limb is in the anatomical position (Fig. 12-28).

Movement. Subject brings the plantar surface of the heel to the opposite knee. In the GM position, the subject slides the heel along the leg to the knee, keeping the lateral surface of the test limb on the table.

Resistance. Applied to the medial malleolus to resist hip lateral rotation and on the lateral surface of the thigh proximal to the knee to resist flexion and abduction.

▼ **Attachments of Psoas Major, Iliacus, and Rectus Femoris Muscles**			
Muscles	**Proximal**	**Distal**	**Innervation**
Psoas major	Transverse processes, bodies, and intervertebral disks of T12 and all lumbar vertebrae	Lesser trochanter of femur	Spinal nerves L1 and L2 (L3)
Iliacus	Iliac fossa and crest, ala of the sacrum	Lesser trochanter of femur	Spinal nerves L2 (L3)
Rectus femoris	Anterior inferior iliac spine (AIIS)	Tibial tuberosity through patellar ligament	Femoral L3 and L4 (L2)

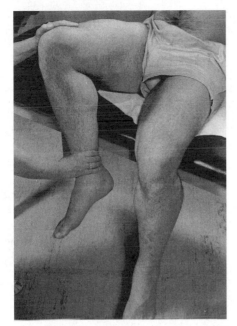

▲ **Figure 12.27** Testing the sartorius muscle in the AG position.

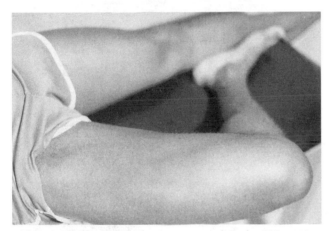

▲ **Figure 12.28** Testing the sartorius muscle in the GM position.

Stabilization. When giving resistance as stated previously, one hand provides counterpressure for the other.

Substitutions

- Iliopsoas and rectus femoris produce straight hip flexion without abduction or lateral rotation.
- Tensor fascia lata produces hip flexion and abduction with medial rather than lateral rotation.

▼ Attachments of Sartorius Muscle			
Muscle	**Proximal**	**Distal**	**Innervation**
Sartorius	ASIS	Proximal medial aspect of tibia	Femoral L2 and L3

GLUTEUS MAXIMUS MUSCLE

The gluteus maximus muscle produces the motion of hip extension from a starting position of hip flexion through a test range of 125 to 140 degrees. The extension action of the gluteus maximus is increased if the hip is laterally rotated and may be tested as a lateral rotator of the hip. With the knee in extension, as the angle of hip flexion decreases, the hamstrings contribute more to the motion. If the knee is flexed, the gluteus maximus contributes more to the action of extension until the hip is flexed less than 45 degrees. Others test the gluteus maximus muscle in the prone position, moving into 15 degrees of hip hyperextension.

Palpation. Palpate between the sacrum and the greater trochanter, with the hip in lateral rotation (Fig. 12-29).

Position

AG: Subject stands with trunk flexed over a table and knee flexed (Fig. 12-30).
GM: Subject is in sidelying position with test limb supported and hip flexed 90 degrees and flexes knee for gluteus maximus action (Fig. 12-31).

Movement. Extension of the hip from a flexed position.

Resistance. Applied proximal to the knee joint on the posterior thigh.

Stabilization. The pelvis is stabilized and hyperextension of the lumbar spine is prevented.

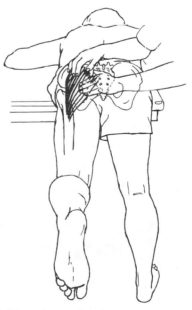

▲ **Figure 12.29** Palpating the gluteus maximus muscle.

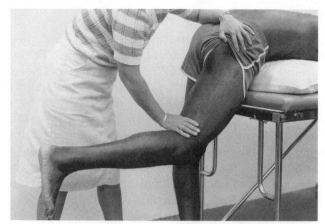

▲ **Figure 12.30** Testing the gluteus maximus muscle in the AG position.

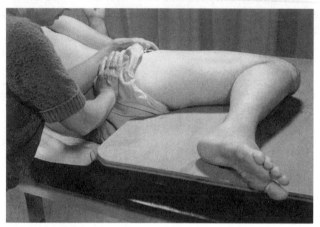

▲ **Figure 12.31** Testing the gluteus maximus muscle in the GM position.

Substitutions

• Hamstrings extend the hip without any action from the gluteus maximus.
• Stabilize the lumbar vertebrae to prevent an increase in lordosis.

GLUTEUS MEDIUS AND MINIMUS MUSCLES

The gluteus medius and minimus muscles produce the movement of hip abduction. The test position is with the hip extended and in neutral rotation. The motion produced is through a test range of 45 degrees. The pelvis should remain motionless. Both muscles may be tested as medial rotators of the hip through a test range of 45 degrees.

Palpation

Gluteus Medius. Only the anterior and middle portions are palpable, either laterally below the crest of the ilium or immediately proximal to the greater trochanter (Fig. 12-32).

Gluteus Minimus. It lies deep to the gluteus maximus and the gluteus medius and therefore is not palpable.

Position

AG: Subject is in sidelying position with the lower hip and knee flexed to 90 degrees. The test limb rests on the table behind the lower limb; the hip is neutral and the knee extended (Fig. 12-33).

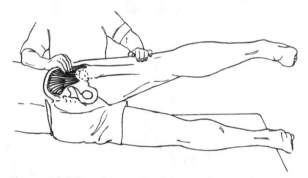

▲ **Figure 12.32** Palpating the gluteus medius muscle.

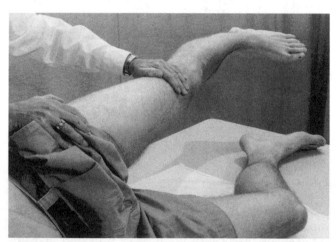

▲ **Figure 12.33** Testing the gluteus medius and minimus muscles in the AG position.

▼ Attachments of Gluteus Maximus Muscle			
Muscle	**Proximal**	**Distal**	**Innervation**
Gluteus maximus	Gluteal line of the ilium, posterior sacrum, coccyx, and sacrotuberous ligament	Iliotibial tract and the gluteal tuberosity of the femur	Inferior gluteal S1 and S2 (L5)

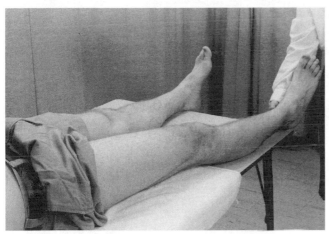

▲ **Figure 12.34** Testing the gluteus medius and minimus muscles in the GM position.

GM: Subject is supine, with the opposite lower limb in neutral and the test lower limb supported on a powder board (Fig. 12-34).

Movement. Abduction of the hip without flexion or lateral rotation.

Resistance. Applied proximal to the knee joint on the lateral side of the thigh.

Stabilization. The pelvis is stabilized.

Substitutions

- The quadratus lumborum and the lateral abdominal muscles tilt the pelvis laterally, giving the appearance of abduction.
- If the subject rolls slightly to the supine position, the tensor fasciae latae is in a more favorable position to abduct the hip because it will be in a flexed position.
- Gluteus maximus (superior portion) is an accessory to hip abduction.

ALTERNATE TESTING OF THE GLUTEUS MEDIUS AND MINIMUS MUSCLES

Alternate testing of the gluteus medius and minimus as medial rotators of the hip is possible.

Position

AG: Subject lies supine or is sitting, with the knees flexed over the edge of the table (Fig. 12-35).
GM: Subject lies supine with the test knee extended and the hip laterally rotated. If the subject is able to stand, then the position is non–weight-bearing on the test

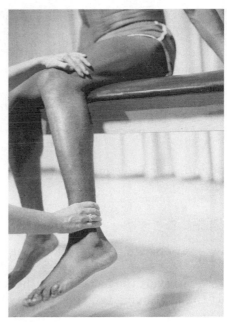

▲ **Figure 12.35** Testing the gluteus medius and minimus muscles during hip medial rotation in the alternate AG position.

limb, the knee is extended, and the hip laterally rotated (Fig. 12-36).

Movement. Medial rotation of the hip joint. In the GM position, the knee must move beyond the midline. In the AG position, the leg moves in a lateral direction.

Resistance. Applied proximal to the lateral malleolus into lateral rotation. If knee pathology is present, resistance should be applied proximal to the knee to prevent torque forces from below.

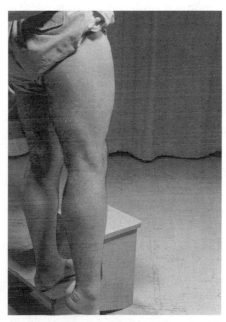

▲ **Figure 12.36** Testing the gluteus medius and minimus muscles during hip medial rotation in the alternate GM position.

▼ Attachments of Gluteus Medius and Minimus Muscles			
Muscle	**Proximal**	**Distal**	**Innervation**
Gluteus medius	Lateral surface of ilium between crest and line	Lateral surface of greater trochanter of femur	Superior gluteal L5 (S1)
Gluteus minimus	External surface of ilium and inferior gluteal line	Anterior surface of greater trochanter of femur	Superior gluteal L5 (S1)

Stabilization. The knee joint is stabilized on the medial side.

Substitutions

- Subject may elevate the buttock on the test side.
- Subject may evert the foot, extend the knee, or abduct the hip, giving the appearance of medial rotation.
- In the GM standing position, the subject may laterally rotate on the supporting limb.

TENSOR FASCIA LATA MUSCLE

The tensor fascia lata muscle produces the motion of hip flexion accompanied by abduction and medial rotation. It may also assist in knee extension.

Palpation. Palpate below and slightly lateral to the ASIS (Fig. 12-37).

Position

AG: Subject is in the sidelying position with the nontest limb in the anatomical position. The test limb is in 45 degrees of hip flex-

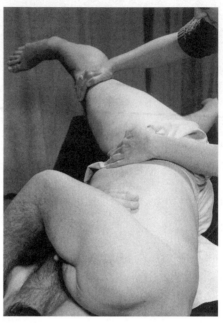

▲ **Figure 12.38** Testing the tensor fascia lata muscle in the AG position.

ion; the knee is extended with the limb resting on the table in front of the nontest limb (Fig. 12-38).

GM: Subject is semisitting with the hips flexed 45 degrees, in neutral rotation, and the arms supporting the trunk. The test leg is on a powder board (Fig. 12-39).

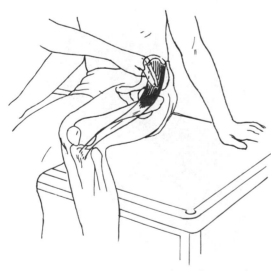

▲ **Figure 12.37** Palpating the tensor fascia lata muscle.

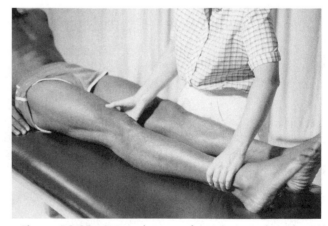

▲ **Figure 12.39** Testing the tensor fascia lata muscle in the GM position.

▼ Attachments of Tensor Fascia Lata Muscle			
Muscle	**Proximal**	**Distal**	**Innervation**
Tensor fascia lata	Lateral surface of anterior superior iliac spine, anterior outer crest of ilium	Iliotibial tract to proximal, lateral aspect of tibia	Superior gluteal L4 and L5

Movement. Abduction of the hip joint while maintaining 45 degrees of hip flexion.

Resistance. Applied to the distal thigh on the lateral side.

Stabilization. The pelvis is stabilized.

Substitutions

- Prevent substitution by stabilizing the pelvis.
- The hip flexors produce only flexion at the hip joint with no abduction.

ADDUCTOR LONGUS, MAGNUS, AND BREVIS AND GRACILIS AND PECTINEUS MUSCLES

The adductor muscles as a group produce adduction of the hip with the hip extended through a test range of 20 to 25 degrees. The adductor longus and brevis and the pectineus may act as synergists in flexion of the hip joint. The adductor magnus muscle (vertical portion) acts as a synergist to hip joint extension. The subject may use the hands on the table to stabilize the trunk.

Palpation. Palpate the adductor longus on the medial side of the thigh immediately below the pubic arch (Fig. 12-40). Palpate the adductor magnus along the medial aspect of the thigh in the middle to lower half (Fig. 12-41). The adductor brevis is too deep for accurate assessment. Palpate the round tendon of the gracilis on the medial aspect of the knee (Fig. 12-42). The pectineus is difficult to palpate and uncomfortable for the subject.

Position

AG: Subject is in the sidelying position with the nontest limb supported in 25 degrees of abduction. The lower limb is the test limb (Fig. 12-43).
GM: Subject lies supine with the opposite limb in 25 degrees of abduction. The test lower limb is in a position of slight abduction, supported on a friction-free surface (Fig. 12-44).

Movement. Abduct the opposite hip on the surface of the table to approximately 25 degrees. Adduct the test hip toward the supported nontest limb approximately 25 degrees.

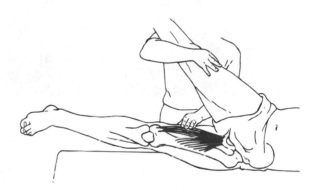

▲ **Figure 12.41** Palpating the adductor magnus muscle.

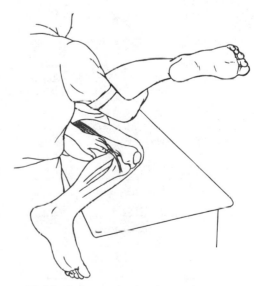

▲ **Figure 12.42** Palpating the gracilis muscle.

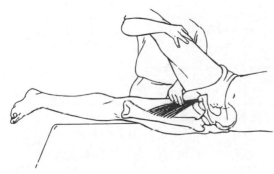

▲ **Figure 12.40** Palpating the hip adductor longus muscle.

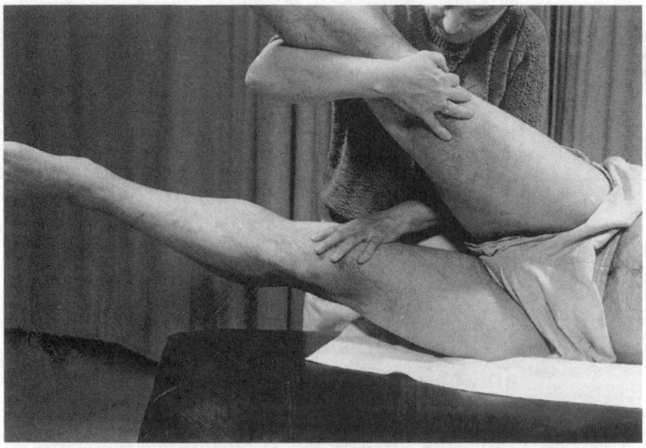

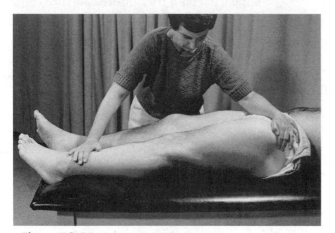

▲ **Figure 12.43** Testing the adductor muscle group in the AG position.

▲ **Figure 12.44** Testing the adductor muscle group in the GM position.

Resistance. Applied proximal to the knee joint into abduction.

Stabilization. The pelvis is stabilized.

Substitutions

- The hamstrings can substitute. Hip adduction is accompanied by lateral rotation of the hip.
- The quadratus lumborum can substitute by elevating the pelvis on the test side.
- Flexing the trunk to the opposite side may give the appearance of hip adduction.
- Medial and lateral rotators allow no rotation during the motion of hip.

OBTURATOR INTERNUS AND EXTERNUS, SUPERIOR AND INFERIOR GEMELLUS, QUADRATUS FEMORIS, AND PIRIFORMIS MUSCLES

The short gluteal, or lateral rotator, muscles produce the motion of lateral rotation of the hip through a test range of 45 degrees.

Palpation. Most of the lateral rotators are too deep to the gluteus maximus to be palpated accurately. The tendon of the piriformis muscle may be palpated as it approaches the greater trochanter posteriorly.

Position

AG: Subject lies supine with the knee flexed over the edge of the table and the opposite

---

▼ **Attachments of the Adductor Longus, Magnus, and Brevis, and Gracilis and Pectineus Muscles**

Muscle	Proximal	Distal	Innervation
Adductor longus	Anterior surface of pubis at crest	Middle third of medial lip of linea aspera of femur	Obturator L3 (L2 and L4)
Adductor magnus	Inferior ramus of pubis and ischium and ischial tuberosity	Gluteal tuberosity, linea aspera, medial supracondylar line, and adductor tubercle of femur	Obturator L3 (L2) Tibial portion of sciatic L3 and L4 (L2)
Adductor brevis	Inferior pubic ramus	Distal pectineal line and superior portion of medial lip of linea aspera of femur	Obturator L3 (L2 and L4)
Gracilis	Inferior pubic ramus and symphysis	Distal to medial condyle of tibia	Obturator L2 (L3)
Pectineus	Superior pubic ramus	Pectineal line of femur	Femoral L2 (L3) Obturator (L2 and L3)

hip and knee flexed with the foot supported on the table (Fig. 12-45).

GM: Subject lies supine with the test limb's knee extended and the hip medially rotated (Fig. 12-46). The subject is standing non–weight-bearing on the test limb with the knee extended and the hip medially rotated (Fig. 12-47).

Movement. Lateral rotation of the hip. In the GM position, the knee must move beyond the midline. In the AG position, the foot and leg move in a medial direction.

Resistance. Applied to the distal leg proximal to the medial malleolus or proximal to the knee joint if pathology exists.

Stabilization. The knee joint is stabilized on the lateral side.

Substitutions

* Subject may elevate the buttock on the opposite side.
* Subject may invert the foot, flex the knee, or adduct the hip, giving the appearance of lateral hip rotation.
* In the standing GM position, the subject may laterally rotate on the supporting lower limb.

CLINICAL ASSESSMENT

Observation and Screening

The biomechanical interrelationship between the lumbosacral spine, sacroiliac joints, hip, and lower extremity necessitates the screening of all areas in patients with complaints in any one region. Pain in the groin or inguinal area is typically associated with true hip joint pathology. However, complaints of pain extending into the anterior thigh and possibly to the knee may also result from hip pathology. The examiner must always be aware of the possibility of referred pain from the lumbosacral spine and sacroiliac joints, not only to these areas, but to the lateral and posterior aspects of the hip as well. Further, a thorough gait analysis may provide relevant information to pathology, areas of muscle weakness, and resultant compensation(s). The reader is referred to the section on gait analysis in Chapter 4 of this text or to other reference sources for more extensive information on gait analysis.

Gross observation of the hip region should include notation of any swelling, muscular atrophy, presence of scars or incision sites, and obvious deformities. The

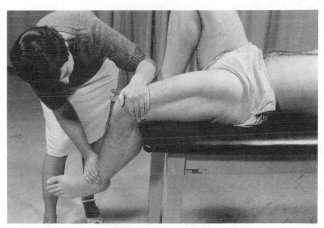

▲ **Figure 12.45** Testing the hip lateral rotator muscles in the AG position.

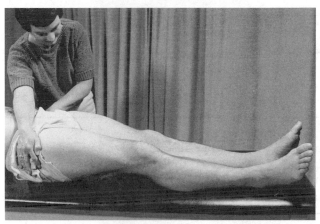

▲ **Figure 12.46** Testing the hip lateral rotator muscles in the GM position.

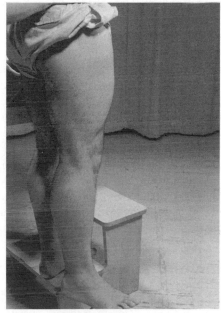

▲ **Figure 12.47** Testing the hip lateral rotator muscles in the GM position.

▼ **Attachments of Obturator Internus and Externus, Superior and Inferior Gemellus, Quadratus Femoris, and Piriformis Muscles**

Muscle	Proximal	Distal	Innervation
Obturator internus	Internal surface of obturator foramen, pelvic surface of ischium, and internal surface of obturator membrane	Medial surface of greater trochanter of femur	Sacral plexus S1 (L5)
Obturator externus	Rami of pubis and ischium and external surface of obturator membrane	Trochanteric fossa of femur	Obturator L4 (L3)
Superior gemellus	Spine of ischium	With obturator internus muscle to greater trochanter of femur	Sacral plexus S1 (L5)
Inferior gemellus	Ischial tuberosity	With obturator internus muscle to greater trochanter of femur	Sacral plexus S1 (L5)
Quadratus femoris	Lateral ischial tuberosity	Intertrochanteric crest	Sacral plexus L5 and S1
Piriformis	Anterior surface of sacrum, border of greater sciatic foramen, and anterior of sacrotuberous ligament	Superior surface of greater trochanter of femur	Sacral plexus S1 (S2)

usual clinical picture associated with a dislocated hip is that of a shortened limb secondary to the superior migration of the femoral head relative to the acetabulum. Additionally, the limb may be postured in some degree of abduction or adduction and internal or external rotation. In cases of a posterior dislocation of the hip, the limb is not only shortened, but usually adducted and internally rotated. Conversely, abduction and external rotation of the limb is commonly associated with an anterior dislocation.

The assessment of symmetry of bony postural landmarks can provide the clinician with important information as to the pathology or dysfunction present. The orientation of postural landmarks, along with the appropriate clinical examination, allows the examiner to assess leg-length discrepancies, pelvic obliquity, sacroiliac dysfunction, limb shortening associated with hip dislocation scoliosis, and certain areas of muscular tightness. For example, tightness of the hip flexors may result in an anterior pelvic tilt and an increase in the lumbar lordosis. Conversely, hamstring tightness may create a posterior pelvic tilt and a subsequent flattening of the lumbar lordosis.

Palpation and Surface Anatomy

Examination of the hip region requires the examiner to observe and palpate certain landmarks to assist in determining the source of pathology (Fig. 12-48). The following structures should be located and identified:

1. Anterior superior iliac spine
2. Anterior inferior iliac spine
3. Iliac crest
4. Umbilicus
5. Posterior superior iliac spine
6. Ischial tuberosity
7. Gluteal fold
8. Greater trochanter
9. Pubic symphysis, both anteriorly and superiorly

Passive and Active Movements and Contractile Testing

The following motions of the hip should be assessed actively and passively and by contractile testing:

1. Flexion
2. Extension
3. Abduction
4. Adduction
5. External rotation
6. Internal rotation

SPECIAL CLINICAL TESTS

THOMAS TEST

Indication. The Thomas test is designed to assess hip flexor tightness/contractures. Some patients may have developed a compensatory lumbar lordosis, masking the flexor contracture.

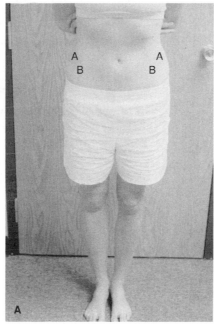
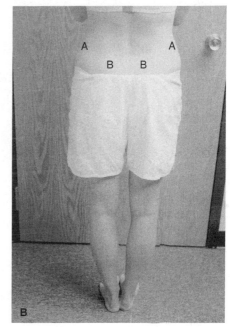

▲ **Figure 12.48** (**A**) Surface anatomy of the anterior hip. (**B**) Surface anatomy of the posterior hip.

A = Iliac Crests   B = ASIS   A = Iliac Crests   B = PSIS

Method. The subject lies supine, and the examiner initially observes the lumbar spine for evidence of an excessive lumbar lordosis or exaggerated hyperextension of the trunk, commonly noted with hip flexor tightness. Next, both hips and knees are flexed toward the chest. While holding one hip in the flexed posture, the subject releases the contralateral limb and extends it toward the table (Fig. 12-49).

Results. Inability of the extended or extending thigh to rest flat on the table is an indication of hip flexor tightness. To be more specific, if the hip and knee of the extended limb remain in a position of flexion, the tightness could be in either the iliopsoas or the rectus femoris muscle.

To delineate the source of tightness, the knee is passively extended. If the limb drops further into

hip extension as it moves closer to the table, the tightness is in the rectus femoris. If passive extension of the knee does not affect the degree of hip flexion, the tightness is not in the rectus femoris but rather in the iliopsoas muscle.

If the hip joint is in a position of abduction and internal rotation while remaining in a flexed posture, tightness of the tensor fasciae latae muscle may be present and further testing of the tensor flexibility with Ober's test is warranted.

In a variation of the Thomas test, the subject lies supine with the test thigh supported on the table and the knee flexed 90 degrees over the table edge. The subject then flexes the contralateral hip and knee to flatten the lumbar lordosis. The examiner observes whether the thigh of the extended hip remains on the table or the knee moves from 90 degrees of flexion toward extension. Movement of the thigh off of the table indicates iliopsoas muscle tightness, while movement of the knee toward more extension represents rectus femoris muscle tightness. If the examiner then attempts to flex the knee passively back to the position of 90 degrees and encounters no resistance or palpable tightness, then the probable cause of restriction is tightness in the joint structures and not the rectus femoris muscle.

ELY'S TEST

Indication. Ely's test is performed in cases of suspected tightness of the rectus femoris muscle.

Method. The subject lies prone while the examiner passively flexes the knee. If passive full knee

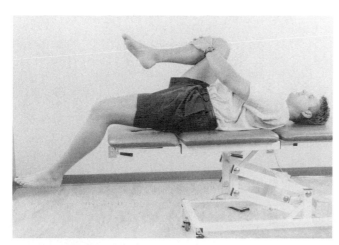

▲ **Figure 12.49** Thomas test.

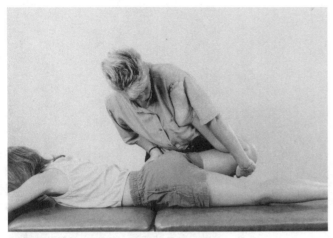

▲ **Figure 12.50** Ely's test.

flexion is achieved, the examiner then passively moves the hip into extension while maintaining the full knee flexion initially achieved (Fig. 12-50).

Results. If, during the passive knee flexion, the subject simultaneously flexes the ipsilateral hip, tightness of the rectus femoris is evident. Limitation of complete full knee flexion and simultaneous full hip extension range of motion also represents tightness of the rectus femoris muscle.

OBER'S TEST

Indication. Ober's test[3] is designed to detect tightness in the tensor fasciae latae muscle and iliotibial band.

Method. The subject is in a sidelying position with the limb to be tested on top. The hip and knee of the lower limb should be flexed to stabilize the subject on the table. The uppermost limb is passively positioned in abduction and some extension so that the iliotibial band crosses over the greater trochanter (Fig. 12-51). The knee may be either flexed or ex-

tended, although greater stretch of the tensor and iliotibial band is elicited in extension. It is important that the examiner stabilize the pelvis in the sidelying position to avoid substitution. The examiner then slowly lowers the uppermost limb, observing to what degree the limb adducts toward the table.

Results. The flexibility of the tensor and iliotibial band is to be considered within normal limits if the uppermost limb adducts and returns to the table. Tightness of this structure is indicated if the limb remains off the table.

PIRIFORMIS TEST

Indication. The piriformis test is indicated in an attempt to determine whether tightness of the piriformis muscle is responsible for pain in the buttocks and possibly down the distribution of the sciatic nerve.

Method. The subject is sidelying with the uppermost test limb positioned in 60 to 90 degrees of hip flexion and 90 degrees of knee flexion. As the examiner stabilizes the pelvis, the hip is passively moved in adduction toward the table (Fig. 12-52).

Results. The production of pain in the buttocks and possibly along the course of the sciatic nerve represents a positive test, resulting from compression of the sciatic nerve by the piriformis muscle.

CONVENTIONAL STRAIGHT LEG RAISE

Indication. The conventional straight leg raise (SLR) is measured to determine the status of the sciatic nerve and the flexibility of the hamstring muscles.

Method. The subject is supine. The examiner passively raises the test limb into hip flexion, making sure to keep the knee extended (Fig. 12-53). The contralateral limb should remain extended during this

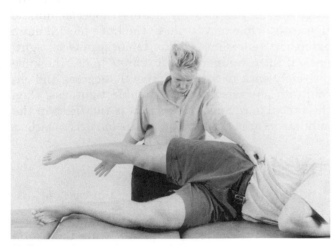

▲ **Figure 12.51** Ober test.

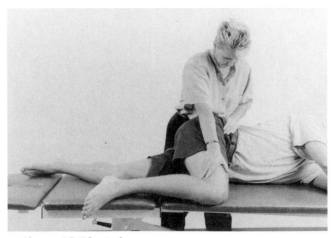

▲ **Figure 12.52** Piriformis test.

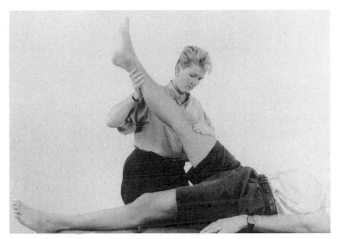

▲ **Figure 12.53** Conventional straight leg raise.

test to prevent posterior tilting of the pelvis, which would allow for some compensation of hamstring tightness.

Results. In assessing hamstring flexibility, the angle of hip flexion necessary to be considered within normal limits is 80 to 90 degrees. A hip flexion angle less than 80 degrees is an indication of hamstring muscle tightness.

90-90 STRAIGHT LEG RAISE

Indication. The 90-90 SLR is an alternate method to assess hamstring flexibility.

Method. The subject is positioned supine with the test hip flexed 90 degrees. The subject maintains this hip flexion position by grasping behind the knee. The examiner then passively extends the knee through its available range of motion (Fig. 12-54).

Results. Knee extension from 20 degrees of flexion to full extension is considered to be within normal limits for hamstring flexibility. Hamstring tightness

is indicated if the knee remains flexed beyond 20 degrees. It is imperative that the motion of knee flexion be done passively because weakness of the quadriceps may prevent the knee from fully extending. This would be misinterpreted as a positive 90-90 SLR for hamstring tightness when actually quadriceps weakness is responsible for the result.

TRENDELENBURG SIGN

Indication. Trendelenburg sign indicates weakness of the gluteus medius muscle during unilateral weight bearing.

Method. The examiner either stands or kneels behind the subject in an optimal position to view the relationship of posterior pelvic structures. The subject stands with weight evenly distributed on the lower limbs. Assuming that there are no postural abnormalities, bony and soft-tissue landmarks should be symmetrical throughout the pelvis and lower limbs. The subject is directed to stand on one limb. A gluteus medius muscle that is functionally strong is able to stabilize the pelvis on the weight-bearing side by maintaining the level of the pelvis on the unsupported side. This balance mechanically is accomplished by the distal attachment of the gluteus medius pulling and holding the pelvis level (Fig. 12-55A and B).

Results. Trendelenburg sign is negative when the pelvis remains level during unilateral weight bearing. A positive sign is indicated when, during unilateral weight bearing, the pelvis drops toward the unsupported limb (see Fig. 12-55C and D). The result of the test is positive, therefore, for the gluteus medius muscle of the weight-bearing limb, indicating that the muscle is either nonfunctional or weak. A Trendelenburg gait, which is evident during unsupported ambulatory activities, is also a positive result.

LEG-LENGTH DISCREPANCIES

True Leg-Length Discrepancy

Indication. Measurement of true leg length assesses whether an actual difference in leg length exists, secondary to bony inequality of the pelvis, femur, or tibia.

Method. The subject lies supine. Care must be taken to ensure that the pelvis is level, the subject is lying relatively straight, and the lower limbs are approximately 15 to 20 cm apart and parallel to one another. If an abduction or adduction contracture is present in one hip, the opposite hip should be assessed in a similar position to ensure accuracy of measurement. Care must also be taken to be consistent in the specific point of the landmarks chosen to measure for discrepancy. Carelessness in replicating

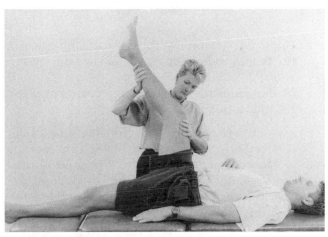

▲ **Figure 12.54** 90-90 straight leg raise.

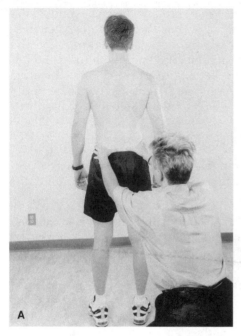

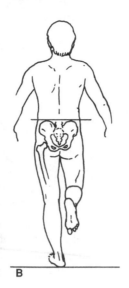

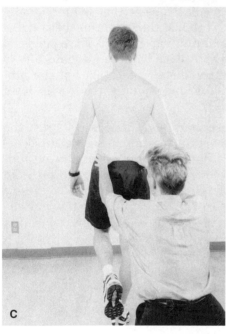

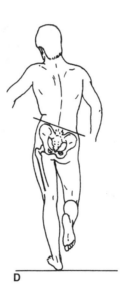

▲ **Figure 12.55** (**A, B**) Trendelenburg sign. Normally, during unilateral weight bearing, the pelvis remains level. (**C, D**) A positive result is present when the pelvis drops toward the unsupported limb during unilateral weight bearing.

points during testing and comparison will yield inaccurate information.

The initial measurement is taken from the ASIS to the medial malleolus (Fig. 12-56). If excessive hypertrophy or atrophy of one thigh is present, the examiner may choose to use the lateral malleolus for measurement rather than the medial malleolus, in hopes of minimizing error due to circumferential soft-tissue differences. If a leg-length discrepancy is found, specific measurements may be taken and compared from various landmarks:

1. ASIS to greater trochanter in assessment of varus or valgus of the hip

2. Greater trochanter to the lateral joint line of the femur, indicating length of the femoral shaft
3. Medial joint line of the knee to medial malleolus, indicating tibial shaft length

Results. Differences between limbs of ¼ to ⅜ in or 1 to 1.5 cm are considered to be within normal limits. Measurement values greater than normal indicate leg-length inequality due to skeletal differences. The specific measurements described previously may allow the examiner to identify the skeletal component responsible for the discrepancy.

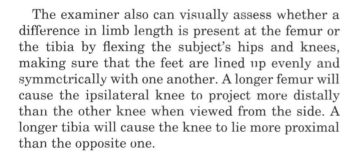

▲ **Figure 12.56** True leg-length measurement. Measure from the ASIS to the medial malleolus.

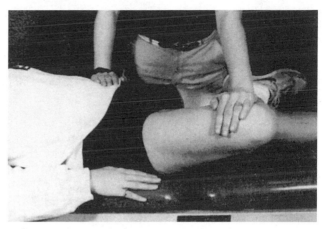

▲ **Figure 12.57** Patrick's test.

The examiner also can visually assess whether a difference in limb length is present at the femur or the tibia by flexing the subject's hips and knees, making sure that the feet are lined up evenly and symmetrically with one another. A longer femur will cause the ipsilateral knee to project more distally than the other knee when viewed from the side. A longer tibia will cause the knee to lie more proximal than the opposite one.

Apparent Leg-Length Discrepancy

Indication. Apparent leg-length discrepancy is assessed to determine whether leg length differences are due to some type of pelvic obliquity, sacroiliac dysfunction, foot pronation or supination, or a postural abnormality. This test is used only after it has been determined that an actual difference in limb length does not exist.

Method. The subject is positioned in the manner described for true leg-length discrepancy. A measurement is taken from the umbilicus to the medial malleolus, indicating the actual distance from a soft tissue to a bony landmark.

Results. Inequality of the measurements between the left and right sides indicates an apparent leg-length discrepancy secondary to pelvic obliquity or postural abnormality.

PATRICK'S TEST (FABER TEST)

Indication. Patrick's test is designed to alert the examiner to the possibility of hip pathology or involvement of the sacroiliac joint. Clinically, this test does not yield useful information regarding specific pathology.

Method. The subject is supine, and the examiner positions the limb to be tested in flexion, abduction,

and external rotation (FABER) so that the foot of the test limb rests on the subject's opposite knee (Fig. 12-57). The examiner then slowly and passively presses the limb being tested toward the table while applying counterpressure to the opposite ilium.

Results. A negative result is indicated if the tested limb drops to the table or comes to lie parallel to the plane of the opposite limb without pain. A positive result is confirmed if there is pain in the back or hip or the tested limb remains in a plane above the opposite limb.

SIGN OF THE BUTTOCK

Indication. The sign of the buttock test is beneficial in determining whether a subject's buttocks pain has its origin in the buttock as a local lesion or is referred from the hip, sciatic nerve, or hamstring muscles.

Method. The examiner performs an SLR test on the subject to the point of buttocks pain and notes the degree of hip flexion. After returning the limb to a neutral position, the limb is subsequently again flexed at the hip but this time with the knee also flexed (Fig. 12-58).

Results. If the amount of hip flexion range of motion is greater with the knee flexed as compared to extended, the test is positive for buttocks pain being referred from the hamstrings or sciatic nerve. However, if the hip range of motion is essentially unchanged with the knee extended or flexed, the test is positive for a local lesion, such as a bursitis, cyst, or neoplasm causing the buttocks pain. Performing SLR causes all of the structures mentioned above to stretch; however, when the knee is allowed to flex as the hip is flexing, stress is taken off the sciatic nerve and hamstrings due to slackening of these structures.

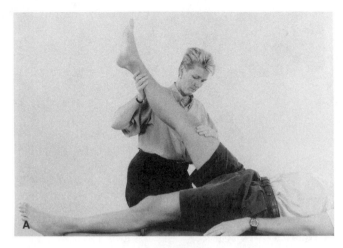

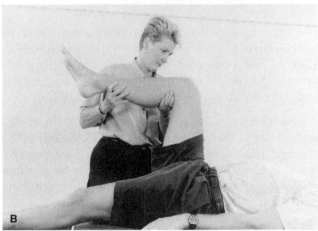

▲ **Figure 12.58** **(A & B)** Sign of the buttock.

NOBLE'S COMPRESSION TEST

Indication. Noble's compression test[2] is performed to determine whether iliotibial band syndrome is present in the knee. As the knee moves through the range of flexion and extension, the iliotibial band moves posterior to the femoral epicondyle during flexion and anterior to the epicondyle during extension. This movement may cause friction between the epicondyle and the band, resulting in reactive inflammation.

Method. The subject lies supine with the knee flexed 90 degrees. The examiner applies pressure immediately proximal (1–2 cm above) to the lateral femoral condyle and maintains that pressure while the knee is slowly extended (Fig. 12-59).

Results. The complaint of pain over the area of the lateral femoral condyle at approximately 30 degrees of knee flexion indicates a positive test for iliotibial band syndrome.

QUADRANT TEST (SCOURING TEST)

Indication. The quadrant test is designed to assess nonspecific hip joint pathology.

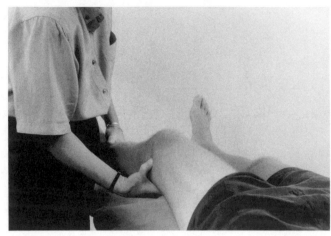

▲ **Figure 12.59** Noble's compression test.

Method. The subject is positioned supine while the examiner flexes the hip and knee of the test limb toward the opposite shoulder (Fig. 12-60). Enough hip flexion and adduction should occur to take up the tissue slack. The examiner then moves the hip through an arc of abduction while maintaining the hip flexion.

Results. A positive test results from any movement irregularities, such as crepitus, glitches, or bumps felt by the examiner. An expression of apprehension or pain by the subject also indicates a positive test.

CRAIG'S TEST

Indication. Craig's test[1,4] is used to assess the angle of femoral neck anteversion.

Method. The subject is positioned prone with the hip and knee of the test limb flexed to 90 degrees. The hip is subsequently internally and externally rotated to find the position where the greater trochanter lies parallel to the table or is in its most

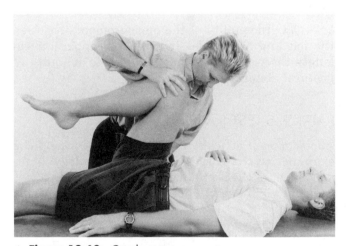

▲ **Figure 12.60** Quadrant test.

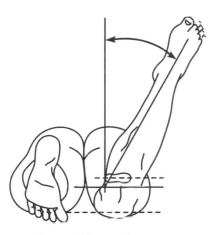

Degree of Anteversion

▲ **Figure 12.61** Craig's test.

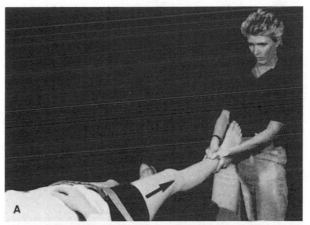

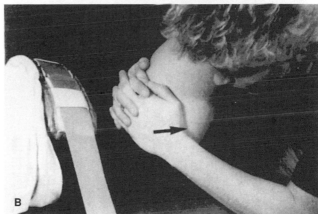

▲ **Figure 12.62** (**A**) Distraction and caudal glide of the hip joint. (**B**) Distraction/caudal glide in cases of knee pathology.

lateral position. The hip is then rotated so that the tibia is vertical or perpendicular to the table top. The angle formed by the two tibial positions is measured (Fig. 12-61).

Results. Normal adult femoral anteversion is between 8 and 15 degrees.

JOINT PLAY (ACCESSORY MOVEMENT)

Distraction and Caudal Glide (Fig. 12-62)

Restriction. General hypomobility; abduction.

Open-Packed Position. Thirty degrees of flexion, 30 degrees of abduction, and slight external rotation.

Positioning. Subject lies supine with a stabilizing strap applied to the pelvis. If the subject has no history of knee pathology, the therapist stands at the bottom of the table facing the subject. A belt is wrapped around the pelvis of the therapist and placed in the web spaces of the therapist's hands. This allows the therapist to apply the distraction force with the body instead of the upper limbs. The therapist's hands are placed around the subject's leg at the ankle.

Movement. The therapist applies a distraction force by leaning backward, thereby creating a pull through the belt to the therapist's hands.

Summary of Hip Joint Play

Table 12-1 provides a summary of joint play of the hip.

REFERENCES

1. Crane L: Femoral torsion and its relation to toeing-in and toeing-out. J Bone Joint Surg 41A:421, 1959
2. Noble HB, Hajek MR, Porter M: Diagnostic treatment of iliotibial band tightness in runners. Physician and Sportsmedicine 10:67, 1982
3. Ober FB: The role of the iliotibial and fascia lata in the causation of low back disabilities and sciatica. J Bone Joint Surg 18:105, 1936
4. Staheli LT: Medial femoral torsion. Orthop Clin North Am 11:39, 1980

TABLE 12.1	**Summary of Hip Joint Play**		
GLIDE	RESTRICTION	FIXED BONE	MOVING BONE
Distraction	General hypomobility	Acetabulum	Femur
Caudal	Abduction and flexion	Acetabulum	Femur
Posterior	Internal rotation and flexion	Acetabulum	Femur
Anterior	External rotation	Acetabulum	Femur
Lateral	Adduction	Acetabulum	Femur

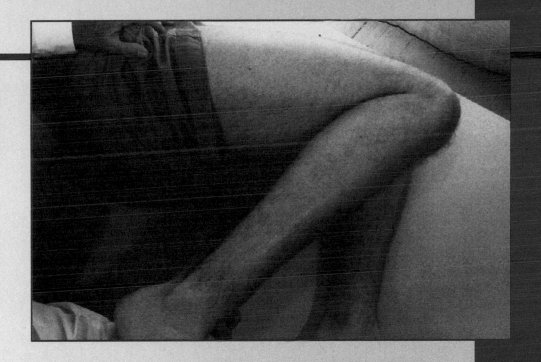

13

Knee

The knee joint, like the elbow, allows shortening and lengthening of the limb. It is a large, complex, and unstable condyloid synovial joint formed by three bones, the distal femur, the proximal tibia, and the patella. There are two degrees of freedom of movement. Motions of flexion and extension occur in the sagittal plane, and axial rotation occurs in the transverse plane. The axis of motion in the coronal plane is located immediately above the joint surfaces through the femoral condyles.

The knee functions in a closed chain, in conjunction with the hip and ankle joints, for supporting the body weight during such activities as squatting, walking, and sitting. In an open kinematic chain, the knee provides mobility for the lower limb. Mobility is provided by bony structures, and stability is provided primarily by soft-tissue structures, such as ligaments and muscles. The knee joint is most stable in the full extended position and least stable in flexion, when the soft-tissue structures are slack and the articular surfaces are least congruent.

GONIOMETRY

KNEE FLEXION

Knee joint motion occurs in the sagittal plane between the condyles of the femur and the tibia. As the tibial condyles flex on the femoral condyles, the tibia glides in a posterior direction. As knee flexion begins, the tibia rotates medially on the femur. If the tibia is fixed, as in ambulation, the femur rotates laterally to provide knee flexion.

Motion. From 0 to 120 to 130 degrees of flexion.

Position

- Preferred: Subject lies supine with the hip flexed 90 degrees (Fig. 13-1).
- Alternate: Subject is in sidelying position on the nontest side. The hip and knee flex simultaneously.

Goniometric Alignment

Axis. Placed over the lateral epicondyle of the femur.

Stationary Arm. Placed parallel to the lateral midline of the femur on a line from the lateral epicondyle to the greater trochanter.

Moving Arm. Placed parallel to the lateral midline of the fibula toward the lateral malleolus.

Stabilization. The thigh is stabilized.

Precautions

- Prevent hip joint rotation and extension and further flexion.

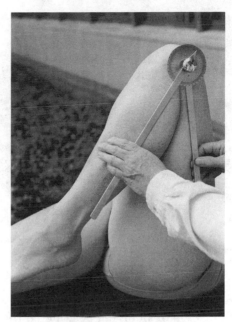

▲ **Figure 13.1** End position for knee flexion measurement.

- Note degree of hip flexion if not 90 degrees.
- Keep the hip joint flexed to prevent stretching of the rectus femoris muscle.

KNEE EXTENSION

The motion of knee joint extension, the return from knee joint flexion, occurs in the sagittal plane. As the knee extends, the tibial condyles glide on the femoral condyles anteriorly. At the end of the range of motion, the tibia rotates laterally on the femoral condyles. If the tibia is fixed, the femur rotates medially on the tibial condyles.

Motion. From 130 to 120 degrees to 0 degrees of extension.

Position

- Preferred: Subject lies supine with the hip joint in extension (Fig. 13-2).

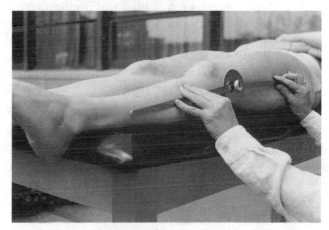

▲ **Figure 13.2** End position for knee extension measurement.

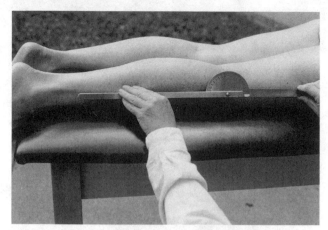

▲ **Figure 13.3** End position for knee extension measurement in the alternate prone position.

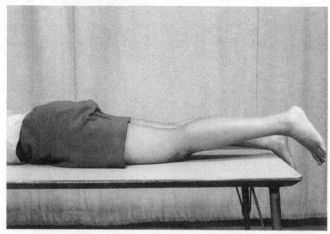

▲ **Figure 13.4** Muscle length test for popliteus and biceps femur (short head) muscles.

- Alternate:
  1. Subject is in sidelying position on the nontest side, with the hip joint in the anatomical position.
  2. Subject is prone, with the hip joint in the anatomical position (Fig. 13-3).

Goniometric alignment and stabilization are the same as for knee flexion.

Precaution

- Prevent hip joint rotation and flexion.

MUSCLE LENGTH TESTING

Knee Flexor Muscles

The short head of the biceps femoris and popliteus muscles are one-joint muscles that lie posterior to the knee joint axis. Both muscles flex the knee joint along with the hamstring muscles. The popliteus muscle is known as the muscle that derotates the knee prior to flexion. If the femur is fixed, then the popliteus muscle will medially rotate the tibia preceding flexion. In the weight-bearing position, the popliteus muscle will laterally rotate the femur preceding knee flexion.

BICEPS FEMORIS—SHORT HEAD AND POPLITEUS MUSCLES

Position. The subject is in the prone position with the hip joints extended. This position places the two-joint hamstring muscles on a slack over the hip and knee joints.

Movement. The examiner extends the knee. The ankle remains relaxed and should be off the end of the table.

Measurement. If the knee joint does not completely extend, then the one-joint knee flexor muscles are tight. A goniometer is used to measure the lack of knee extension using the identical bony landmarks for assessing knee flexion/extension joint range (Fig. 13-4).

Considerations

- Limitations may also exist in the posterior capsule of the joint and the posterior muscles.
- The ankle must remain relaxed in plantar flexion. The gastrocnemius muscle crosses the knee and ankle joints. A shortness of this muscle may present with a knee flexor tightness.

Knee Extensor Muscles

The knee joint extensor muscles include the quadriceps femoris and tensor fasciae latae. The quadriceps femoris muscles cross anterior to the axis of the knee joint and are powerful extensors. Three of the quadriceps femoris muscles are one joint, the vastus lateralis, vastus medialis, and vastus intermedius. The two-joint muscles crossing the anterior knee joint are the rectus femoris and the tensor fasciae latae. The length assessment for these two muscles is described with the hip joint.

VASTUS LATERALIS, VASTUS MEDIALIS, AND VASTUS INTERMEDIUS MUSCLES

Position. The subject assumes a sidelying position on the nontest lower limb or supine with the hip joint flexed approximately 90 degrees. The hip position must take into account the tension from the two-joint muscles that cross the hip anteriorly and posteriorly.

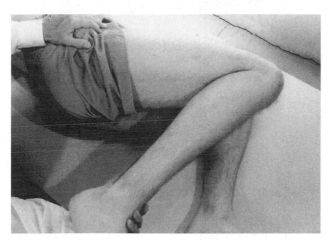

▲ **Figure 13.5** Muscle length test for knee extensor muscles.

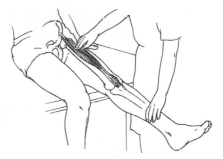

▲ **Figure 13.6** Palpating the rectus femoris muscle.

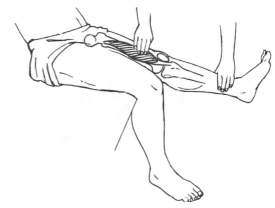

▲ **Figure 13.7** Palpating the vastus medialis muscle.

Movement. The knee joint is flexed until the soft-tissue structures of the calf and thigh are juxtaposed.

Measurement. A goniometer is used and aligned with the bony landmarks designated for goniometry. The range of motion normally is 125 degrees (Fig. 13-5).

Considerations

- The anterior capsular structures may be shortened, along with the one-joint quadriceps muscles crossing the joint.
- Flexion of the hip joint is critical to allow slack in the two-joint muscles crossing the hip anteriorly.

MANUAL MUSCLE TESTING

QUADRICEPS FEMORIS MUSCLES (RECTUS FEMORIS, VASTUS INTERMEDIUS, MEDIALIS, AND LATERALIS)

The quadriceps femoris muscles produce the motion of knee joint extension from a starting position of 90 degrees of flexion. In the break test method of evaluating knee joint extension, the knee is unlocked to approximately 10 degrees short of full extension.

Palpation. Palpate the rectus femoris in the V-shaped area between the sartorius and tensor fasciae latae muscles (Fig. 13-6). The vastus intermedius lies deep to the rectus femoris and is difficult to palpate with accuracy. Lift the rectus femoris muscle, and palpate beneath it from the medial or lateral side.

Palpate the vastus medialis along the medial thigh. The bulky portion is proximal to the patella (Fig. 13-7).

Palpate the vastus lateralis along the lateral thigh (Fig. 13-8).

Position

Against gravity (AG): Subject is semisitting with the hip flexed 45 degrees and the knee flexed 90 degrees over the edge of the table with support under the knee (Fig. 13-9).

Gravity minimized (GM): Subject is in sidelying position with the test leg supported on a friction-free surface. The hip is flexed 45 degrees and the knee 90 degrees (Fig. 13-10).

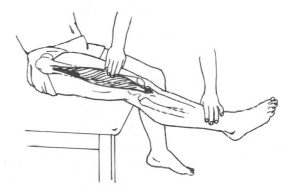

▲ **Figure 13.8** Palpating the vastus lateralis muscle.

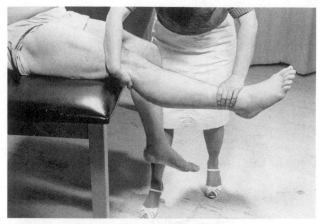

▲ **Figure 13.9** Testing the quadriceps femoris muscles in the AG position.

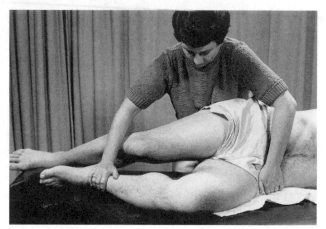

▲ **Figure 13.10** Testing the quadriceps femoris muscles in the GM position.

Movement. Extend the knee joint to 0 degrees, or complete extension.

Resistance. Applied to the anterior surface, proximal to the ankle joint.

Stabilization. The thigh is stabilized.

Substitutions

* In the GM position, the subject may extend the hip, causing passive extension of the knee joint.
* The subject may quickly flex the knee, then relax.
* The articularis genu is an accessory muscle for knee extension and pulls the joint capsule superiorly during the motion to prevent the capsule from becoming trapped in the joint.

HAMSTRING MUSCLES (BICEPS FEMORIS, SEMIMEMBRANOSUS, AND SEMITENDINOSUS)

The hamstring muscles produce the motion of knee flexion from a starting position of 10 degrees of knee flexion, which unlocks the knee joint. The test range is approximately 90 degrees, and the hip may or may not be flexed on a pillow or over the edge of the table. Hip flexion is necessary if the rectus femoris muscle shows tightness. If one of the hamstring muscles is weak, the tibia will rotate toward the strong side.

Palpation. Palpate the biceps femoris along the lateral posterior thigh; the tendon lies immediately proximal to the back of the knee (Fig. 13-11).

Palpate the semimembranosus immediately proximal to the knee posteriorly on either side of the semitendinosus tendon (Fig. 13-12). This muscle is best palpated during the initial 45 degrees of knee flexion.

Palpate the semitendinosus tendon immediately proximal to the knee joint posteriorly on the medial side (Fig. 13-13).

Position

AG: Subject lies prone with the hip flexed and in neutral rotation and the knee flexed 10 degrees (Fig. 13-14).

▼ Attachments of Quadriceps Femoris Muscles

Muscle	Proximal	Distal	Innervation
Rectus femoris	Anterior inferior iliac spine; superior rim of acetabulum	Tibial tuberosity through patellar ligament	Femoral L3 and L4 (L2)
Vastus intermedius	Anterior and lateral proximal two thirds of femoral shaft, distal half of linea aspera	Tibial tuberosity through patellar ligament	Femoral L3 and L4 (L2)
Vastus medialis	Distal intertrochanteric line, medial lip of linea aspera, proximal supracondylar line, and tendon of adductor longus and magnus muscles	Tibial tuberosity through patellar ligament	Femoral L3 and L4 (L2)
Vastus lateralis	Proximal aspect of intertrochanteric line, inferior greater trochanter, and proximal half of lateral lip of linea aspera of femur	Tibial tuberosity through patellar ligament	Femoral L3 and L4 (L2)

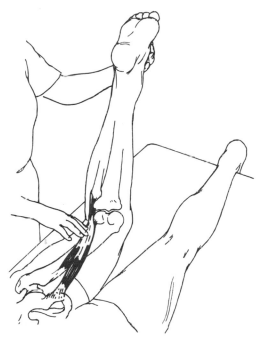

▲ **Figure 13.11** Palpating the biceps femoris muscle.

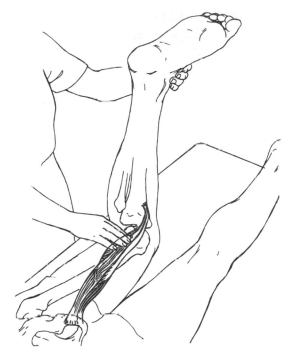

▲ **Figure 13.13** Palpating the semitendinosus muscle.

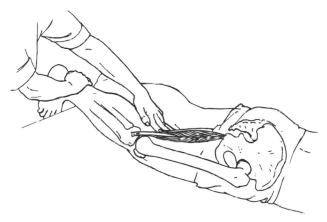

▲ **Figure 13.12** Palpating the semimembranosus muscle.

GM: Subject is in sidelying position with the test leg on a friction-free surface. The hip is slightly flexed, and the knee is flexed 10 degrees (Fig. 13-15).

Movement. Flex the knee joint to 90 degrees.

Resistance. Applied posteriorly, proximal to the ankle joint with the tibia in lateral rotation for the biceps femoris and in medial rotation for the semimembranosus and the semitendinosus muscles.

Stabilization. The thigh is stabilized. If weakness exists, the subject will increase flexion of the hip.

Substitutions

• The gastrocnemius is an accessory knee flexor. To minimize its action, do not allow the ankle to plantar flex.

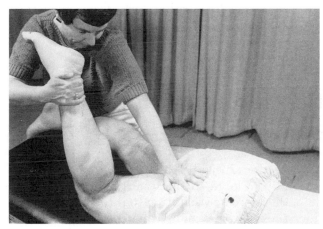

▲ **Figure 13.14** Testing the hamstring muscles in the AG position.

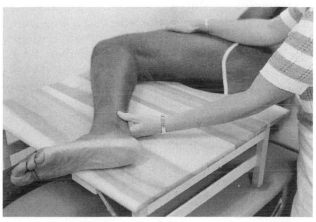

▲ **Figure 13.15** Testing the hamstring muscles in the GM position.

▼ **Attachments of Hamstring Muscles**

Muscle	Proximal	Distal	Innervation
Biceps femoris, long head	Ischial tuberosity and sacrotuberous ligament	Head of fibula and lateral tibial condyle	Tibial portion of sciatic nerve S1 (L5 and S2)
Biceps femoris, short head	Lateral lip of linea aspera, proximal supracondylar line of the femur	Head of fibula and lateral tibial condyle	Peroneal portion of sciatic nerve S1 (L5 and S2)
Semimembranosus	Ischial tuberosity	Posteromedial aspect of medial tibial condyle	Tibial portion of sciatic nerve L5 and S1 (S2)
Semitendinosus	Ischial tuberosity	Proximal medial tibial shaft	Tibial portion of sciatic nerve L5 and S1 (S2)

- The gracilis is an accessory knee flexor; therefore, do not allow the hip to adduct.
- The sartorius is an accessory knee flexor; therefore, prevent the hip from flexing and abducting.
- The gastrocnemius muscle is an accessory muscle to knee flexion; therefore, do not allow the ankle to plantar flex.
- In the GM position, the subject may flex the hip, causing passive flexion of the knee.

CLINICAL ASSESSMENT

Observation and Screening

As with the hip joint, the knee complex is biomechanically related to the other joints of the lower limb, therefore necessitating that the examiner consider these other regions when assessing symptom complaints in and around the knee. Also, the possibility of referral of symptoms from the lumbosacral spine must be considered in patients with knee symptomatology. Gait analysis may also provide information about specific problems of the knee, antalgia, and range-of-motion and strength limitations.

In gross observation of the knee complex, the examiner should look for evidence of tissue damage in the form of abrasions, contusions, or ecchymoses. Localized swelling usually indicates localized inflammation, such as a bursitis or tendinitis. Generalized swelling that occurs immediately after an insult is typical of hemarthrosis or intra-articular derangements. Conversely, generalized swelling that occurs more gradually 8 to 24 hours postinjury often is associated with synovial irritation or meniscal damage. Girth measurements are especially important and should be taken at thigh level, at the joint, and into the calf. These measurements provide the clinician with information regarding muscular atrophy and swelling. The knee region should also be checked for tissue temperature, areas of point tenderness, the popliteal pulse, and any clicking or crepitis, which may indicate a meniscal tear or arthritis, respectively.

Anterior observation of the knee allows for identification of genu valgum (knock knees) and genu varum (bow legs). The normal adult exhibits approximately 7 degrees of valgus at the knee. Patellar abnormalities, such as patella alta (high-riding patella), patella baja (low-riding patella), and "winking patellas" may be appreciated from this view. Winking patellas, a result of internal femoral torsion or excessive external tibial torsion, can quickly and grossly be evaluated with the subject standing. The subject is asked to stand with the feet pointing directly forward, and the orientation of the patellas is examined. Normally, the patellas should both be facing forward in the same direction as the feet. In cases of winking patellas, the patellas will face inward toward one another while the feet are pointing forward. Finally, enlargement of the tibial tubercle is often associated with the presence of Osgood Schlatter's disease.

A lateral view of the knee enables assessment of genu recurvatum (hyperextended knees), and the patellar abnormalities described previously can also be appreciated in this position.

A posterior perspective enables visualization of valgus and varus deformities of the knee, but, more importantly, it allows for direct observation of the popliteal area. Swelling of the popliteal area may be associated with internal derangement or a Baker's cyst. Distal thigh swelling is often seen with insertional hamstring tendinitis, whereas proximal calf swelling may result from inflammation of the gastrocnemius muscle heads.

Palpation and Surface Anatomy

Examination of the knee joint requires that the therapist be familiar with the location of various structures and landmarks. The following are among the structures to be observed or palpated (Fig. 13-16):

1. Medial tibial plateau
2. Tibial tuberosity
3. Medial femoral condyle
4. Adductor tubercle
5. Lateral tibial plateau
6. Lateral femoral condyle
7. Head of the fibula
8. Patella
9. Quadriceps tendon
10. Prepatellar bursae
11. Suprapatellar bursae
12. Infrapatellar bursae
13. Pes anserine bursae
14. Medial meniscus
15. Medial collateral ligament
16. Semitendinosus tendon
17. Semimembranosus tendon
18. Lateral meniscus
19. Lateral collateral ligament
20. Biceps femoris tendon
21. Iliotibial band
22. Common peroneal nerve
23. Popliteal fossa
24. Popliteal artery
25. Origin of the heads of the gastrocnemius muscle

Active and Passive Movements and Contractile Testing

The active and passive movements that need to be assessed during examination of the knee and contractile testing include the following:

1. Flexion
2. Extension
3. External tibial rotation
4. Internal tibial rotation

SPECIAL CLINICAL TESTS

PATELLAR TENDON REFLEX

Indication. The patellar tendon reflex is assessed to determine the integrity of the neurological function of the L4 level.

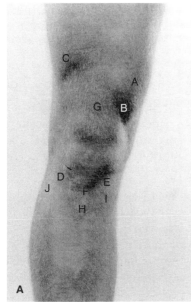

A

A = Vastus Medialis
B = Vastus Medialis Obliquis
C = Vastus Lateralis
D = Lateral Joint Line
E = Medial Joint Line
F = Patellar Tendon
G = Quadriceps Tendon
H = Tibial Tubercle
I = Pes Anserine Bursa
J = Fibular Head

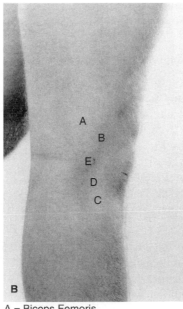

B

A = Biceps Femoris
B = Iliotibial Band
C = Fibular Head
D = Lateral Collateral Ligament
E = Lateral Femoral Condyle

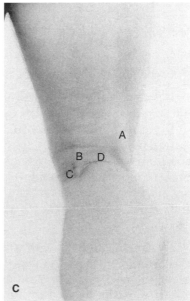

C

A = Biceps Femoris
B = Semitendinosus
C = Gracilis
D = Popliteal Fossa

▲ **Figure 13.16** Surface anatomy of the knee. **(A)** Anterior knee. **(B)** Lateral knee. **(C)** Posterior knee.

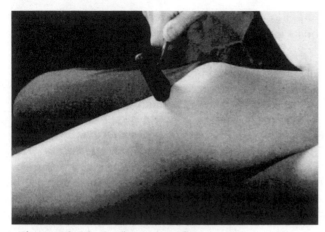

▲ **Figure 13.17** Patellar tendon reflex.

Method. The subject may be either supine or seated for this test. In either case, the knee should be in a position of flexion and the quadriceps muscle relaxed. The examiner taps the patellar tendon with the broad side of the reflex hammer and observes the response (Fig. 13-17).

Results. The normal response should be one of a jerking into knee extension. As in other reflex tests, one should compare the reaction of the uninvolved side. A diminished or heightened response indicates similar findings, as noted in previous reflex tests.

WILSON'S TEST

Indication. Wilson's test is performed in suspected cases of osteochondritis dissecans.

Method. The subject sits, with the knee to be examined flexed over the edge of the table. The subject is asked to rotate the tibia inward and to maintain that rotation while actively extending the knee. The subject is instructed to stop extending the knee at approximately 30 degrees from full extension, where the pain noticeably increases. The subject is then asked to rotate the tibia outward, and the examiner observes for fluctuation of pain.

Results. If, during the outward tibial rotation, the subject's pain disappears, the test for osteochondritis dissecans is positive. The pain experienced during this test must be located in the medial femoral condyle. Pain felt in any other area of the knee during the course of this examination is not representative of osteochondritis dissecans.

PATELLOFEMORAL TESTS

Q Angle

Indication. The Q angle test should be performed in all evaluations of knee pathology, especially in cases of patellofemoral pathomechanics and dysfunction. The Q angle is also extremely important in the biomechanical examination of the lower limb for determining postural malalignment syndromes.

Method. The Q angle is a static measurement of the angle that the patellar tendon makes with the rectus femoris. It provides an indication of the lateral vector force applied to the patella.

The subject lies supine with the lower limb relaxed and in the anatomical position. Positioning is important because it has been demonstrated that various positions of the hip and foot may alter the Q angle. The examiner places the axis of the goniometer over the midpoint of the patella with the proximal arm positioned over the thigh, citing the anterior superior iliac spine (Fig. 13-18). The distal arm lies over the tibial tubercle. The Q angle may be measured with the subject in the long sitting position if the subject cannot lie supine.

Results. Normally, the Q angle in men should range from 10 to 15 degrees and in women from 10 to 19 degrees. Typically, women's Q angles fall toward the higher end of the range, while those of men fall toward the lower end. Angles found to be lower than the norms may be related to chondromalacia patellae and patella alta, while angles greater than the norms are associated with patellofemoral dysfunction, increased femoral anteversion, genu valgum, or increased external tibial torsion. If assessed in the sitting position, the Q angle should measure 0 degrees.

Patellofemoral Grinding Test (Clarke's Sign)

Indication. The patellofemoral grinding test should be performed in suspected cases of patellofemoral dysfunction and is designed to determine the integrity of the posterior patella and the trochlear groove of the femur.

Method. The subject lies supine with the knee extended and the lower limb in a relaxed posture. The examiner places the web space of the hand around the superior pole of the patella (Fig. 13-19).

The subject is then asked to do a "quad set" (isometric quadriceps contraction) while the examiner resists the tendency of the patella to glide superiorly. It is important that the examiner not exert a posteriorly directed force on the patella, which would push the patella against the femur, thereby causing pain and a false-positive test.

Results. A negative result is one in which the subject is able to sustain the contraction without pain while the examiner is applying force. A positive result is manifested in retropatellar pain and the subject's inability to maintain the contraction. Because

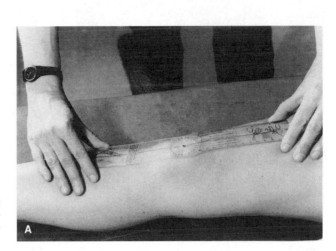
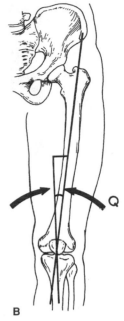

▲ **Figure 13.18** **(A)** Measurement of Q angle. **(B)** Q angle is the difference in measurement between the anatomical and mechanical axes of the knee.

subjects normally experience pain if the examiner's force is too great, this test should be repeated a few times and compared with responses elicited in the uninvolved knee.

Waldron's Test

Indication. Waldron's test helps diagnose chondromalacia patellae.

Method. The subject begins this test in the standing position. While the examiner palpates the patella, the subject is instructed to do several deep knee bends or squats in a slow, controlled manner.

Results. The examiner should be palpating the patella, noting where in the range pain is felt and crepitus is detected. For this test to be positive for chondromalacia, the pain and crepitus must occur

simultaneously. Patellar tracking should also be observed during this procedure.

Patellar Apprehension Test

Indication. The patellar apprehension test[8] is used to assess patellofemoral subluxation or dislocation.

Method. The subject lies supine with the knee in a slightly flexed posture of approximately 30 degrees. With the knee relaxed, the examiner places the thumbs along the medial patellar border and applies a laterally directed force (Fig. 13-20A).

Results. If the subject feels as though the knee is beginning to dislocate, the quadriceps will suddenly contract to pull the patella back in line, and the subject will look apprehensive (see Fig. 13-20B). These findings constitute a positive result.

McConnell's Test

Indication. McConnell's test may be performed when patellofemoral pain is suspected.

Method. The subject is asked to perform an activity that creates patellofemoral compressive forces, thereby reproducing pain. This activity may be a quadriceps contraction while the knee is in a flexed position, ascending and descending stairs, or squatting. Once the pain is reproduced, the examiner gently glides the patella medially while the subject performs the activity.

Results. A positive test result for patellofemoral pain is diminished pain response when the patella

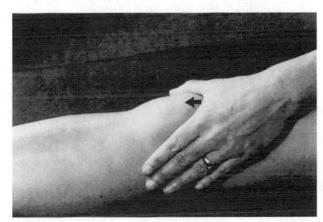

▲ **Figure 13.19** Patellofemoral grinding test.

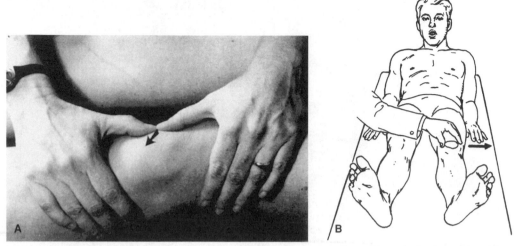

▲ **Figure 13.20** **(A)** Patellar apprehension test. **(B)** Positive test is indicated by a look of apprehension on the subject's face.

has been glided medially. One must be aware that a positive result yields no information regarding the specific source or etiology of the pain; it tells only that patellofemoral pathology is present.

Frund's Sign

Indication. This test may be used in conjunction with more definitive tests for chondromalacia patellae.

Method. The subject is seated while the examiner percusses or taps over the patella in various degrees of knee flexion.

Results. A positive test is indicated by pain.

Passive Patellar Tilt Test

Indication. This test may be helpful in the assessment of chondromalacia patellae.

Method. The subject lies supine with the lower limb extended and relaxed. The examiner lifts the lateral edge of the patella off of the lateral femoral condyle while maintaining the patella within the trochlear groove of the femur. The angle between the transverse line from lateral to medial through the patella and a line parallel to the table is measured (Fig. 13-21).

Results. The normal angle is 15 degrees, although this angle may be 5 degrees less in males as compared with females. Subjects with angles less than normal may be predisposed to chondromalacia patellae.

Lateral Pull Test

Indication. This test is helpful in determining the role of excessive lateral pull of the quadriceps on patellofemoral pain.

Method. The subject is supine with the lower limb extended and relaxed. As the subject performs a quadriceps set, the examiner observes for abnormal lateral patellar displacement.

Results. During quadriceps contraction, the patella should normally move symmetrically in a superior or superior and lateral direction. Excessive lateral patellar movement indicates a positive test.

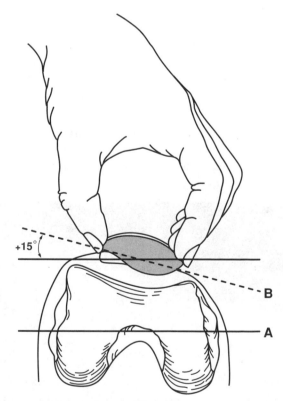

▲ **Figure 13.21** Passive patellar tilt test. (From Kolowich, P. A., et al.: Am. J. Sports Med. 18:361, 1990.)

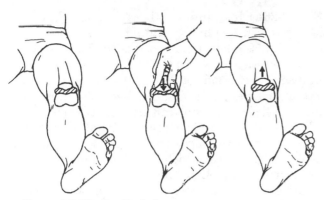

▲ **Figure 13.22** Patellar ballotement test.

TESTS FOR EFFUSION OF THE KNEE

Patellar Ballottement Test (Patellar Tap Test)

Indication. The patellar ballottement test may be used with people whose presenting symptom is gross effusion of the knee.

Method. The subject is supine with the knee in extension or as close to extension as the subject can comfortably tolerate. The examiner gently pushes the patella in a posterior direction and then releases it (Fig. 13-22).

Results. When the examiner releases the patella of a subject with significant effusion, it will spring back or rebound anteriorly. This rebound effect is due to the dispersion of the fluid from between the patella and the femur when the examiner pushes posteriorly, followed by a rapid flush of fluid back beneath when the patella is released.

Fluctuation Test

Indication. The fluctuation test is indicated for people with subtle, minimal effusion.

Method. The subject is positioned as for the patellar ballottement test. The examiner milks the fluid caudally from the suprapatellar pouch, simultaneously pushing it from the medial side of the knee to the lateral side (Fig. 13-23). One or two fingers are placed without pressure along the lateral aspect of the knee to be examined.

Results. As the fluid is milked first inferiorly and then laterally, the examiner feels a slight bulging or an increase in pressure laterally, secondary to flushing of the fluid to the lateral side.

TESTS FOR PLICA

Hughston's Plica Test[8]

Indication. Plica testing is performed when symptoms suggest involvement of the synovial plica. Plica

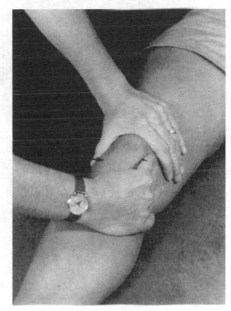

▲ **Figure 13.23** Fluctuation test.

testing should also be done to differentiate between plica pathology and questionable meniscal lesions.

Method. The subject lies supine. The examiner's one hand flexes the knee and medially rotates the leg, and the heel of the other hand is placed along the lateral aspect of the patella (Fig. 13-24).

The examiner then pushes the patella medially while simultaneously palpating the medial femoral condyle with the fingers. The knee is then passively flexed and extended while the examiner palpates the plica.

Results. Palpable "popping" of the plica under the examiner's fingers while the testing maneuver is being performed indicates pathology.

Mediopatellar Plica Test[13]

Indication. The indication is suspected inflammation of the synovial plica.

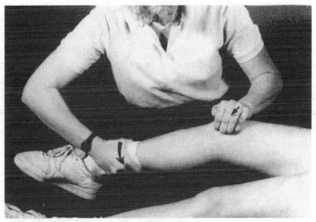

▲ **Figure 13.24** Hughston's plica test.

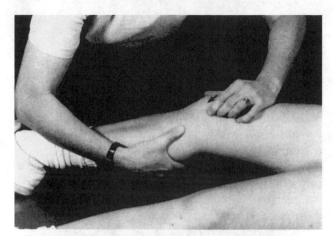

▲ **Figure 13.25** Mediopatellar plica test.

Method. The subject lies supine. The examiner passively flexes the knee to approximately 30 degrees and attempts to move the patella in a medial direction, noting any pain response (Fig. 13-25).

Results. Pain indicates that the edge of the mediopatellar plica is becoming pinched between the medial femoral condyle and the patella.

Stutter Test

Indication. The "stutter" test is indicated when plica involvement is suspected and the subject shows no evidence of joint effusion.

Method. The subject is seated with both knees flexed over the edge of the table to 90 degrees. The examiner instructs the subject to extend one knee slowly as the examiner palpates the patella during the movement.

Results. Pathology is present if the patella jumps, or stutters, at some point in the range between 60 and 45 degrees from full extension, interrupting what would normally be smooth, fluid motion.

MENISCAL TESTS

All procedures described in the following eight tests are indicated when a subject's history or mechanism of injury leads the examiner to suspect damage to the medial or lateral meniscus. These tests, although clinically diagnostic of meniscal tears, are often not definitive. Therefore, arthrography, magnetic resonance imaging, or arthroscopic examination is necessary for definitive diagnosis.

McMurray's Test[12]

Method. The subject relaxes supine, and the examiner places the knee being examined into as much flexion as the subject's range of motion will allow

(Fig. 13-26A). In examining the right knee, the examiner grasps the subject's right heel with the right hand while the left hand controls the joint. The left hand is positioned so that the thumb and index finger firmly grip either side of the joint posterior to the lateral and medial ligaments. The heel is then rotated, causing relative internal and external tibial rotation.

This test has many variations, including the addition of an abduction-adduction force and gradual extension of the knee, which may be combined or imposed separately. Lateral tibial rotation with an abduction or valgus force is associated with testing the medial meniscus, while internal rotation with an adduction or varus force stresses the lateral meniscus (see Fig. 13-26B and C).

Results. The examiner may palpate and listen over the meniscus for evidence of clicking or snapping, often accompanied by pain, which indicates pathology. Structures other than menisci may produce the clicking or snapping, so the test result may be false-positive.

Apley's Grinding Test[1]

Method. The subject lies prone with the knee joint flexed to 90 degrees (Fig. 13-27). The examiner stabilizes the posterior distal thigh with one hand while the other hand grasps the plantar surface of the calcaneus. The examiner transmits a compressive force through the calcaneus and the leg to the knee while simultaneously rotating the leg laterally and medially.

Results. Pain reproduced with compression and lateral tibial rotation may indicate a positive finding for a lateral meniscal tear, while pain associated with compression and medial rotation may indicate medial meniscal pathology. Pain evident on tibial distraction and rotation has been associated with ligament injury.

O'Donoghue's Test

Method. The examiner flexes the supine subject's knee to 90 degrees and then rotates the leg inward and outward a few times. The examiner then fully flexes the subject's knee and again rotates it in both directions.

Results. Increased pain on rotation with the knee fully flexed as compared with 90-degree flexion indicates a meniscal tear or capsule irritation.

Helfet's Test (Screw Home Mechanism)[6]

Indication. The screw home mechanism provides information on the normal biomechanical lateral rotation of the tibia on the femur during extension in an open kinematic chain. Absence of this normal ro-

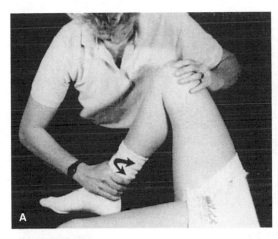

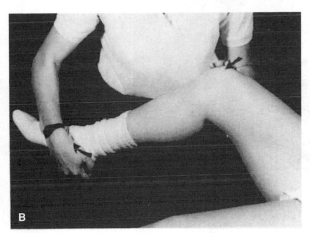

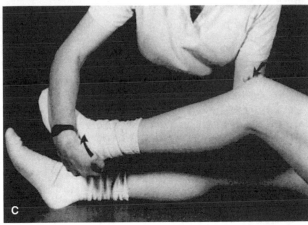

▲ **Figure 13.26** (**A**) McMurray's test. (**B**) Lateral tibial rotation combined with a valgus force to the knee during knee extension assesses the medial meniscus. (**C**) Medial tibial rotation combined with a varus force to the knee during knee extension assesses the lateral meniscus.

tation may be associated with a torn meniscus or patellofemoral dysfunction.

Method. The subject sits with the knees flexed approximately 90 degrees over the edge of the table. A skin pencil is used to mark the midpoint of the patella and the tibial tuberosity. In this sitting position, the two markings should align vertically. The subject then slowly extends the knee, and at full extension, the landmarks are palpated and marked again (Fig. 13-28). The relationship between the first set of markings and the second set is examined.

Results. During normal biomechanical extension of the knee, the leg moves from a relatively neutral position to one of external rotation. Therefore, the second mark on the tibial tuberosity should lie lateral to the first mark on the tibia. If this is not the finding, normal lateral tibial rotation during extension is decreased or absent. This abnormal biomechanical situation may be related to the torn meniscus or to patellofemoral pathology.

Bounce Home Test

Indication. The bounce home test is used to determine whether a structure (the meniscus) may be preventing complete extension of the joint.

Method. The subject is supine as the examiner cups the heel of the foot with the hand. The examiner then maximally flexes the subject's knee and from that position, allows passive motion into extension.

Results. Normally, the knees move smoothly into full extension. In a knee with a meniscal tear, extension is either not complete or has a springy end feel, which is classically associated with meniscal tears.

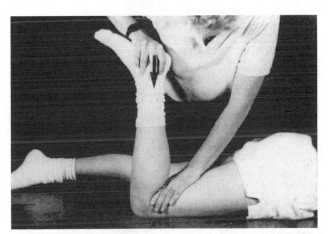

▲ **Figure 13.27** Apley's grinding test: Compression force through the leg combined with medial tibial rotation assesses the medial meniscus; lateral tibial rotation during compression tests the lateral meniscus.

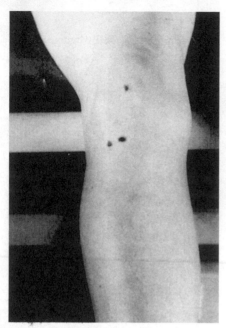

▲ **Figure 13.28** Screw home mechanism: In the position of knee extension, the second mark on the tibial tubercle should lie lateral to the initial mark made with the knee in flexion.

Test for Retracting Meniscus[6]

Indication. This test is indicated in suspected cases of a retracting meniscus.

Method. The subject lies supine as the examiner flexes the knee 90 degrees. The examiner palpates the area of the tibial plateau corresponding to the anatomical location of the medial meniscus. The subject's leg is then rotated laterally and medially while the examiner carefully palpates for the meniscus.

Results. In a normal biomechanical situation, the medial meniscus should be impalpable during lateral tibial rotation and should reappear during medial rotation. A torn medial meniscus will not be felt to disappear during lateral rotation.

Payr's Test

Indication. This test is helpful in the assessment of a medial meniscus tear, primarily in the body or posterior horn.

Method. The subject lies supine with the limb of the test knee positioned in a figure-four position (Fig. 13-29).

Results. Pain along the medial joint line represents a positive test.

Bragard's Sign

Bragard's sign can be used in the diagnosis of medial meniscal lesions.

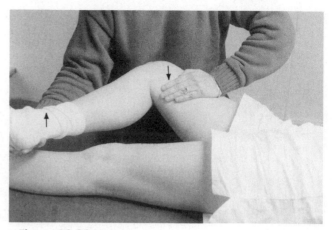

▲ **Figure 13.29** Payr's test.

Method. As the subject lies supine, the examiner initially flexes the knee and then externally rotates the tibia while extending the knee. The examiner then internally rotates the tibia while flexing the knee.

Results. Pain and tenderness along the medial joint line during knee extension with tibial external rotation that decreases with knee flexion and internal tibial rotation indicates a positive test for medial meniscal involvement.

Ligamentous Testing

Ligamentous testing of the knee is an integral part of the total joint assessment. For ease in organization, the examination of the ligamentous structures may be divided into the following classifications: straight-plane medial, lateral, anterior, and posterior instability and anteromedial, anterolateral, posterolateral, and posteromedial rotatory instability.

TESTS FOR STRAIGHT-PLANE INSTABILITY

Apley's Distraction Test

Indication. Apley's test is indicated in suspected cases of medial or lateral collateral ligament injury.

Method. The subject lies prone with the knee flexed 90 degrees. The examiner stabilizes the femur by placing the leg on the distal posterior surface of the thigh. The examiner grasps the distal portion of the leg with both hands, using the malleoli as prominences to which leverage may be applied. The leg is distracted and simultaneously moved into lateral and medial tibial rotation (Fig. 13-30).

Results. Pain on the medial aspect of the knee joint during distraction and lateral tibial rotation may indicate a lesion of the medial collateral ligament. Lat-

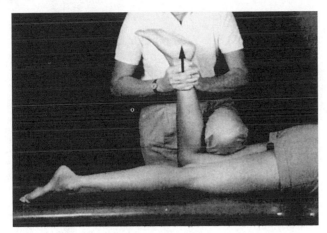

▲ **Figure 13.30** Apley's distraction test.

eral knee pain experienced during distraction and internal tibial rotation may represent a lateral collateral ligament injury.

Valgus (Abduction) Stress Test[16]

Indication. The valgus and abduction stress test is used to assess the integrity of the structures responsible for medial stability of the joint.

Method. The subject lies supine with the limb in a relaxed position.

This test should be performed in full extension and in an unlocked position of about 20 to 30 degrees of flexion to allow testing of both the primary and secondary restraints. In the position of flexion, the posterior capsule is relaxed, thereby allowing for isolated testing of the medial collateral ligament.

The examiner places one hand along the lateral side of the knee joint and the other medially on the subject's leg (Fig. 13-31). Using the lateral hand as a fulcrum, the examiner applies a valgus force to the knee by pulling the leg from the midline of the body.

Results. Medial gapping or pain during the procedure is evidence of dysfunction. A positive result

with the knee in the unlocked flexed position could mean dysfunction of the medial collateral ligament, the middle third of the medial capsule, the posterior cruciate ligament, or the posterior oblique ligament.

Gapping or pain noted when testing the knee in full extension represents more extensive joint damage in terms of stability. Structures that may be damaged in association with this instability may include superficial and deep fibers of the medial collateral ligament, the posteromedial capsule, the posterior oblique ligament, the anterior and posterior cruciate ligaments, the semimembranosus muscle, and the medial quadriceps expansion.

Varus (Adduction) Stress Test

Indication. The varus stress test[16] is indicated in people who may have sustained damage to the lateral stabilizing structures of the knee.

Method. The subject is relaxed and supine. The examiner places one hand along the medial aspect of the joint and the other on the lateral side of the leg (Fig. 13-32). With the hand on the knee acting as a fulcrum, the examiner imparts a varus force on the joint by pulling the leg into adduction.

This test is performed with the knee in extension and in an unlocked position of 20 to 30 degrees. As in the valgus stress test, laxity in the completely extended position represents a more serious injury.

Results. Gapping or pain while the test is performed in the unlocked position indicates possible injury to the lateral collateral ligament, the middle third of the lateral capsule, the posterolateral capsule, the arcuate complex (lateral collateral ligament, short lateral ligament, arcuate ligament, tendinous aponeurotic expansion of the popliteus muscle), the iliotibial band, and the biceps femoris tendon.

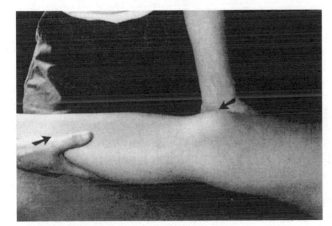

▲ **Figure 13.31** Valgus stress test of the knee.

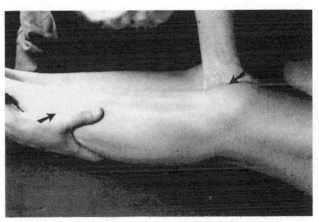

▲ **Figure 13.32** Varus stress test of the knee.

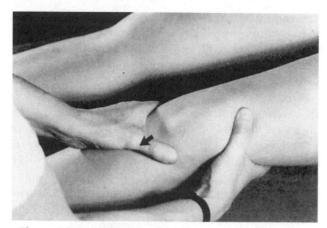

▲ **Figure 13.33** Lachman's test.

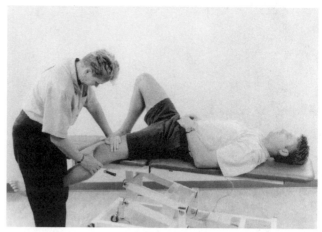

▲ **Figure 13.34** Drop leg Lachman test.

Lachman's Test

Indication. Lachman's test[2,10,16] is the most reliable clinical assessment of anterior cruciate insufficiency, especially of the posterolateral band.

Method. The subject lies supine with the limb in slight external rotation and the knee in approximately 30 degrees of flexion (Fig. 13-33). This position allows the posterior meniscal horns to clear the femoral condyles, thereby obviating a false-negative finding for anterior cruciate ligament tear. The examiner stabilizes the distal thigh with one hand while creating an anterior "drawer" force on the proximal tibia with the other.

Results. The lack of firm end feel while drawing the tibia forward or more draw on the test leg than on the normal limb represents a positive test for anterior cruciate ligament insufficiency. The following structures may be involved: the anterior cruciate ligament, the arcuate complex, or the posterior oblique ligament.

Drop Leg Lachman Test[10]

Indication. This test for anterior cruciate ligament deficiency is a variation of the Lachman test and may be easier to do for clinicians with small hands.

Method. The subject lies supine with the thigh of the test knee supported on the table and the leg stabilized between the examiner's legs in 30 degrees of flexion. The examiner's one hand stabilizes the thigh against the table while the other hand applies an anterior force to the posterior aspect of the proximal tibia (Fig. 13-34).

Results. The same findings as seen with the Lachman test represent a positive test.

Alternate Lachman Test[16]

This is an alternate test for anterior cruciate ligament insufficiency.

Method. The subject is positioned prone with the test knee flexed 30 degrees and supported by the examiner's thigh under the subject's ankle. As the examiner palpates the anterior joint line medially and laterally with one hand, the other hand applies an anterior force to the proximal posterior calf (Fig. 13-35).

Results. The same findings as seen with the Lachman test represent a positive test.

Dynamic Extension Test (Active Lachman Test)

Indication. The dynamic extension test[16] may also be used to evaluate a knee with anterior cruciate ligament insufficiency. It is a variation of Lachman's

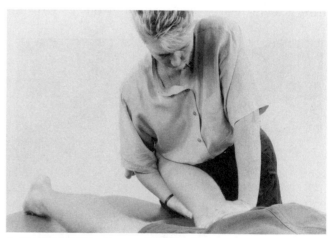

▲ **Figure 13.35** Alternate Lachman test.

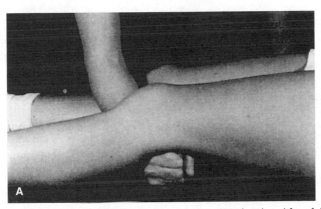
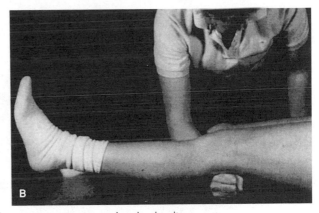

▲ **Figure 13.36** Dynamic extension test: **(A)** The closed fist of the examiner is positioned under the distal femur of the subject, whose knee is extended. **(B)** Closed fist of examiner under distal femur while subject extends knee.

test, performed dynamically with a quadriceps contraction.

Method. The subject lies supine, with the knee extended and the examiner's closed fist under the distal thigh (Fig. 13-36A). The subject raises the leg from the table as the examiner observes the tibial movement (see Fig. 13-36B); the subject then lowers the leg back onto the examiner's fist, and again tibial motion is noted.

Results. If the anterior cruciate ligament is deficient, as the subject extends the knee, the tibia moves anteriorly onto the femur. When the leg is then lowered and relaxed on the closed fist, the tibia falls backward onto the femur into its resting position. This test may prove beneficial for the acutely injured knee where more intricate assessment methods are difficult, if not impossible, to perform.

Anterior Drawer Test

Indication. Suspicion of anterior cruciate ligament laxity or rupture is an indication for the anterior drawer examination. This test may yield a false-negative result.

Method. The subject lies supine with the knee flexed to 90 degrees. The examiner stabilizes the foot on the table in neutral rotation by sitting on it (Fig. 13-37). The examiner grasps the proximal tibia, ensuring relaxation of the hamstrings, and attempts to pull the tibia anteriorly on the femur. Simultaneous palpation of the anterior joint line with the thumbs allows the examiner to feel the forward translation of the tibia accurately.

Results. Approximately 6 mm anterior translation of the tibia on the femur is normal. A positive straight drawer test is one in which there is excessive, equal forward displacement of both tibial condyles on the femoral condyles. The examiner must be sure that the posterior cruciate ligament is not lax or torn, because such a condition may result in a false-positive anterior drawer test (see drop back sign, below).

Excessive anterior displacement of the tibia may represent involvement of any of the following structures: the anterior cruciate ligament (notably the anteromedial band), the posterolateral or posteromedial capsule, the deep fibers of the medial collateral ligament, the posterior oblique ligament, the iliotibial band, or the arcuate complex.

Anterior Drawer in External Rotation

Method. The subject is positioned as in the anterior drawer test, but the foot and leg are stabilized in external rotation. This externally rotated position causes tightening of the medial structures. The examiner imposes an anterior "drawing" force on the tibia.

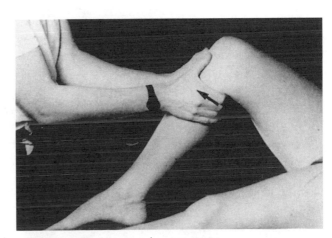

▲ **Figure 13.37** Anterior drawer test.

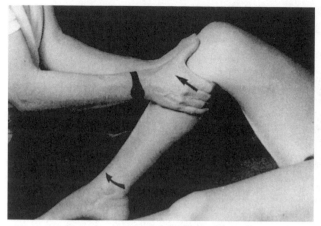

▲ **Figure 13.38** Anterior drawer in external rotation.

Results. If any laxity of the medial compartment structures exists—most notably in the medial collateral ligament—the medial tibial condyle displaces farther forward than the lateral condyle of the tibia (Fig. 13-38). This movement is associated with external tibial rotation, which is present with anteromedial rotary instability.

Anterior Drawer in Internal Rotation

Method. The subject is positioned as for the straight anterior drawer, except that the foot and tibia are placed in internal rotation. This position tightens the lateral collateral ligament and other lateral compartment structures.

Results. If, during this drawer test, the lateral tibial condyle displaces anteriorly and medially with respect to the medial tibial condyle and the femoral condyles, anterior cruciate and lateral compartment laxity are evident (Fig. 13-39). The combined anterior motion and internal tibial rotation is typical of anterolateral rotatory instability.

Posterior Drawer Test[2,16]

Indication. The posterior drawer examination technique should be performed in cases of suspected posterior cruciate ligament tear.

Method. The subject lies supine, with the knee being examined flexed to 90 degrees and the foot resting on the examining table (Fig. 10-40). The examiner sits on the foot to stabilize it, grasps the proximal tibia, and pushes the tibia posteriorly on the femur.

Results. Excessive posterior translation of the tibia backward on the femur represents a positive result. Any of the following structures may be damaged and associated with a positive finding: the posterior cruciate or posterior oblique ligament, the arcuate complex, or the anterior cruciate ligament.

Daniels Quadriceps Neutral Angle Test[16]

Indication. This test is used primarily in instrumented testing for posterior cruciate ligament insufficiency.

Method. The neutral position of the injured knee is determined by initial testing of the noninjured knee. The subject is placed supine with the noninjured limb in 45 degrees of hip flexion and 90 degrees of knee flexion with the foot lying flat on the table. The examiner stabilizes the subject's foot against the table while asking the subject to extend the knee isometrically. As the contraction is occurring, the examiner observes the knee for a decrease or increase in the knee flexion angle as a result of tibial displacement. A reduction in the knee flexion angle represents posterior tibial displacement, while an increase in the knee flexion angle results from anterior tibial displacement. This process is repeated at varying positions of knee flexion until no

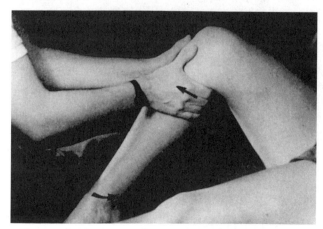

▲ **Figure 13.39** Anterior drawer in internal rotation.

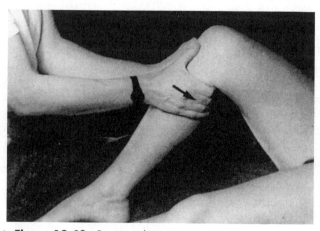

▲ **Figure 13.40** Posterior drawer test.

tibial displacement is observed, usually in the range of 60 to 90 degrees. The position of no tibial displacement represents the quadriceps neutral angle position. Next, the injured knee is positioned at the identified neutral angle, and the test is repeated in this position.

Results. Anterior tibial displacement at the quadriceps neutral angle position indicates a positive test for insufficiency of the posterior cruciate ligament.

Godfrey's Test

Indication. Godfrey's test[16] is designed to assess posterior instability of the knee.

Method. The subject lies supine, and the examiner flexes the hips and knees approximately 90 degrees, supporting the limbs beneath the legs (Fig. 13-41).

Results. A posterior sagging of the leg indicates posterior instability of the knee.

Drop Back Sign (Posterior "Sag" Sign)

Indication. The drop back sign should be assessed in all cases of suspected anterior or posterior cruciate ligament laxity or rupture.

Method. The subject is placed in the drawer test position of 90 degrees of knee flexion with the foot resting on the table. In this position, the relationship of the tibia to the femur is examined.

Results. If the posterior cruciate ligament is intact, a normal biomechanical relationship will exist between the tibia and femur. With ligament laxity or a tear, gravity in this testing posture will cause the tibia to "drop back" and come to lie farther posterior than normal with respect to the femur (Fig. 13-42).

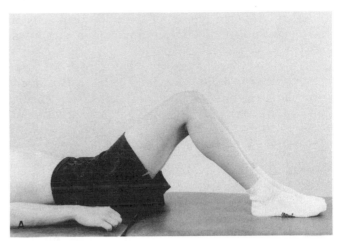

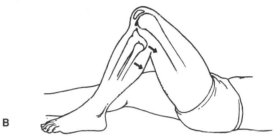

▲ **Figure 13.42** (**A & B**) Sag sign.

In the subject with a drop back sign, accuracy of the assessment of the anterior cruciate ligament becomes important. The examiner must first restore the normal femoral and tibial alignment before performing the anterior drawer test. If the normal relationship is not established prior to assessment of the anterior cruciate ligament, it will result in a false-positive result for the anterior drawer.

ANTEROMEDIAL ROTARY INSTABILITY TEST

Slocum's Test

Indication. Slocum's test may be performed to diagnose anteromedial rotary instability.

Method. The subject is positioned supine, with the knee flexed about 85 degrees and the foot resting on the table with the leg in 15 degrees of lateral rotation. The external tibial rotation causes increased tension in the intact posteromedial structures and thereby diminishes anterior tibial displacement, even with a lax anterior cruciate ligament. The examiner grips the proximal tibia and attempts to draw it forward.

An alternate testing position is sitting with the knees flexed over the table edge. Again the leg is rotated laterally 15 degrees, and an anterior drawing force is applied to the proximal tibia.

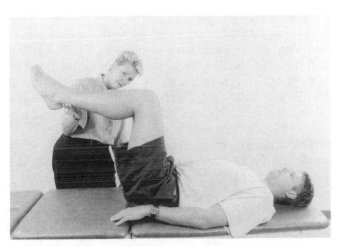

▲ **Figure 13.41** Godfrey's sign.

Results. Anterior motion of the tibia, primarily on the medial side, indicates anteromedial rotary instability.

Structures that may be implicated with this type of instability include the medial collateral ligament (especially the superficial fibers), the posteromedial capsule, the posterior oblique ligament, and the anterior cruciate ligament.

ANTEROLATERAL ROTARY INSTABILITY TESTS

Slocum's Test

Indication. Slocum's test is indicated when assessing anterolateral rotatory instability of the knee.

Method. The subject may be either supine or seated, with the knee flexed 80 to 90 degrees. The leg, with the foot resting on the table, is placed in 30 degrees of medial rotation, and the examiner imposes an anterior force on the proximal tibia.

Results. When the lateral aspect of the tibia displaces farther anteriorly than the uninvolved side of the knee, anterolateral rotary instability is indicated.

The following structures may be involved with this type of instability: the anterior or posterior cruciate ligament, the lateral collateral ligament, the posterolateral capsule, the arcuate complex, and the iliotibial band.

Losee's Test

Indication. Losee's test[11] is indicated in suspected anterolateral rotary instability.

Method. The subject lies supine. The examiner laterally rotates the leg by grasping the foot and ankle (Fig. 13-43). This tibial rotation reduces the

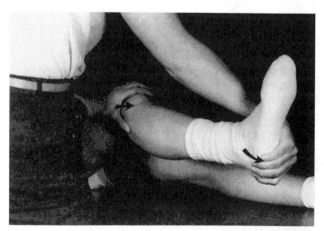

▲ **Figure 13.43** Losee's test: The examiner applies a valgus force to the knee while extending the joint and applies anterior force to the head of the fibula.

subluxation of the knee. Stabilizing the leg against the trunk, the examiner flexes the subject's knee to 30 degrees to relax the hamstring muscle. The examiner places the other hand anterolaterally on the knee so that the fingers lie over the patella, and the thumb wraps around the fibular head. The examiner applies a valgus force to the knee using the examiner's trunk as a fulcrum while extending the subject's knee and applying an anterior force to the fibular head. The purpose of the valgus stress is to make any anterior subluxation more pronounced by compressing the structures of the lateral side. Simultaneously, the ankle and foot are allowed to move into medial rotation, which ensures the anterior subluxation of the lateral tibial condyle.

Results. As the examiner goes through the testing maneuver, a "clunk" of the knee just prior to full extension indicates anterior tibial subluxation typical of anterolateral rotary instability. Structures implicated in this instability may include the anterior cruciate and lateral collateral ligaments, the posterolateral capsule, the arcuate complex, and the iliotibial band.

Lateral Pivot Shift

Indication. The pivot shift[4,5,17] is the test of choice in the assessment of anterolateral rotary instability of the knee.

Method. The subject is relaxed and supine with the hip flexed 20 degrees and held in slight internal rotation. The examiner flexes the knee approximately 5 degrees by placing the heel of one hand behind the fibula, over the lateral gastrocnemius muscle. The examiner's other hand holds the leg in slight internal rotation by grasping the ankle. A valgus stress is then applied to the knee while maintaining the medial tibial rotation (Fig. 13-44*A*). If the leg is then passively moved into flexion, the tibia will reduce posteriorly at about 30 or 40 degrees (see Fig. 13-44*B*).

Results. Tibial reduction at 30 to 40 degrees represents anterolateral rotary instability. The reduction is a result of the iliotibial bands becoming a flexor as it moves posterior to the axis of the knee. Because of its distal attachment, the flexion moment causes the tibia to be pulled posteriorly with contraction of the tensor muscle and iliotibial band.

The same structures that are implicated as being damaged in Losee's test are associated with the pivot shift.

Active Pivot Shift

Indication. The active pivot shift may be used in the assessment of anterolateral instability of the knee.

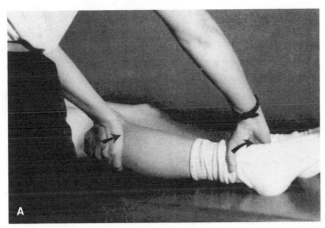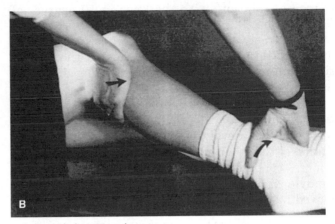

▲ **Figure 13.44** **(A)** Lateral pivot shift: While maintaining the tibia in slight medial rotation, the examiner flexes the knee about 5 degrees and applies valgus force. **(B)** The knee is then moved into flexion, where reduction of the tibia occurs at 30 to 40 degrees.

Method. The subject is seated with the knee between 80 and 90 degrees of flexion and the tibia neutrally rotated with the foot resting on the floor. The examiner stabilizes the foot on the floor while directing the subject to perform an isometric quadriceps contraction.

Results. Anterolateral subluxation of the lateral tibial plateau represents a positive test.

Hughston's Jerk Test [8]

Indication. Anterolateral rotary instability is an indication for this test.

Method. The subject and examiner are positioned as described for the pivot shift, except that the subject's hip is flexed 45 degrees (Fig. 13-45). At 90 degrees of knee flexion, the leg is then extended while maintaining the valgus stress and internal tibial rotation.

Results. In a positive test, the lateral tibial condyle shifts anteriorly with a sudden movement at approximately 25 degrees of knee flexion. If the knee is extended more, the tibia reduces spontaneously. Structures named in Losee's test are associated with a positive finding here.

Slocum's Anterolateral Rotary Instability Test

Indication. Slocum's anterolateral rotary instability test provides another means of assessment of anterolateral rotary instability.

Method. The subject is positioned between supine and sidelying, with the uppermost limb being involved (Fig. 13-46). The bottom limb is flexed to provide stabilization during the test. The foot of the test limb rests on the table in a position

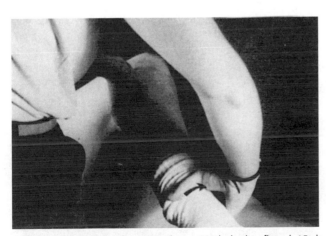

▲ **Figure 13.45** Hughston's jerk test: With the hip flexed 45 degrees and slightly medially rotated and the knee flexed 90 degrees, valgus stress is applied as the knee is extended.

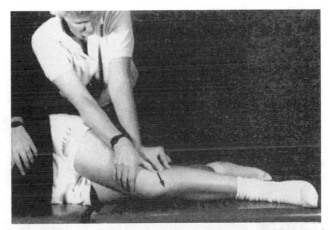

▲ **Figure 13.46** Slocum's anterolateral rotary instability test: With even anteriorly directed pressure applied to the lateral femoral condyle and fibular head, the knee is moved into flexion. A clunk felt as the knee passes through the range of 25 to 45 degrees indicates lateral tibial condyle reduction.

of medial rotation, with the knee in 10 degrees of flexion. The valgus force is created by the knee hanging freely as a result of the leg position. When anterior tibial subluxation is present, the lateral tibial condyle may be palpated as being displaced forward on the femur.

The examiner stands behind the subject and positions a thumb and index finger behind the fibular head and the lateral tibial plateau, respectively. The thumb of the other hand is placed behind the lateral femoral condyle. As even pressure is applied to the condyle and the fibular head, the knee is gently moved into flexion.

Results. A positive test result is demonstrated when the lateral tibial condyle reduces as the knee flexes through the range between 25 and 45 degrees. As reduction occurs, a clunk can be felt by the examiner.

The Slocum anterolateral rotary instability test may prove useful in the subject who is unable to relax the hamstrings or in the overweight person who may be difficult to handle in other testing positions. Damaged structures associated with other tests of anterolateral rotary instability are tested by this examination.

Flexion-Rotation Drawer Test

Indication. The flexion-rotation drawer test[14] is a variation of the pivot shift for the assessment of anterolateral rotary instability. It is a combination of Lachman's test and the lateral pivot shift.

Method. While keeping the tibia in neutral rotation, the examiner flexes the subject's knee to 15 degrees by supporting the calf and grasping the ankle (Fig. 13-47A). In this position, the examiner observes any abnormal tibial motion. The knee is then gently flexed an additional 15 degrees, and again, the tibial motion is noted (see Fig. 13-47B).

Results. In the knee with anterolateral rotary instability, the initial position of 15 degrees of flexion causes the lateral portion of the femur to move posteriorly and rotate laterally. After the knee is flexed another 15 degrees, the tibia drops from its position of relative anterior subluxation to neutral. The structures associated with anterolateral rotary instability are also involved here.

Crossover Test of Arnold

Indication. This test may be included in the battery of tests for anterolateral rotary instability and is a modification of the pivot shift.

Method. The subject is standing and crosses the uninjured leg in front of the injured leg. The examiner stabilizes the foot of the injured knee by gently stepping on it and directs the subject to rotate the trunk away from the injured knee approximately 90 degrees from the stabilized foot (Fig. 13-48). Once in this position, the subject isometrically contracts the quadriceps.

Results. Similar results as seen with the pivot shift indicate a positive test.

POSTEROLATERAL ROTARY INSTABILITY TESTS

Jakob's Test (Reverse Pivot Shift)

Indication. Jakob's test[9] is indicated in suspected cases of posterolateral rotary instability.

Method. The subject lies supine with the knee muscles relaxed. The examiner stands at the end of the table facing the subject's leg, lifts it with one hand, and stabilizes it against the pelvis. The other hand, placed proximally on the fibula, supports the lateral side of the leg. The knee is flexed 70 to 80 de-

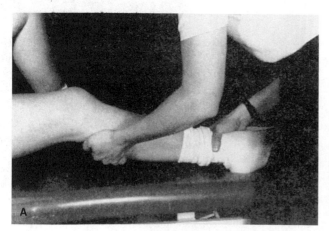
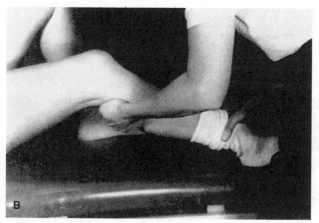

▲ **Figure 13.47** Flexion-rotation drawer test: Testing involves knee flexion to 15 degrees with neutral tibial rotation (**A**), followed by additional knee flexion another 15 degrees with observation of tibial motion (**B**).

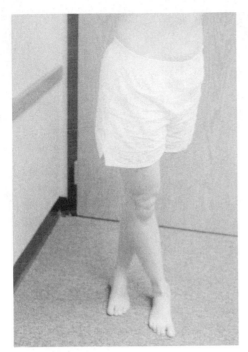

▲ **Figure 13.48** Crossover test of Arnold.

grees, and the tibia is externally rotated at the ankle, producing posterolateral subluxation of the lateral tibial condyle (Fig. 13-49A). The knee is then allowed to move passively into extension, aided by gravity and the weight of the leg. As the knee moves into extension, the examiner leans into the foot, creating a valgus force transmitted through the leg to the knee (see Fig. 13-49B).

Results. In posterolateral rotary instability, the lateral tibial condyle reduces by shifting anteriorly to the neutral position at about 20 degrees from full extension. As the knee is again flexed, the lateral tibial condyle moves into posterior subluxation and lateral rotation.

The following structures may be damaged, thereby contributing to posterolateral rotary instability: the posterior or anterior cruciate or the lateral collateral ligament, the posterolateral capsule, the arcuate complex, or the biceps femoris tendon.

External Rotational Recurvatum Test

Indication. The external rotational recurvatum test[3,7] assesses posterolateral rotary instability.

Method 1. The subject lies supine. The examiner places one hand around the subject's foot or heel, while the other hand holds the posterolateral portion of the knee (Fig. 13-50A and B). Beginning in a flexion of 30 to 40 degrees, the knee is slowly extended while the examiner palpates for a response.

Results. Hyperextension and lateral rotation of the lateral tibial condyle not palpable on the uninvolved side indicate posterolateral rotary instability.

Method 2. The subject lies supine with both lower limbs extended. The examiner lifts both limbs from the table by grasping the great toe (see Fig. 13-50C).

Results. Subjects with posterolateral rotary instability demonstrate relative hyperextension of the knee and external tibial rotation in the test limb compared with the uninvolved side. As a result of the external tibial rotation, the tibial tuberosity lies more laterally on the affected side. There is also noticeable bowing of the medial side of the involved limb.

Hughston's Posterolateral Drawer Sign[7]

Indication. Suspicion of anterolateral rotary instability is an indication for this test.

Method. The subject is supine with the hip flexed 45 degrees and the knee flexed 80 to 90 degrees. The

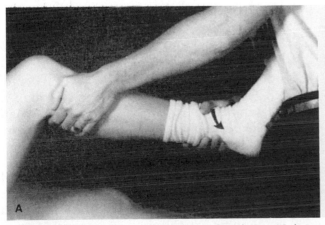 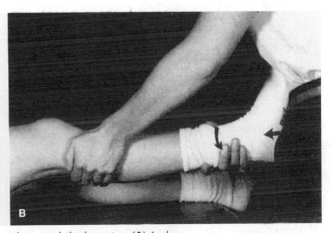

▲ **Figure 13.49** Jakob's test: The knee is flexed 70 to 80 degrees with external tibial rotation. (**A**) As the knee is passively moved into extension, the examiner leans into the foot, putting valgus force on the knee (**B**).

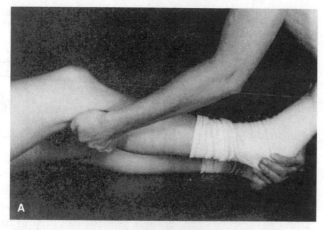

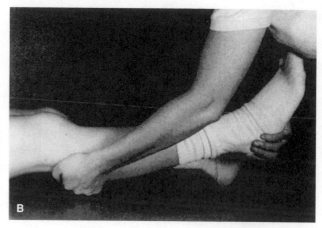

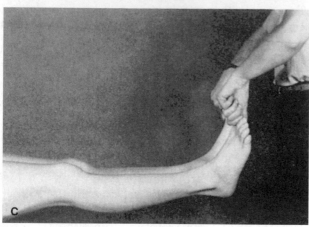

▲ **Figure 13.50 (A)** External rotational recurvatum test: One method is with the knee flexed 30 to 40 degrees and supported by the examiner. **(B)** The knee is slowly extended as the examiner palpates for a response of hyperextension and lateral tibial rotation. **(C)** In an alternate method the examiner grasps the great toes and lifts the extended limbs off the table.

examiner rotates the tibia laterally at the ankle and then sits on the foot to stabilize it. The examiner pushes the tibia posteriorly as in the drawer test.

Results. If, during the posterior drawer test, the lateral tibial condyle of the test leg rotates excessively or moves posteriorly as compared with the uninvolved knee, the result is positive. This test can only be positive in the presence of anterior cruciate ligament rupture. Other structures that when damaged produce this form of instability include those described with Jakob's test.

Dynamic Posterior Shift Test[15]

Indication. This test can be used in the assessment of posterior and posterolateral instability.

Method. As the subject lies supine, the examiner flexes the hip and knee of the test limb to 90 degrees, keeping the femur in neutral rotation. One hand of the examiner stabilizes the anterior thigh, while the other hand moves the knee into extension.

Results. A clunk as the knee approaches full extension represents the anterior reduction of the tibia and a positive test.

POSTEROMEDIAL ROTARY INSTABILITY TESTS

Hughston's Posteromedial Drawer Sign

Indication. Hughston's posteromedial drawer sign is used in the assessment of posteromedial rotary instability.

Method. The subject is positioned as for Hughston's posterolateral drawer sign, except that the tibia is internally rotated. The examiner performs a posterior drawer to the proximal tibia.

Results. Excessive posterior movement or rotation of the medial tibial condyle on the test leg as compared with the uninvolved knee indicates posteromedial rotary instability. The structures listed below may be involved with this form of rotary instability: posterior and anterior cruciate, medial collateral, and posterior oblique ligaments; posteromedial capsule; and semimembranosus muscle.

If the posterior cruciate is intact, the tibia will demonstrate only posterolateral rotation. If the posterior cruciate is torn, the tibia will not only rotate posterolaterally, but will sublux posteriorly.

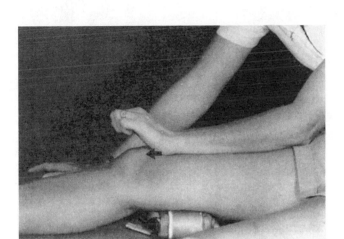

▲ **Figure 13.51** Inferior glide of the patella.

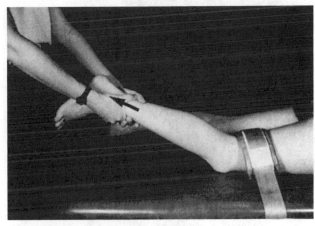

▲ **Figure 13.52** Distraction of the tibiofemoral joint.

JOINT PLAY (ACCESSORY MOVEMENT)

Patellofemoral Joint

INFERIOR GLIDE (FIG. 13-51)

Restriction. Knee flexion.

Open-Packed Position. Slight knee flexion.

Positioning. The subject lies supine with the knee slightly flexed over a small roll beneath the joint. The examiner places the heel of the mobilizing hand on the superior border of the patella, with the palm and fingers resting over the patellar area. The other hand is placed on top of the mobilizing hand to assist in the movement.

Movement. The examiner moves the patella in an inferior direction.

Tibiofemoral Joint

Distraction (Fig. 13-52)

Restriction. General hypomobility.

Open-Packed Position. Twenty-five degrees of knee flexion.

Positioning. The subject lies prone with the distal thigh stabilized by a strap. The examiner stands at the foot of the table facing the subject. The examiner grasps the distal leg of the subject above the malleoli.

Movement. The examiner applies a distraction force to the subject's knee as the examiner leans backward, pulling on the subject's leg.

Anterior Glide (Fig. 13-53)

Restriction. Knee extension.

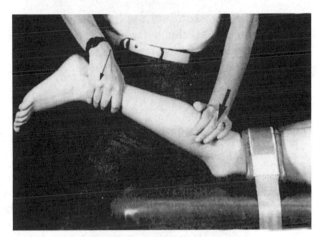

▲ **Figure 13.53** Anterior glide of the tibia.

Positioning. The subject lies prone so that the distal thigh rests at the edge of the treatment table. A wedge is placed beneath the distal thigh to help support the distal thigh. The examiner stands beside the knee being treated with one hand on the posterior proximal leg as close to the joint line as possible. The other hand holds the distal leg to provide support and to maintain the resting position.

Movement. The examiner applies an anterior force to the proximal posterior leg.

Posterior Glide (Fig. 13-54)

Restriction. Knee flexion.

Positioning. The subject lies supine so that the distal thigh rests at the edge of the treatment table. A wedge is placed beneath the distal thigh to support the distal femur. The examiner stands beside the knee being treated. One hand is placed on the anterior proximal leg as close to the joint line as possible. The other hand holds the distal leg to provide support and to maintain the resting position.

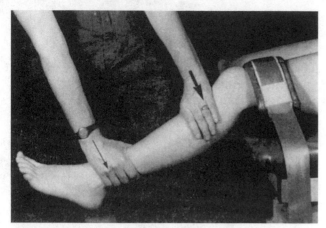

▲ **Figure 13.54** Posterior glide of the tibia.

Movement. The examiner applies a posterior force to the proximal posterior leg.

Superior Tibiofibular Joint

Anterior Glide (Fig. 13-55)

Restriction. Foot pronation.

Open-Packed Position. Anatomical position.

Positioning. The subject is placed in a weight-bearing position of knee flexion to 90 degrees. The examiner places the thenar eminence of one hand on the posterior proximal fibula of the subject. The other hand may be positioned on top of the mobilizing hand to assist in the movement.

Movement. The examiner applies an anteriorly directed force to the posterior surface of the proximal fibula.

Posterior Glide (Fig. 13-56)

Restriction. Foot supination.

Positioning. The subject lies supine with the knee joint resting in extension. The examiner places the

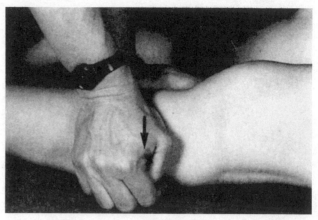

▲ **Figure 13.56** Posterior glide of the fibula.

thenar eminence of the mobilizing hand on the anterior surface of the proximal fibula. The other hand may be used to assist in the movement by placing it on top of the mobilizing hand.

Movement. The examiner applies a posteriorly directed force to the anterior surface of the proximal fibula.

Inferior Tibiofibular Joint

Anterior Glide (Fig. 13-57)

Restriction. Foot pronation.

Open-Packed Position. Anatomical position.

Positioning. The subject lies prone. A wedge may be placed beneath the distal tibia to aid in stabilization. The examiner places the thenar eminence of one hand posteriorly on the subject's lateral malleolus to apply the mobilizing force. The other hand may be positioned on top of the mobilizing hand to assist in the movement.

Movement. The examiner applies an anteriorly directed force to the posterior surface of the distal fibula.

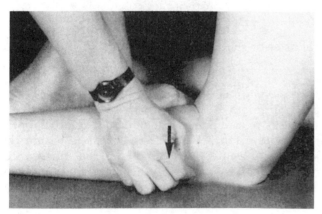

▲ **Figure 13.55** Anterior glide of the fibula.

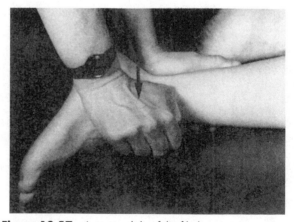

▲ **Figure 13.57** Anterior glide of the fibula.

TABLE 13.1 **Summary of Joint Play of the Knee**			
GLIDE	RESTRICTION	FIXED BONE	MOVING BONE
Patellofemoral Joint			
Inferior	Flexion	Femur	Patella
Superior	Extension	Femur	Patella
Medial	General hypomobility	Femur	Patella
Tibiofemoral Joint			
Distraction	General hypomobility	Femur	Tibia
Anterior	Extension	Femur	Tibia
Posterior	Flexion	Femur	Tibia
Superior/Inferior Tibiofibular Joints			
Posterior	Supination of foot	Tibia	Fibula
Anterior	Pronation of foot	Tibia	Fibula

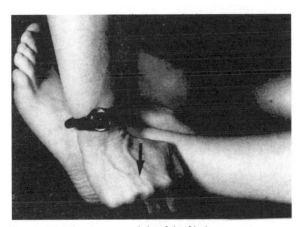

▲ **Figure 13.58** Posterior glide of the fibula.

Posterior Glide (Fig. 13-58)

Restriction. Foot supination.

Positioning. The subject lies supine. The examiner places the thenar eminence of the mobilizing hand on the anterior surface of the lateral malleolus to apply the mobilizing force. The other hand may be used to assist in the movement by placing it on top of the mobilizing hand.

Movement. The examiner applies a posteriorly directed force to the anterior surface of the distal fibula.

Summary of Joint Play of the Knee

Table 13-1 provides a summary of joint play of the patellofemoral, tibiofemoral, superior tibiofibular, and inferior tibiofibular joints.

REFERENCES

1. Apley AG: The diagnosis of meniscus injuries—Some new clinical methods. J Bone Joint Surg 29B:78, 1947
2. Davies GJ, Larson R: Examining the knee. Phys Sports Med 6(4):49–67, 1978
3. Delee JC, Riley MB, Rockwood CA: Acute posterolateral rotatory instability of the knee. Am J Sports Med 11:199–206, 1983
4. Feto JF, Marsall JL: Injury to the anterior cruciate ligament producing the pivot shift sign. An experimental study on cadaver specimens. J Bone Joint Surg 61A:710, 1979
5. Galway HR, MacIntosh DL: The lateral pivot shift: A symptom and sign of anterior cruciate ligament insufficiency. Clin Orthop 147:45, 1980
6. Helfet A: Disorders of the Knee. Philadelphia, JB Lippincott, 1974
7. Hughston JC, Norwood LA: The posterolateral drawer test and external rotational recurvatum test for posterolateral rotary instability of the knee. Clin Orthop 147:82, 1980
8. Hughston JC, Walsh WM, Puddu G: Patellar Subluxation and Dislocation. Philadelphia, WB Saunders, 1991
9. Jakob RP, Hassler H, Staeubli HU: Observations on rotary instability of the lateral compartment of the knee. Acta Orthop Can 52(Suppl 191):1, 1981
10. Jensen K: Manual laxity tests for anterior cruciate ligament injuries. J Orthop Sports Phys Ther 11:474–481, 1990
11. Losee RE: Diagnosis of chronic injury to the anterior cruciate ligament. Orthop Clin North Am 16:1, 1985
12. McMurray TP: The semilunar cartilages. Br J Surg 29:407, 1942
13. Mital MA, Hayden J: Pain in the knee in children: The medial plica shelf syndrome. Orthop Clin North Am 10:713, 1979
14. Noyes FR, Butler DL, Grood ES, et al: Clinical paradoxes of anterior cruciate instability and a new test to detect its instability. Orthop Trans 2:36, 1978
15. Shelbourne KD, Benedict F, McCarroll JR, Rettig AC: Dynamic posterior shift test—An adjunct in evaluation of posterior tibial subluxation. Am J Sports Med 17:275, 1989
16. Strobel M, Stedtfeld HW: Evaluation of the Knee. Berlin, Springer-Verlag, 1990
17. Tamea CD, Henning CE: Pathomechanics of the pivot shift maneuver. Am J Sports Med 9:31, 1981

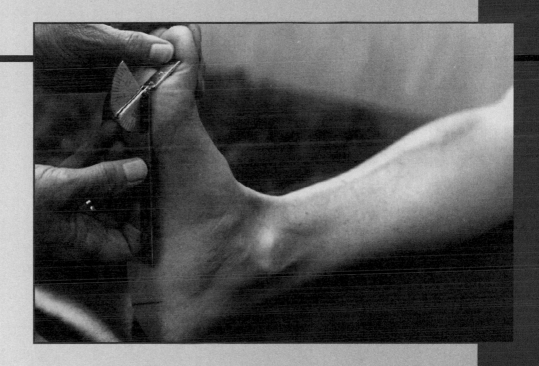

14

Ankle and Foot

The ankle and foot are flexible enough to adapt to uneven terrain but sufficiently stable to bear the body's weight. Ankle injuries occur frequently. The ankle and foot have to make continuous adjustments to the ground during ambulation to compensate for the motion of deviation at the knee and hip joints and keep the center of gravity over the relatively small base of support.

The talocrural joint is composed of the distal ends of the tibia and fibula and the trochlea of the talus. As a hinge joint, it permits one degree of freedom of motion. The medial and lateral surfaces of the joint are guarded by the medial malleolus of the tibia and the lateral malleolus of the fibula. The axis of motion lies transversely and passes through the talus, connecting the two malleoli. The plane of the axis is oblique in that the lateral malleolus extends more distally and is posterior to the medial malleolus. The posterior alignment of the lateral malleolus is due to the torsion of the tibia. Movements at the talocrural joint are described as dorsiflexion and plantar flexion. During the motion at the talocrural joint, the fibula moves on the tibia superiorly and inferiorly.

The superior surface of the calcaneus and the inferior surface of the talus form the subtalar joint. The talus also articulates with the tarsal navicular anteriorly. The motions of supination and pronation occur around an oblique axis, allowing the foot to conform to the surface of the terrain. The axis for supination and pronation motion is described by a line that begins on the lateral posterior aspect of the heel and proceeds anterior, superior, and medial.

The bones that form the articulation for the midtarsal joint are the talus and calcaneus proximally and the navicular and cuboid distally. This joint permits coordinated movement of the forefoot with the rearfoot.

The structure of the transtarsal joint has been analyzed frequently, but the joint axis has not been agreed upon. Manter and Hicks have suggested longitudinal and oblique axes around a relatively fixed naviculocuboid unit. The longitudinal axis is nearly horizontal, permitting the motion of pronation and supination. The oblique axis is relatively transverse, also permitting supination and pronation with dorsiflexion and plantar flexion and accompanying abduction and adduction. The two axes provide the total range of motion for supination and pronation.

Triplanar movement occurs at the talocrural, subtalar, and midtarsal joints. In an open kinematic chain, the movement of supination includes the components of plantar flexion, adduction, and inversion, while pronation includes the components of dorsiflexion, abduction, and eversion. Clinicians often measure goniometric triplanar motion as subtalar inversion and eversion.

The metatarsophalangeal (MTP) joints of the foot are condyloid synovial joints with two degrees of freedom of motion, allowing flexion and extension and abduction and adduction. The motion of flexion is limited, and extension and hyperextension motion is 90 degrees or more in combination with plantar flexion of the first ray. This motion is important for the weight-bearing functions of the foot. Great toe hyperextension is important for toe-off during ambulation.

The interphalangeal (IP) joints of the toes are hinge synovial joints with one degree of freedom of motion, permitting flexion and extension.

GONIOMETRY

ANKLE JOINT DORSIFLEXION

The motion of ankle joint dorsiflexion occurs in the sagittal plane between the distal ends of the tibia and fibula and the articular surface of the talus. The talus moves on the tibia into ankle dorsiflexion, and the motion is accompanied by an accessory gliding motion in a posterior direction. There is an accompanying motion between the superior and inferior tibiofibular joints. The fibula moves superiorly, abducts, and rotates medially with the tibia during ankle dorsiflexion.

Motion. From 0 to 20 degrees of ankle dorsiflexion.

Position

• Preferred: Subject lies supine with the knee joint flexed 20 to 30 degrees and supported by a pillow or towel roll. The ankle joint is in the anatomical position (Figs. 14-1 and 14-2).
• Alternate: Subject is sitting or in any position that allows the knee to be slightly flexed, and the ankle is in the anatomical position (Fig. 14-3).

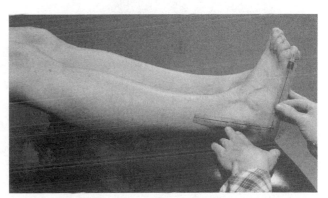

▲ **Figure 14.1** Starting position for measuring ankle dorsiflexion.

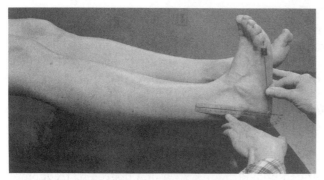

▲ **Figure 14.2** End position for measuring ankle dorsiflexion.

Goniometric Alignment

Axis. Placed 1 in distal to the lateral malleolus of the fibula.

Stationary Arm. Placed parallel to the lateral midline of the fibula, projecting toward the fibular head.

Moving Arm. Placed parallel to the lateral midline of the calcaneus.

Stabilization. The leg is stabilized.

Precautions

- Prevent hip and knee joint motion.
- Avoid inversion and eversion.
- Keep the knee flexed to prevent stretching of the gastrocnemius muscle.
- Align the moving arm of the goniometer with the lateral calcaneus, not with the forefoot.

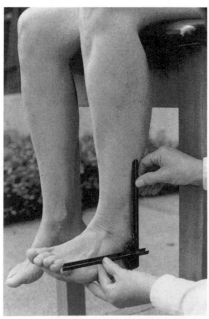

▲ **Figure 14.3** End position for measuring ankle dorsiflexion in the alternate sitting position.

ANKLE JOINT PLANTAR FLEXION

The motion occurs in the sagittal plane between the distal tibia and fibula and the superior surface of the talus. As the motion of plantar flexion occurs, the talus glides anteriorly on the tibia. During ambulation, the tibia glides posteriorly on the talus. Motion at the tibiotalar joint is accompanied by motion at the superior and inferior tibiofibular joints. The fibula adducts and glides inferiorly on the tibia during plantar flexion.

Motion. From 0 to 45 degrees of plantar flexion at the talotibial (talocrural) joint.

Position

- Preferred: Subject lies supine with the hip and knee joints extended and the ankle in the anatomical position (Fig. 14-4).
- Alternate: Subject sits with the knee flexed and the foot in the anatomical position (Fig. 14-5).

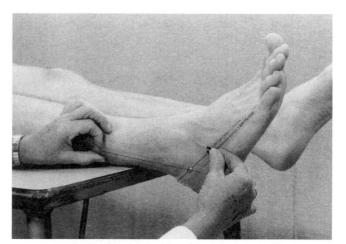

▲ **Figure 14.4** End position for measuring ankle plantar flexion.

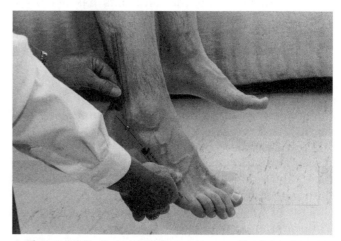

▲ **Figure 14.5** End position for measuring ankle plantar flexion in the alternate sitting position.

Goniometric alignment and stabilization are the same as for ankle joint dorsiflexion.

Precautions

- Avoid forefoot flexion.
- Prevent hip joint rotation.
- Prevent inversion and eversion of the foot.

MIDTARSAL-SUBTALAR SUPINATION (INVERSION)

Midtarsal-subtalar motion occurs between talus and calcaneus, talus and navicular, and calcaneus and cuboid. The motion occurs in the transverse, sagittal, and frontal planes.

Motion. From 0 to 30 degrees of inversion.

Position

- Preferred: Subject lies supine with the hip in the anatomical position and the ankle relaxed. The knee may be either flexed or extended (Fig. 14-6).
- Alternate: Subject sits with the knee flexed 90 degrees (Figs. 14-7 and 14-8).

Goniometric Alignment

Axis

- Preferred: Placed over the dorsal surface of the foot, midway between the malleoli.
- Alternate: Placed on the lateral side of the foot, at the level of the fifth MTP joint.

Stationary Arm

- Preferred: Placed along the anterior surface over the crest of the tibia in line with the tibial tuberosity.

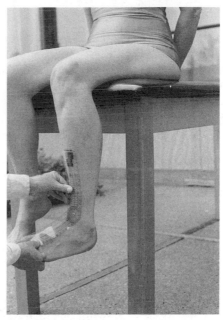

▲ **Figure 14.7** End position for measuring triplanar inversion in the alternate sitting position.

- Alternate: Placed parallel to the longitudinal axis of the tibia laterally.

Moving Arm

- Preferred: Placed along the dorsal surface of the second metatarsal shaft.
- Alternate: Placed parallel to the plantar surface of the heel.

Stabilization. The leg is stabilized.

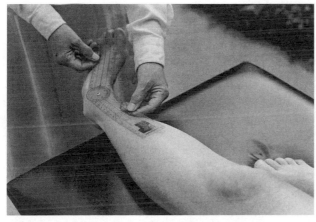

▲ **Figure 14.6** End position for triplanar inversion measurement.

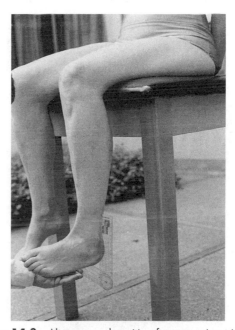

▲ **Figure 14.8** Alternate end position for measuring triplanar inversion in the sitting position.

Precautions

- Prevent medial rotation and extension of the knee joint.
- Prevent hip joint lateral rotation and abduction.
- Allow ankle joint plantar flexion.

MIDTARSAL (TRANSTARSAL)-SUBTALAR PRONATION (EVERSION)

In the test position, the motion is assessed in the frontal plane between talus and calcaneus, talus and navicular, and calcaneus and cuboid.

Motion. From 0 to 25 degrees of foot eversion.

Position, goniometric alignment, and stabilization are the same as for midtarsal-subtalar supination (Figs. 14-9, 14-10, and 14-11)

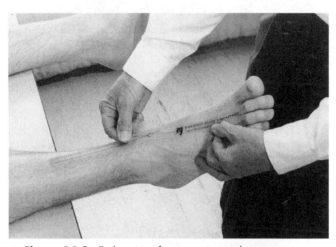

▲ **Figure 14.9** End position for measuring triplanar eversion.

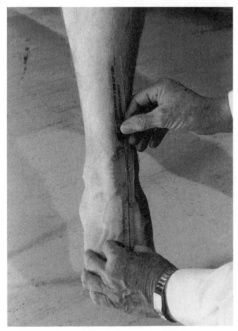

▲ **Figure 14.10** End position for measuring triplanar eversion in the alternate sitting position.

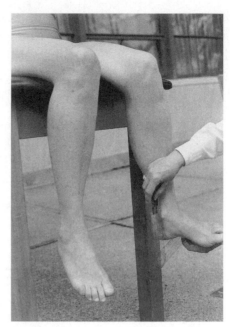

▲ **Figure 14.11** Alternate end position for measuring triplanar eversion in the sitting position.

Precautions

- Prevent lateral rotation of the knee.
- Prevent hip joint medial rotation and abduction.
- Allow for dorsiflexion at the ankle.

The Toes

The position for measurement of toe motion may be any comfortable position for the subject in which the ankle is in the anatomical position. It is best if the subject is able to see the procedure. Usually the mobility of the toes is measured not specifically, but grossly. Observations should identify deformities, such as hallux valgus and hammer toes. Extension and hyperextension motion of all toes is important for ambulation.

FLEXION OF THE FIRST METATARSOPHALANGEAL JOINT

Great toe flexion occurs in the sagittal plane between the head of the first metatarsal and the base of the proximal phalanx. As the motion of flexion occurs, the base of the proximal phalanx glides in a plantar direction.

Motion. From 0 to 45 degrees of flexion.

Goniometric Alignment

Axis. Placed over the dorsal aspect of the MTP joint (Fig. 14-12).

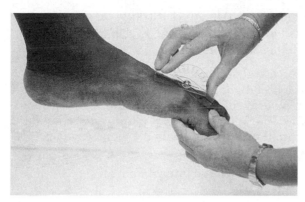

▲ **Figure 14.12** End position for metatarsophalangeal joint flexion measurement of the first digit.

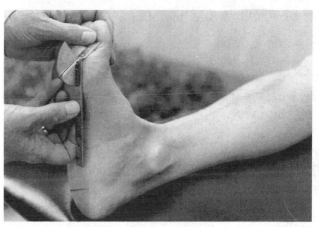

▲ **Figure 14.13** End position for metatarsophalangeal joint extension and hyperextension measurements.

Stationary Arm. Placed over the dorsal aspect of the shaft of the first metatarsal bone.

Moving Arm. Placed along the dorsal surface of the shaft of the proximal phalanx.

Stabilization. The metatarsal bones are stabilized.

Precautions

- Prevent ankle joint plantar flexion.
- Prevent midtarsal motions.
- Allow the lateral toes to flex.

EXTENSION AND HYPEREXTENSION OF THE FIRST METATARSOPHALANGEAL JOINT

Extension of the great toe is the return from flexion, whereas hyperextension moves beyond the anatomical position. As the base of the proximal phalanx extends on the first metatarsal bone, the motion is accompanied by a dorsal glide.

Motion. From 45 to 0 degrees of extension and 0 to 90 degrees of hyperextension at the first MTP joint.

Goniometric Alignment

Axis. Placed over the plantar aspect of the first MTP joint (Fig. 14-13).

Stationary Arm. Placed over the plantar midline shaft of the first metatarsal bone.

Moving Arm. Placed along the plantar shaft of the proximal phalanx.

Stabilization. The metatarsal bones are stabilized.

Precautions

- Prevent ankle joint dorsiflexion.
- Prevent forefoot inversion or eversion.

- Allow the lateral four digits to extend.
- Permit IP joint flexion.

FLEXION OF THE LATERAL FOUR METATARSOPHALANGEAL JOINTS

Flexion of the MTP joints in the lateral four digits occurs in the sagittal plane between the metatarsals and the proximal phalanges. As the proximal phalanx moves into flexion, it glides in a plantar direction. Each joint is measured individually.

Motion. From 0 to 40 degrees of MTP joint flexion.

Goniometric Alignment

Axis. Placed over the dorsal aspect of the MTP joints (Fig. 14-14).

Stationary Arm. Placed along the dorsal midline longitudinal shaft of each metatarsal bone.

Moving Arm. Placed along the dorsal midline longitudinal shaft of each proximal phalanx.

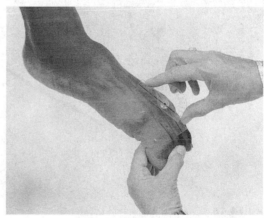

▲ **Figure 14.14** End position for measuring metatarsophalangeal joint flexion of the second digit.

Stabilization. The metatarsal bones are stabilized.

Precautions

- Prevent ankle joint and forefoot motions.
- Allow toes not being tested to flex.

EXTENSION AND HYPEREXTENSION OF THE LATERAL FOUR METATARSOPHALANGEAL JOINTS

Extension of the MTP joint occurs between the proximal phalanges and the metatarsal bones. As the motion occurs, the bases of the proximal phalanges glide in a dorsal direction.

Motion. From 40 to 0 degrees of extension and 0 to 45 degrees of hyperextension.

Goniometric Alignment

Axis. Placed over the plantar aspect of the MTP joint (Fig. 14-15).

Stationary Arm. Placed along the plantar midline shaft of the metatarsals.

Moving Arm. Placed along the plantar midline aspect of the shaft of the proximal phalanx of each digit.

Stabilization. The metatarsals are stabilized.

Precautions

- Prevent ankle joint and forefoot motion.
- Permit IP joint flexion.
- Allow the other digits to extend or hyperextend.

FLEXION OF THE FIRST INTERPHALANGEAL JOINT AND THE LATERAL FOUR PROXIMAL INTERPHALANGEAL JOINTS

As the distal phalanx flexes on the proximal phalanx of the first digit, the base of the distal phalanx glides in a plantar direction. The middle phalanges of the lateral four digits glide in a plantar direction during proximal interphalangeal (PIP) joint flexion.

Motion. From 0 to 90 degrees for the great toe; 0 to 35 degrees for the lateral four toes.

Goniometric Alignment

Axis. Placed over the dorsal aspect of the IP joints (Fig. 14-16).

Stationary Arm. Placed on the dorsal midline shaft of the proximal phalanges for each digit.

Moving Arm. Placed on the dorsal midline shaft of the distal phalanx of the great toe and the dorsal midline shaft of the middle phalanges of the lateral four toes.

Stabilization. The proximal phalanges and metatarsals are stabilized.

Precautions

- Prevent ankle and forefoot motion.
- Avoid MTP joint motion.
- Allow the distal IP joint to flex.

EXTENSION AND HYPEREXTENSION OF THE FIRST INTERPHALANGEAL JOINT AND EXTENSION OF THE LATERAL FOUR JOINTS

Extension of the IP joints is the return from flexion. Hyperextension is a motion in the sagittal plane beyond the anatomical position. The distal phalanx of

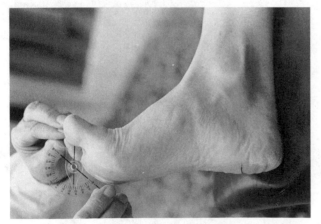

▲ **Figure 14.15** End position for measuring metatarsophalangeal joint extension for the second digit.

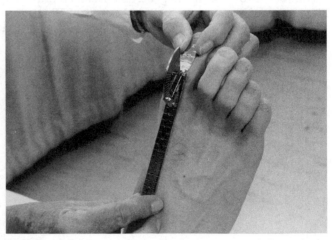

▲ **Figure 14.16** End position for measuring interphalangeal joint flexion for the first digit.

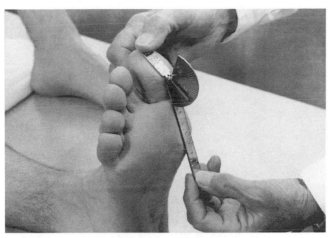

▲ **Figure 14.17** End position for measuring interphalangeal joint extension for the first digit.

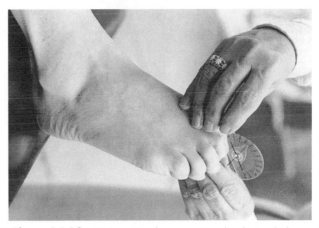

▲ **Figure 14.18** End position for measuring distal interphalangeal flexion of the second digit.

the first digit glides in a dorsal direction during extension and hyperextension. The middle phalanges of the lateral four digits also glide in a dorsal direction during extension and hyperextension.

Motion. From 90 to 0 degrees for the great toe and 35 to 0 degrees for the lateral four toes. Hyperextension is minimal at the IP joints.

Goniometric Alignment

Axis. Placed over the plantar aspect of the IP joints (Fig. 14-17).

Stationary Arm. Placed over the plantar midline shaft of the proximal phalanges.

Moving Arm. Placed over the plantar midline shaft of the distal phalanx of the great toe and over the middle phalanges of the other toes.

Stabilization. The proximal phalanges are stabilized.

Precautions

- Prevent ankle joint and forefoot motions.
- Avoid MTP joint motion.
- Allow the distal IP joints to extend.

FLEXION OF THE LATERAL FOUR DISTAL INTERPHALANGEAL (DIP) JOINTS

Flexion occurs between the middle and distal phalanges of the lateral four digits. The accessory motion that occurs during flexion is plantar gliding of the distal phalanges on the middle phalanges.

Motion. From 0 to 60 degrees of DIP joint flexion.

Goniometric Alignment

Axis. Placed over the dorsal aspect of the DIP joints.

Stationary Arm. Placed along the dorsal midline shaft of the middle phalanges.

Moving Arm. Placed along the dorsal midline shaft of the distal phalanges (Fig. 14-18).

Stabilization. The metatarsals and the proximal and middle phalanges.

Precautions

- Prevent ankle joint and forefoot motions.
- Avoid MTP and PIP joint motion of the digit being measured.

EXTENSION AND HYPEREXTENSION OF THE LATERAL FOUR DISTAL INTERPHALANGEAL JOINTS

The motion of extension and hyperextension of the DIP joint is the return from the flexion motion and beyond the anatomical position for hyperextension. As the extension motion occurs, the bases of the distal phalanges glide in a dorsal direction.

Motion. From 60 to 0 degrees of extension; hyperextension is minimal.

Goniometric Alignment

Axis. Placed over the dorsal aspect of the DIP joint.

Stationary Arm. Placed along the dorsal midline shaft of the middle phalanges.

Moving Arm. Placed along the dorsal midline shaft of the distal phalanges.

Stabilization. The proximal and middle phalanges are stabilized.

Precautions

- Prevent ankle and forefoot motions.
- Prevent MTP and PIP joint motions.
- Allow the digits that are not being tested to extend.

MUSCLE LENGTH TESTING

Ankle Joint

The plantar flexors of the ankle lie posterior to the transverse axis and function in the sagittal plane. The action of the ankle plantar flexion is one of the most powerful movements in the body. The most powerful is the one-joint soleus muscle, accompanied by the two-joint gastrocnemius and plantaris muscles. The two-joint plantar flexor muscles also function in knee joint flexion. Limitation in dorsiflexion due to shortening of the gastrocnemius and plantaris muscles is not uncommon.

SOLEUS MUSCLE

Position. The subject is in a supine position or short sitting with the knee flexed.

Movement. The examiner dorsiflexes the ankle joint with the knee joint maintained in flexion.

Measurement. A goniometer is used to measure any limitation in dorsiflexion. The arms of the goniometer are aligned as in measuring dorsiflexion range of motion (Fig. 14-19).

Considerations

- The knee joint remains flexed to eliminate the effect of the two-joint gastrocnemius and plantaris muscles.
- The posterior joint capsular structures may also show tightness, along with the soleus muscle.

GASTROCNEMIUS AND PLANTARIS MUSCLES

Position. The subject is supine or sitting with the knee joint extended.

Movement. The examiner dorsiflexes the ankle joint with the knee joint remaining extended.

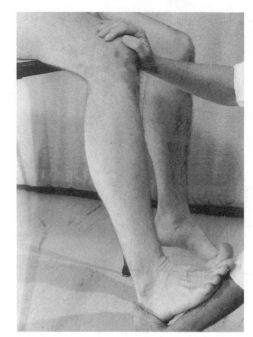

▲ **Figure 14.19** Length testing for the soleus muscle.

Measurement. The goniometric dorsiflexion measurement at the ankle joint will usually be less with the knee joint extended due to a common tightness of the gastrocnemius and plantaris muscles. Use the same bony landmarks as indicated in the goniometry section (Fig. 14-20).

Considerations

- From 0 to 20 degrees for range of motion in dorsiflexion is an average range with the knee flexed; with the knee joint extended, 10 degrees is an average dorsiflexion range of motion.
- If excessive range is noted due to the muscles being too lengthened, instability at the ankle

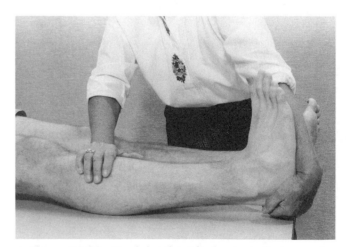

▲ **Figure 14.20** Muscle length test for the plantar flexion muscles.

joint may result. Adequate support is necessary for proper function in a weight-bearing position.

- Limitation of dorsiflexion with the knee extended includes both the two-joint and one-joint muscles. The examiner must flex the knee joint to eliminate the tightness of the gastrocnemius muscle. If limitations continue to exist, it may be as a result of either the posterior capsular structures or the soleus muscle.

Dorsiflexor Tightness. These muscles do not commonly show tightness. They cross the ankle anterior to the joint axis and if tight, would limit plantar flexion. Lengthening of the dorsiflexors would be necessary following immobilization of the ankle joint.

MANUAL MUSCLE TESTING

Ankle

GASTROCNEMIUS AND
PLANTARIS MUSCLES

The gastrocnemius and plantaris muscles produce 45 degrees of plantar flexion with the knee extended. The motion is tested in the prone position. If no weakness is apparent, a test is performed in the functional position (standing).

Palpation. Palpate the gastrocnemius, with its short, bulky medial and lateral heads immediately distal to the posterior knee joint (Fig. 14-21). (The plantaris is not palpable.)

Position

Against gravity (AG):
Preferred (weight-bearing test): The subject stands with the knee extended and the opposite foot off the floor (Fig. 14-22).

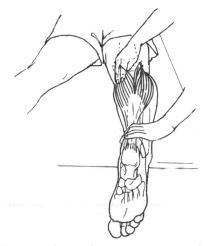

▲ **Figure 14.21** Palpating the gastrocnemius muscle.

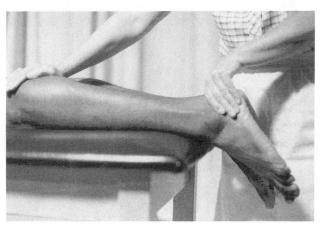

▲ **Figure 14.22** Testing the gastrocnemius muscle in the AG position.

Alternate (non–weight-bearing test): Subject lies prone with the foot over the edge of the table (Fig. 14-23).
Gravity minimized (GM): Subject is in sidelying position with the ankle in the anatomical position (Fig. 14-24).

Movement. Plantar flexion of ankle; the heel moves up toward the back of the leg, as in standing on tiptoes.

Resistance. Applied to the plantar surface of the rearfoot. Standing, the body weight provides the resistance.

Stabilization. The leg is stabilized, or the standing subject may balance by placing the hands on the table but may not bear weight on them.

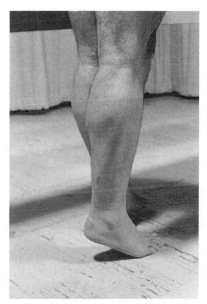

▲ **Figure 14.23** Testing the gastrocnemius muscle in the AG standing position.

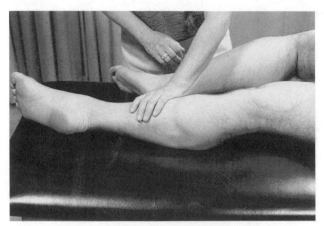

▲ **Figure 14.24** Testing the gastrocnemius muscle in the GM position.

Grades

Non–weight-bearing

P+: Moves through less than half the range
F−: Moves through more than half the range
F: Moves through full range
F+: Cannot take maximal resistance
G: Takes maximal resistance

Standing

P+: Less than half the range
F−: More than half the range
F: 1 repetition
F+: 2 to 3 repetitions
G: 4 to 6 repetitions
G+: 7 to 9 repetitions
N: 10 repetitions

Substitutions

- Do not allow toe flexors to contract.
- Do not allow inversion to occur with the plantar flexion using the tibialis posterior muscle.
- Do not allow eversion with the plantar flexion by using the peroneal muscles.
- Soleus is a plantar flexor muscle in any position of the knee joint.
- Subject may quickly dorsiflex, then relax.

SOLEUS MUSCLE

The soleus muscle produces plantar flexion of the ankle joint regardless of the position of the knee. To determine the individual functioning of the soleus as a plantar flexor, the knee is flexed to minimize the effect of the gastrocnemius muscle.

Palpation. The soleus muscle is covered largely by the gastrocnemius muscle, but it is easily palpated distal to the gastrocnemius bulk on either side (Fig. 14-25).

Position

AG: Subject lies prone with the knees flexed 90 degrees (Fig. 14-26).
GM: Subject is in sidelying position with the knee flexed 90 degrees (Fig. 14-27).
    Alternate: Subject stands with some degree of knee flexion, while rising up on toes (Fig. 14-28).

Movement. Plantar flexion of the ankle; the heel moves toward the back of the leg, as in pointing the toes.

Resistance. Applied to the plantar surface of the rearfoot, unless subject is standing, in which case the body weight provides the resistance.

Stabilization. Stabilize the leg. A standing subject may balance by placing the hands on the table but may not bear weight on the hands.

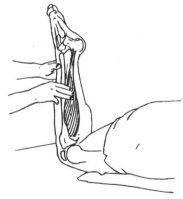

▲ **Figure 14.25** Palpating the soleus muscle.

▼ Attachments of Gastrocnemius and Plantaris Muscles			
Muscle	**Proximal**	**Distal**	**Innervation**
Gastrocnemius	Medial and lateral condyle of femur	Posterior surface of calcaneus through Achilles' tendon	Tibial S2 (S1)
Plantaris	Lateral supracondylar line of femur	Posterior surface of calcaneus through Achilles' tendon	Tibial S2 (S1)

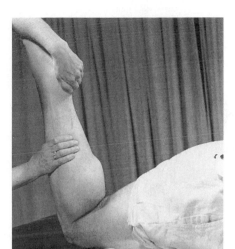

▲ **Figure 14.26** Testing the soleus muscle in the AG position.

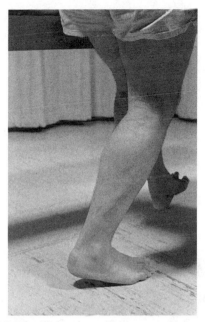

▲ **Figure 14.28** Alternate standing position for testing the soleus muscle against gravity.

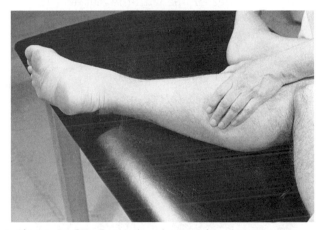

▲ **Figure 14.27** Testing the soleus muscle in the GM position.

Substitutions

- The gastrocnemius will also plantar flex the foot. To minimize its action, flex the knee.
- Do not allow inversion to occur with the plantar flexion using the tibialis posterior muscle.
- Do not allow eversion with the plantar flexion using the peroneal muscles.
- The subject may quickly dorsiflex, then relax.

TIBIALIS ANTERIOR MUSCLE

The tibialis anterior muscle produces the motion of dorsiflexion and inversion through a test range of 15 degrees from the starting (anatomical) position. The knee must remain flexed to allow complete dorsiflexion. If dorsiflexion does not appear to be limited, the test may be conducted with the knee extended.

Palpation. Palpate the tibialis anterior along its course from the lateral side of the tibia. The tendon is also palpated as it crosses the dorsum of the foot from the lateral to the medial side (Fig. 14-29).

Position

AG: Subject sits with the knee flexed over the edge of the table. The ankle is in the anatomical position (Fig. 14-30).
GM: Subject is in sidelying position with the test leg uppermost.

Movement. Dorsiflexion and inversion of the ankle.

Resistance. Applied to the medial dorsal aspect of the forefoot into plantar flexion and eversion.

▼ Attachments of Soleus Muscle			
Muscle	**Proximal**	**Distal**	**Innervation**
Soleus	Head of fibula, proximal third of shaft, soleal line and midshaft of posterior tibia	Posterior surface of calcaneus through Achilles' tendon	Tibial S2 (S1)

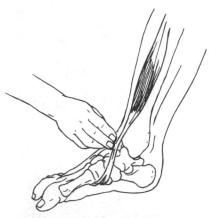

▲ **Figure 14.29** Palpating the tibialis anterior muscle.

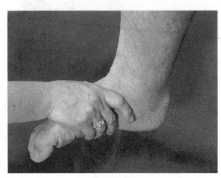

▲ **Figure 14.30** Testing the tibialis anterior muscle in the AG position.

Stabilization. The leg is stabilized.

Substitutions

- The extensor hallucis longus, maintain the big toe in flexion.
- The extensor digitorum longus dorsiflexes and everts.
- Tibialis posterior will invert without dorsiflexing.
- Together, posterior tibialis and extensor hallucis longus will produce dorsiflexion and inversion.
- The subject may quickly plantar flex, then relax.

TIBIALIS POSTERIOR MUSCLE

The tibialis posterior muscle produces the motion of inversion in a plantar flexed position through a test range of 20 degrees.

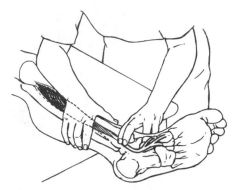

▲ **Figure 14.31** Palpating the tibialis posterior muscle.

Palpation. Palpate the tibialis posterior tendon as it crosses the medial malleolus (Fig. 14-31).

Position

AG: Subject is in sidelying position with the leg to be tested off the edge of the table (Fig. 14-32).

GM: Subject lies supine with the foot over the edge of the table. The leg and ankle are in the anatomical position (Fig. 14-33).

Movement. Inversion of the foot while keeping the ankle in slight plantar flexion.

Resistance. Applied to the medial border of the forefoot into eversion and dorsiflexion.

Stabilization. The leg is stabilized.

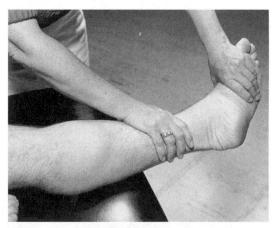

▲ **Figure 14.32** Testing the tibialis posterior muscle in the AG position.

▼ Attachments of Tibialis Anterior Muscle			
Muscle	**Proximal**	**Distal**	**Innervation**
Tibialis anterior	Distal to lateral tibial condyle, proximal half of lateral tibial shaft, and interosseous membrane	First cuneiform bone, medial and plantar surfaces and base of first metatarsal	Deep peroneal L4 (L5)

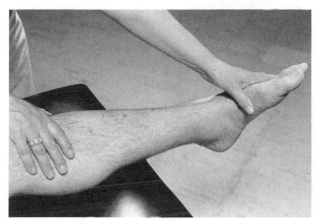

▲ **Figure 14.33** Testing the tibialis posterior muscle in the GM position.

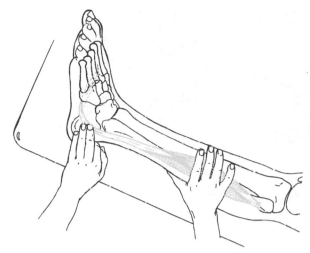

▲ **Figure 14.34** Palpating the peroneus longus muscle.

Substitutions

- The ankle dorsiflexes as it inverts using the tibialis anterior muscle.
- The medial toe flexors contribute to inversion and plantar flexion; keep them relaxed.
- Gastrocnemius and soleus muscles cause plantar flexion.
- Subject may quickly evert, then relax.
- Extensor hallucis longus is an accessory muscle to inversion but not plantar flexion.
- Flexor hallucis longus, flexor hallucis brevis, and abductor hallucis muscles invert the forefoot.

PERONEUS LONGUS, PERONEUS BREVIS, AND PERONEUS TERTIUS MUSCLES

The lateral compartment muscles and the peroneus tertius muscle produce the motion of eversion from a starting position of the ankle in the anatomical position through a test range of 20 degrees.

Palpation. Palpate the tendon of the peroneus longus immediately distal to the lateral malleolus descending to the plantar surface of the foot. Because the two peroneal tendons may not appear separated at this point, observe for depression of the great toe (Fig. 14-34).

The peroneus brevis is covered by the peroneus longus muscle. However, the tendon immediately distal to the lateral malleolus is directed anteriorly toward the fifth metatarsal and is easily identified from the peroneus longus muscle (Fig. 14-35).

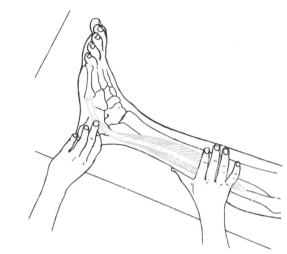

▲ **Figure 14.35** Palpating the peroneus brevis muscle.

Peroneus tertius may be absent. The tendon is a slip from the extensor digitorum longus muscle. If present, it is palpated laterally on the forefoot toward the fifth metatarsal.

Position

AG: Subject is in sidelying position. The upper leg is the test leg, with the ankle in the anatomical position (Fig. 14-36).

GM: Subject lies supine with the foot over the edge of the table and the ankle in the anatomical position (Fig. 14-37).

▼ Attachments of Tibialis Posterior Muscle			
Muscle	**Proximal**	**Distal**	**Innervation**
Tibialis posterior	Posterior surface of tibia, proximal two thirds posterior of fibula, and interosseous membrane	Tuberosity of navicular bone, tendinous expansion to other tarsals and metatarsals	Tibial L4 and L5

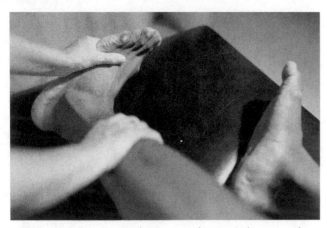

▲ **Figure 14.36** Testing the peroneus longus and peroneus brevis muscles in the AG position.

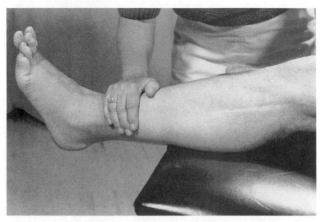

▲ **Figure 14.37** Testing the peroneus longus and peroneus brevis muscles in the GM position.

Movement. Eversion of the foot while maintaining the ankle in a neutral position.

Resistance. Applied to the lateral border of the forefoot.

Stabilization. The leg is stabilized.

Substitutions

- The extensor digitorum longus dorsiflexes the foot while everting.
- The flexor digitorum longus everts the foot, with some plantar flexion.
- Subject may quickly invert the foot, then relax.
- The abductor digiti minimi everts the forefoot.

Digits

Because of the shortness of the digits, gravity is not an important factor in the function of the toe muscles. Therefore, all toes are tested with the subject sitting or supine so that the subject can see the toes and observe the movements. The ankle is in the anatomical position.

Grades for the toes differ from the standard format because gravity is not considered a factor.

O: No contraction occurs.
T or 1: Muscle contraction is palpated, but no movement occurs.
P or 2: Subject can partially complete the range of motion.
F or 3: Subject can complete the test range.
G or 4: Subject can complete the test range but is able to take less resistance on the test side than on the opposite side.
N or 5: Subject can complete the test range and take maximal resistance on the test side as compared with the normal side.

FLEXOR HALLUCIS BREVIS AND LONGUS MUSCLES

The flexor hallucis brevis and flexor hallucis longus muscles produce MTP joint flexion through a test range of 30 to 45 degrees and IP joint flexion through a test range of 90 degrees. The foot must be maintained in midposition.

Palpation. Palpate the flexor hallucis brevis along the medial arch of the foot, adjacent to the first metatarsal head (Fig. 14-38).

Palpate the flexor hallucis longus tendon as it crosses the plantar surface of the proximal phalanx of the great toe (Fig. 14-39).

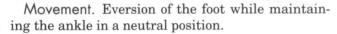

▼ Attachments of Peroneus Longus, Brevis, and Tertius Muscles

Muscle	Proximal	Distal	Innervation
Peroneus longus	Lateral condyle of tibia, head and proximal two thirds of fibula	Base of first metatarsal and first cuneiform, lateral side	Superficial peroneal L5 and S1 (S2)
Peroneus brevis	Distal two thirds of lateral fibular shaft	Tuberosity of fifth metatarsal	Superficial peroneal L5 and S1 (S2)
Peroneus tertius	Lateral slip from extensor digitorum longus	Tuberosity of fifth metatarsal	Deep peroneal L5 and S1

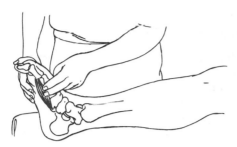

▲ **Figure 14.38** Palpating the flexor hallucis brevis muscle.

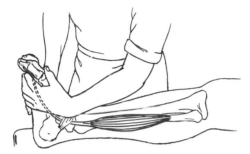

▲ **Figure 14.39** Palpating the flexor hallucis longus muscle.

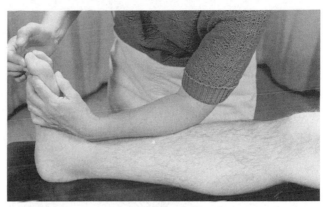

▲ **Figure 14.40** Testing the flexor hallucis longus muscle.

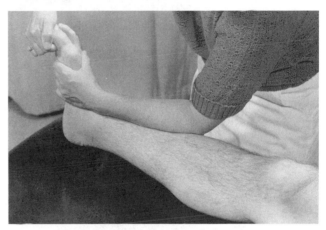

▲ **Figure 14.41** Testing the flexor hallucis brevis muscle.

Position. Subject is sitting or supine (Figs. 14-40 and 14-41).

Movement. Flexion of the MTP and IP joints.

Resistance. Applied beneath the proximal and distal phalanx of the great toe.

Stabilization. The foot is kept in the anatomical position, and the first metatarsal is stabilized.

Substitutions

- The flexor hallucis longus flexes the IP and MTP joints.
- The subject may quickly extend the toe, then relax.

FLEXOR DIGITORUM BREVIS AND LONGUS MUSCLES

The flexor digitorum longus and brevis muscles produce IP joint flexion through a test range of 75 to 80 degrees. The motion is tested with the foot in the anatomical position. If the gastrocnemius muscle is shortened, preventing the ankle from assuming the anatomical position, the knee is flexed. The toes may be tested simultaneously.

Palpation. The flexor digitorum brevis muscle is difficult to palpate. However, the tendon is palpable on the plantar surface of the proximal phalanx of each of the lateral four toes.

Palpate the flexor digitorum longus tendons on the plantar surface of each middle phalanx of the lateral four toes (Fig. 14-42).

Position. Subject is sitting or supine (Fig. 14-43).

Movement. Flexion of the IP joints of the lateral four toes.

Resistance. Applied beneath the distal and proximal phalanges. The toes may be tested simultaneously.

▼ Attachments of Flexor Hallucis Brevis and Longus Muscles			
Muscle	**Proximal**	**Distal**	**Innervation**
Flexor hallucis brevis	Plantar surface of cuboid and third cuneiform bones	Base of proximal phalanx of great toe	Medial plantar S3 (S2)
Flexor hallucis longus	Posterior distal two thirds of fibula	Base of distal phalanx of great toe	Tibial S2 (S3)

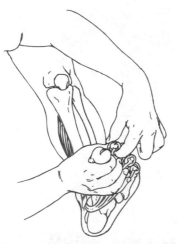

▲ **Figure 14.42** Palpating the flexor digitorum longus muscle.

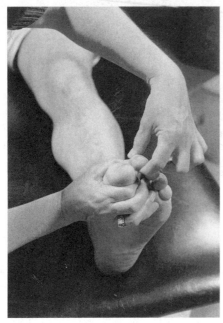

▲ **Figure 14.43** Testing the flexor digitorum longus muscle.

Stabilization. The foot is held in the midposition, and the metatarsals are stabilized.

Substitution

• Alone, the flexor digitorum longus flexes all the joints of the toes.

EXTENSOR HALLUCIS LONGUS AND BREVIS MUSCLES

The extensor hallucis longus and the extensor hallucis brevis muscles produce the motion of extension of the IP and MTP joints through a test range of 75 degrees of hyperextension at the MTP joint and from a flexed position to 0 degrees extension at the IP joint. The foot is maintained in midposition.

Palpation. Palpate the extensor hallucis longus tendon on the dorsum of the foot, lateral to the tibialis anterior tendon and as it crosses the dorsum of the first metatarsal (Fig. 14-44).

The extensor hallucis brevis muscle lies deep to the extensor digitorum longus tendons and is difficult to palpate. The tendon is a medial slip from the extensor digitorum brevis. Palpate the muscle belly on the dorsal lateral surface of the foot.

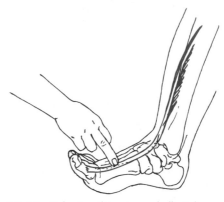

▲ **Figure 14.44** Palpating the extensor hallucis longus muscle.

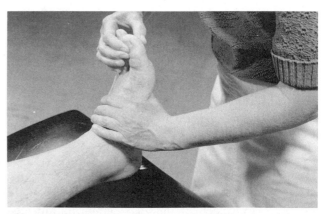

▲ **Figure 14.45** Testing the extensor hallucis longus muscle.

▼ Attachments of Flexor Digitorum Brevis and Longus Muscles

Muscle	Proximal	Distal	Innervation
Flexor digitorum brevis	Tuberosity of calcaneus	One tendon slip into base of middle phalanx of each of the lateral four toes	Medial and lateral plantar S3 (S2)
Flexor digitorum longus	Middle three fifths of tibia	Base of distal phalanx of lateral four toes	Tibial S2 (S3)

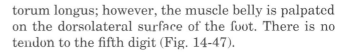

▼ **Attachments of Extensor Hallucis Longus and Brevis Muscles**

Muscle	Proximal	Distal	Innervation
Extensor hallucis longus	Middle half of anterior shaft of fibula	Base of distal phalanx of great toe	Deep peroneal L5 and S1
Extensor hallucis brevis	Distal superior and lateral surfaces of calcaneus	Dorsal surface of proximal phalanx	Deep peroneal S1 and S2

Position. Subject is sitting or supine (Fig. 14-45).

Movement. Extension of the MTP and IP joints of the first digit.

Resistance. Applied to the dorsum of both phalanges of the first digit.

Stabilization. The foot and the first metatarsal are stabilized.

Substitutions

• Plantar flexion of the ankle may stretch the extensor tendons and produce extension of the toes by tendon action.
• The subject may quickly flex the toe, then relax.

EXTENSOR DIGITORUM LONGUS AND BREVIS MUSCLES

The extensor digitorum longus and the extensor digitorum brevis muscles produce the motion of extension at the MTP and IP joints of the lateral four digits from a flexed position. The test range for the MTP joints is to 45 degrees of hyperextension and that of the IP joints, to 0 degrees of extension. The foot is in the anatomical position.

Palpation. Palpate the four tendons of the extensor digitorum longus as they cross the dorsolateral surface of the foot to each of the lateral four digits (Fig. 14-46).

The extensor digitorum brevis tendons are difficult to palpate as they lie deep to the extensor digi-

torum longus; however, the muscle belly is palpated on the dorsolateral surface of the foot. There is no tendon to the fifth digit (Fig. 14-47).

Position. Subject is sitting or supine (Figs. 14-48 and 14-49).

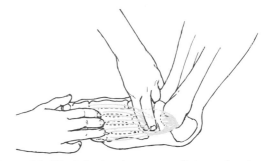

▲ **Figure 14.47** Palpating the extensor digitorum brevis muscle.

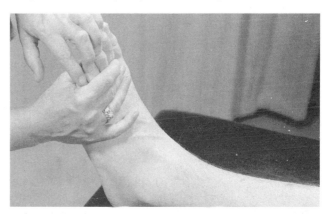

▲ **Figure 14.48** Testing the extensor digitorum longus muscle.

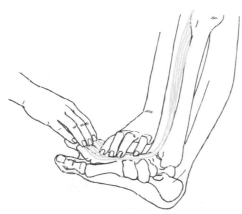

▲ **Figure 14.46** Palpating the extensor digitorum longus muscle.

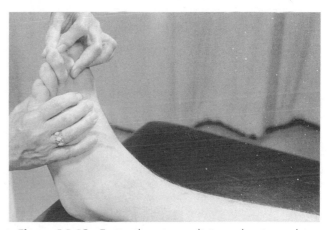

▲ **Figure 14.49** Testing the extensor digitorum brevis muscle.

▼ Attachments of Extensor Digitorum Longus and Brevis Muscles

Muscle	Proximal	Distal	Innervation
Extensor digitorum longus	Lateral condyle of tibia, proximal anterior surface of shaft of fibula	One tendon to each lateral four toes, to middle phalanx, and extending to distal phalanges	Deep peroneal L5 and S1
Extensor digitorum brevis	Distal, superior surface of calcaneus	Dorsal surface of second through fourth toes, base of proximal phalanx	Deep peroneal S1 and S2

Movement. Extension of the MTP and IP joints of the lateral four digits.

Resistance. Applied to the dorsal surface of the proximal and distal phalanges.

Stabilization. The ankle and the metatarsals are stabilized.

Substitutions

- The toes deviate laterally as they extend using the extensor digitorum brevis.
- Plantar flexion of the ankle may stretch the extensor tendons and produce extension of the toes by tendon action.
- The subject may quickly flex the toes, then relax.

Intrinsic Muscles of the Foot

The intrinsic muscles of the foot are tested with the subject in either the supine or sitting position. Most subjects are unable voluntarily to contract the intrinsic muscles of the foot individually. The second digit and the second metatarsal are the reference structures for movements of the digits.

ABDUCTOR HALLUCIS MUSCLE

Palpation. Palpate the medial side of the first metatarsal.

Position. Subject is sitting or supine.

Movement. Abduction at the MTP joint of the first digit.

Resistance. Applied medially to the distal end of the first phalanx.

Stabilization. The metatarsals are stabilized.

Substitutions

- The first digit moves in the sagittal plane by using the flexor hallucis longus and brevis.
- The first digit moves in the sagittal plane by contracting the extensor hallucis longus and brevis.

ADDUCTOR HALLUCIS MUSCLE

Palpation. The muscle is too deep to palpate accurately.

Position. Subject is sitting or supine.

Movement. Adduction of the proximal phalanx of the first digit toward the second digit.

Resistance. Applied to the lateral side of the proximal phalanx of the first digit.

Stabilization. The metatarsals are stabilized.

Substitutions

- The first digit may flex or extend in the sagittal plane.
- Subject may abduct then relax, giving the appearance of adduction.

LUMBRICAL MUSCLES

Palpation. The four muscles are too deep to palpate with accuracy.

Position. Subject is sitting or supine.

Movement. Extension of the IP joints and assistance in flexion of the MTP joints of the lateral four digits.

▼ Attachments of Abductor Hallucis Muscle

Muscle	Proximal	Distal	Innervation
Abductor hallucis	Tuberosity of calcaneus and plantar aponeurosis	Base of proximal phalanx, medial side	Medial plantar L5 and S1 (L4)

▼ Attachments of Adductor Hallucis Muscle

Muscle	Proximal	Distal	Innervation
Adductor hallucis	Base of second, third, and fourth metatarsals and deep plantar ligaments	Proximal phalanx of first digit lateral side	Medial and lateral plantar S1 and S2

▼ Attachments of Lumbrical Muscles

Muscle	Proximal	Distal	Innervation
Lumbricals	Medial and adjacent sides of flexor digitorum longus tendon to each lateral digit	Medial side of proximal phalanx and extensor hood	Medial and lateral plantar L5, S1, and S2 (L4)

Resistance. Applied to the middle and distal phalanges of the lateral four digits.

Stabilization. The lateral four metatarsals are stabilized.

Substitution

- The dorsal and plantar interossei assist in extension of the IP joints.

PLANTAR INTEROSSEI MUSCLES

Palpation. The three muscle bellies are too deep to palpate with accuracy; however, the tendinous expansion onto the medial side of the extensor hood of the lateral three digits is palpable.

Position. Subject is sitting or supine.

Movement. Extension of the IP joints of the lateral three digits. Adduction of the digits is not practical for most individuals.

Resistance. Applied to the middle and distal phalanges.

Stabilization. Stabilize the lateral three metatarsals.

Substitution

- Extension of the MTP joints of the lateral three digits can substitute by contracting the extensor digitorum longus and brevis.

DORSAL INTEROSSEI AND ABDUCTOR DIGITI MINIMI MUSCLES

Palpation. The muscle bellies of the four dorsal interossei are too deep to palpate with accuracy; however, the tendinous expansion onto the extensor hood of the middle three digits is palpable.

Palpate the abductor digiti minimi along the lateral side of the fifth metatarsal.

Position. Subject is sitting or supine.

Movement. Extension of the IP joints and abduction at the MTP joints of the lateral four digits.

Resistance

Dorsal Interossei. Applied to the middle and distal phalanges.

Abductor Digiti Minimi. Applied to the lateral side of the proximal phalanx of the fifth digit.

Stabilization. The metatarsals are stabilized.

▼ Attachments of Plantar Interossei Muscles

Muscle	Proximal	Distal	Innervation
Plantar interossei			
First	Base and medial side of third metatarsal	Base of proximal phalanx and extensor hood of third digit	Medial and lateral plantar S1 and S2
Second	Base and medial side of fourth metatarsal	Base of proximal phalanx and extensor hood of fourth digit	
Third	Base and medial side of fifth metatarsal	Base of proximal phalanx and extensor hood of fifth digit	

▼ Attachments of Dorsal Interossei and Abductor Digiti Minimi Muscles

Muscle	Proximal	Distal	Innervation
Dorsal interossei			
First	First and second metatarsal bones	Proximal phalanx and extensor hood of second digit medially	
Second	Second and third metatarsal bones	Proximal phalanx and extensor hood of second digit laterally	Medial and lateral plantar S1 and S2
Third	Third and fourth metatarsal bones	Proximal phalanx and extensor hood of third digit laterally	
Fourth	Fourth and fifth metatarsal bones	Proximal phalanx and extensor hood of fourth digit laterally	
Abductor digiti minimi	Lateral side of fifth metatarsal bone	Proximal phalanx of fifth digit	Lateral plantar S1 and S2

Substitution

• The extensor digitorum longus and brevis muscles extend the MTP joints of the middle digits.

CLINICAL ASSESSMENT

Observation and Screening

As with the other joints of the lower limb and the lumbosacral spine, symptomatology in the ankle and foot may result from localized pathology or trauma but also may be referred from other regions. Conversely, abnormalities in the ankle and foot often play a significant role in the initiation of symptoms further up the kinetic chain and into the sacroiliac and lumbosacral areas.

The ankle and foot should be examined in a weight-bearing and non–weight-bearing position, without shoes and socks. Weight bearing allows the examiner to observe the entire lower limb and trunk for compensation secondary to abnormalities in the foot and ankle. Examination in the non–weight-bearing position permits assessment of structural and functional abilities of the foot and ankle without compensation occurring.

As with other regions of the body, the ankle and foot should be examined for swelling, skin temperature, ecchymosis, scars, open areas or ulcerations, and bony and soft-tissue abnormalities. Localized swelling usually indicates localized trauma, such as perimalleolar swelling associated with ankle sprains. More generalized swelling tends to be seen with vascular or lymphatic abnormalities and certain medical conditions. Transient lower leg and foot swelling are also commonly seen in the lower extremity of postsurgical subjects. Areas of corns and calluses should be noted as sites of abnormal or excessive pressure.

Deformities of the foot that should be noted include gross pes planus (flat foot), pes cavus (high arch), claw toes, hammer toes, hallux valgus, and Morton's toe. Pes planus can be grossly assessed by the observation of the medial longitudinal arch, which will appear flattened. Conversely, pes cavus presents with an abnormally high medial longitudinal arch. Claw toes are characterized by extension of the MCP joint and flexion of the PIP and DIP joints. Hammer toes provide a clinical appearance of MCP joint extension and PIP joint flexion. The DIP joint may present in a position of flexion, extension, or neutral. In both deformities, the examiner should expect to see evidence of callus formation dorsally over the flexed joints and plantarly under the extended joints. Hallux valgus is defined as a lateral deviation of the proximal phalanx of the great toe relative to the first metacarpal at the MCP joint. Individuals with hallux valgus typically exhibit callus formation on the medial aspect of the first MTP joint. Morton's toe is identified as the second toe being longer than the great toe, resulting in greater stresses to the second toe.[3]

Examination of the patient's shoes may provide the examiner with a wealth of information about abnormalities of the foot and ankle. The pattern of heel wear should reveal wearing of the lateral posterior aspect of the heel, correlating with the appropriate position of initial contact during the gait cycle. Breakdown of the heel counter medially is commonly seen in individuals who pronate, whereas lateral breakdown is evident with supinators. Evidence of a normal toe crease running from distal medial to proximal lateral across the top of the shoe should be present. Lack of a toe crease indicates lack of normal heel off through push off during the gait cycle. Scuffing of the tip of the shoe is commonly observed in patients with weak or absent dorsiflexion of the ankle or insufficient hip or knee flexion during the swing phase of gait.

Palpation and Surface Anatomy

The following structures and landmarks should be observed or palpated during assessment of the ankle and foot complex (Fig. 14-50):

1. Navicular tuberosity
2. Sustentaculum tali
3. Heads of the talus
4. Medial malleolus
5. Tarsal bones

6. Base of the fifth metatarsal
7. Lateral malleolus

Active and Passive Movements and Contractile Testing

The following motions of the ankle and foot are assessed as part of the evaluation process for active and passive movements and contractile testing:

1. Ankle dorsiflexion
2. Ankle plantar flexion
3. Triplanar inversion
4. Triplanar eversion
5. MTP joint flexion
6. MTP joint extension
7. IP joint flexion
8. IP joint extension

SPECIAL CLINICAL TESTS

DRAWER TEST

Indication. The drawer test[1,2] is performed on subjects who have sustained an ankle sprain or other trauma that could result in ankle instability. The integrity of the structures involved in preventing forward displacement of the tibia on the talus is assessed.

Method. The subject is supine or sitting. The test ankle is relaxed and in approximately 20 degrees of plantar flexion. The examiner stabilizes the distal leg with one hand, while the other hand grips the calcaneus (Fig. 14-51). By pulling the calcaneus forward and causing it to impact the talus, the examiner attempts to displace the talus anteriorly.

Results. Straightforward displacement of the talus on the tibia indicates both medial and lateral liga-

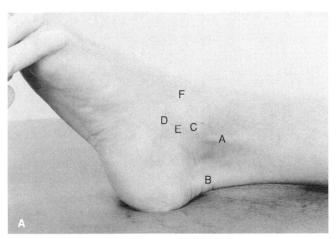

A - Tibialis Posterior Muscle D - Navicular
B - Achilles Tendon E - Sustentaculum Talus
C - Medial Malleolus F - Medial Talar Head

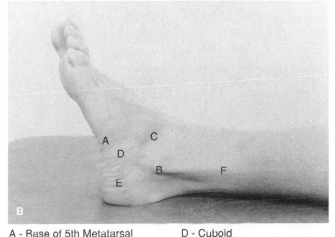

A - Base of 5th Metatarsal D - Cuboid
B - Lateral Malleolus E - Calcaneus
C - Lateral Talar Head F - Peroneus Longus Muscle

▲ **Figure 14.50** (**A**) Surface anatomy of the lateral ankle and foot. (**B**) Surface anatomy of the medial ankle and foot.

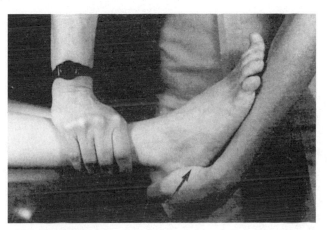

▲ **Figure 14.51** Drawer test.

ment instability involving the superficial and deep deltoid ligaments, the anterior talofibular ligament, and the anterolateral capsule. If there is instability and laxity on one side only, then only that side will displace forward. For example, if only the lateral side is involved, the lateral talus will displace forward and internally, resulting in anterolateral rotary instability of the ankle (anterolateral drawer test). The examiner may also feel a clunk as the talus slides from under cover of the ankle mortise.

VARUS STRESS TEST

Indication. The varus stress test[1,2] is used to assess the integrity of the lateral ligaments of the ankle (anterior and posterior talofibular and calcaneofibular).

Method. The subject is either seated or supine with the ankle in a relaxed slightly plantar flexed position. The examiner stabilizes the lower leg and grips and inverts the calcaneus maximally (Fig. 14-52). The examiner should palpate all three lateral ligaments with the stabilizing hand as the inversion force is applied.

Results. Lateral gapping and rocking of the talus beneath the mortise indicates instability. All three ligaments must be lax or torn for gross instability to be present.

VALGUS STRESS TEST (KLEIGER'S TEST)

Indication. Valgus stress test[1,2] assesses instability of the medial side of the ankle, most notably the deltoid ligament.

Method. The subject is positioned as for the varus stress test. The examiner stabilizes the lower leg with one hand and grips the calcaneus with the other (Fig. 14-53). A maximal eversion force is ap-

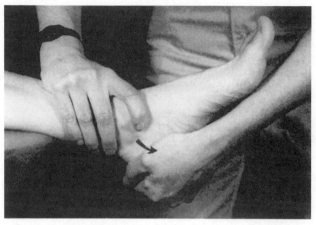

▲ **Figure 14.53** Valgus stress test.

plied to the calcaneus as the lower leg is stabilized. The stabilizing hand should palpate over the deltoid ligament as the eversion force is applied.

TALAR TILT TEST

Indication. The talar tilt test[2] assesses the integrity of the calcaneofibular ligament.

Method. The subject is either supine or in a side-lying position with the foot relaxed. Maintaining the foot in an anatomical position brings the calcaneofibular ligament perpendicular to the long axis of the talus. The talus is then tilted into abduction and adduction (Fig. 14-54).

Results. Excessive tilting associated with adduction of the talus is associated with laxity or tearing of the calcaneofibular ligament, because in this position, the ligament is maximally stressed.

THOMPSON'S TEST

Indication. Thompson's test[4] should always be performed in cases of suspected Achilles' tendon rupture.

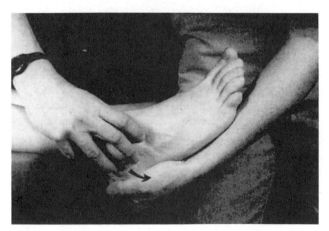

▲ **Figure 14.52** Varus stress test.

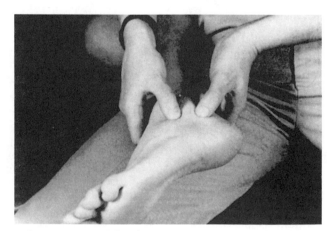

▲ **Figure 14.54** Talar tilt test.

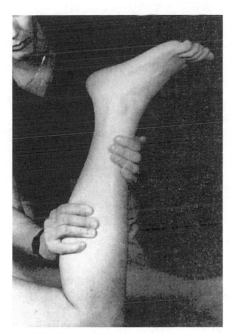

▲ **Figure 14.55** Thompson's test.

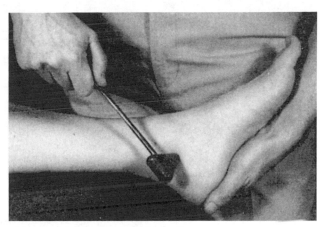

▲ **Figure 14.56** Posterior tibial reflex.

Method. The subject is prone, and the knee is flexed to 90 degrees. The examiner squeezes the calf of the leg being tested and observes the response (Fig. 14-55).

Results. Normally, when the calf with an intact gastrocsoleus muscle complex is squeezed, the response is one of passive plantar flexion. In the case of a ruptured Achilles' tendon, there will be no associated plantar flexion as the calf is squeezed.

HOMANS' SIGN

Indication. Homans' sign test is indicated in suspected cases of deep vein thrombosis.

Method. The subject may be tested supine, prone, or sitting. The examiner passively extends the knee and then dorsiflexes the ankle. The calf also may be palpated concurrently.

Results. Pain in the calf during ankle dorsiflexion is suggestive of thrombophlebitis, but other signs of inflammation must be present in the calf area before this test is interpreted as positive. The examiner must also be aware that tightness of the gastrocnemius may be responsible for discomfort during this test. For this reason, both legs should be tested and a distinction made between pain arising from a possible thrombophlebitis or that due to muscle tightness.

POSTERIOR TIBIAL REFLEX

Indication. The posterior tibial reflex is tested to evaluate the integrity of the L5 nerve root level.

Method. The subject lies supine with the test ankle crossed over and resting on the opposite leg. The ankle is placed in a position of mild dorsiflexion by the examiner. The examiner uses the pointed end of the reflex hammer to tap the posterior tibial tendon where it crosses behind the medial malleolus (Fig. 14-56).

Results. A response of plantar flexion combined with inversion will be noted. This response should be compared with that in the opposite ankle to evaluate the normal response for that subject. A hyperactive reflex may indicate an upper motor neuron problem, whereas a hypoactive response may represent lower motor neuron pathology.

ACHILLES' TENDON REFLEX

Indication. The Achilles' tendon reflex is assessed to determine the integrity of the S1 nerve root level.

Method. The Achilles' tendon reflex can be tested with the subject prone, supine, or seated, although the prone position is preferred. The examiner flexes the subject's knee approximately 90 degrees and applies gentle stretch to the ankle into dorsiflexion. It is important not to hold the ankle forcefully in dorsiflexion because this may mask the reflex response. As the gentle pressure into dorsiflexion is maintained, the examiner taps the Achilles' tendon with the broad end of the reflex hammer (Fig. 14-57).

Results. The normal response should be plantar flexion when the tendon is struck. The response of the involved ankle should be compared to that of the uninvolved ankle. Less response on the involved side represents a hypoactive reflex, whereas an exaggerated response is considered hyperactive.

TINEL'S SIGN

Indication. Tinel's sign is indicated in individuals with a suspected neuroma of the anterior tibial

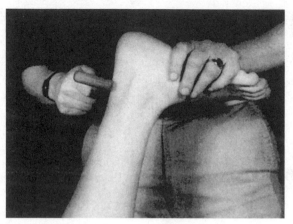

▲ **Figure 14.57** Achilles tendon reflex.

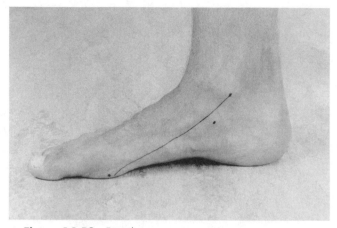

▲ **Figure 14.58** Feiss line.

branch of the deep peroneal nerve or of the posterior tibial nerve.

Method. Assessment of the deep peroneal nerve is accomplished by the examiner tapping over the nerve on the dorsum of the ankle. Percussing over the tibial nerve where it passes posterior to the medial malleolus assesses that structure.

Results. A positive test is indicated by tingling or paresthesias down the distribution of the respective nerve.

FUNCTIONAL TESTS

Indication. Functional tests involving the foot and ankle are indicated when there is suspicion of weakness of the L5 or S1 musculature.

Method. The subject stands for both tests. To assess the functional ability of the L5 musculature, have subject walk on the heels. The S1 musculature is tested by having the subject walk on the toes.

Results. Inability to walk on the heels represents weakness or paralysis of the L5 musculature that controls dorsiflexion of the ankle. S1 weakness or paralysis of the ankle plantar flexors is manifested by the subject's inability to walk on tiptoes.

FEISS LINE

Indication. The Feiss line serves as a gross means of assessing pronation of the foot, manifested by a flattening of the medial longitudinal arch. The relative position of the navicular tuberosity in the weight-bearing and non–weight-bearing positions is examined.

Method. The subject is examined both standing and seated, with approximately 3 to 6 in between the feet. A line is drawn from the tip of the medial malleolus to the plantar aspect of the first MTP joint (Fig. 14-58).

Results. Ideally, the navicular tuberosity should lie on or very close to the line drawn. If the navicular falls one third of the distance to the floor, the condition is called first-degree flatfoot. If the navicular falls two thirds of the distance to the floor, the condition represents second-degree flatfoot. If it rests on the floor, the condition is third-degree flatfoot. The Feiss line should be assessed with the subject in both weight-bearing and non–weight-bearing postures, because it is an indication of the rigidity of flatfoot and of whether the subject will be able to wear orthotics.

JOINT PLAY (ACCESSORY MOVEMENT)

Talocrural Joint

Distraction (Fig. 14-59)

Restriction. General hypomobility.

Open-Packed Position. Ten degrees of ankle plantar flexion; midway between inversion and eversion.

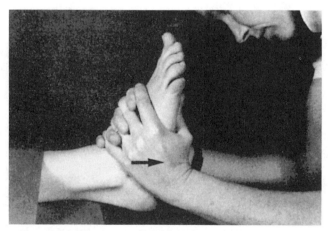

▲ **Figure 14.59** Distraction of the talocrural joint.

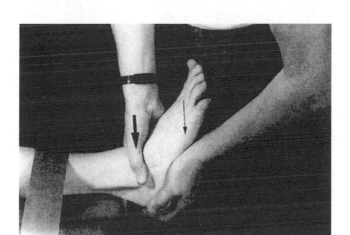

▲ **Figure 14.60** Posterior glide of the talus.

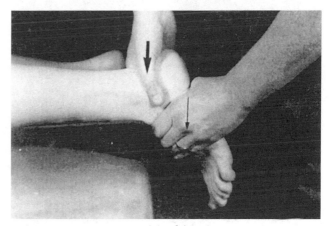

▲ **Figure 14.61** Anterior glide of the talus.

Positioning. The subject lies supine with the distal leg stabilized by a strap. The examiner stands at the end of the table facing the subject. The examiner clasps the hands together and places them on the dorsum of the foot with the ulnar borders on the talus as close to the joint line as possible.

Movement. The examiner applies a distraction force to the subject's talus. The focus of the application of the force is through the medial aspect of the examiner's hands.

Posterior Glide (Fig. 14-60)

Restriction. Dorsiflexion.

Positioning. Subject lies supine with the distal leg placed at the edge of the table and stabilized with a strap. The examiner places the mobilizing hand with the web space on the dorsum of the foot over the anterior talus. The other hand cups the calcaneus to provide support and to maintain the open packed position.

Movement. The examiner directs a posterior force through the web space to the subject's anterior talus.

Anterior Glide (Fig. 14-61)

Restriction. Plantar flexion.

Positioning. The subject lies prone with the distal leg at the edge of the table and stabilized by a wedge beneath it. The examiner places the web space of the mobilizing hand on the posterior aspect of the foot over the Achilles' tendon, with the thumb and index fingers below the respective malleoli on the talus. The other hand grasps the proximal foot to provide support and to maintain the open-packed position.

Movement. The examiner applies an anterior force to the posterior aspect of the talus.

Subtalar Joint

Distraction (Fig. 14-62)

Restriction. General hypomobility.

Open-Packed Position. Midway between inversion and eversion.

Positioning. The subject lies prone with a wedge or small roll beneath the talus for stabilization. The examiner places one hand on the anterior surface of the subject's leg for additional stability. The mobilizing hand is placed so that the heel and palm cup the calcaneus.

Movement. The examiner applies an inferior or distraction force to the subject's calcaneus.

Distal Glide (Fig. 14-63)

Restriction. General hypomobility.

Positioning. Same as for distraction.

Movement. The examiner applies a distal force along the long axis of the foot to the subject's calcaneus.

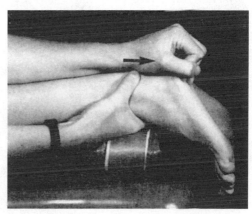

▲ **Figure 14.62** Distraction of the subtalar joint.

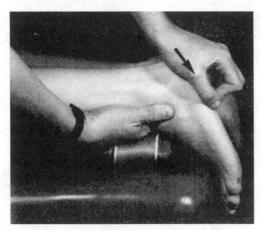

▲ **Figure 14.63** Distal glide of the calcaneus.

Midtarsal Joint

TALONAVICULAR JOINT

Dorsal and Plantar Glide (Fig. 14-64)

Restriction. General hypomobility.

Open-Packed Position. Anatomical position.

Positioning. The subject may be either supine or long sitting, with the knee joint flexed. The examiner places the thumb, web space, and index finger of the stabilizing hand over the medial aspect of the talus. The thumb and index finger of the mobilizing hand are placed on the plantar and dorsal surfaces of the navicular.

Movement. The examiner applies a dorsal-plantar force to the navicular in the direction of hypomobility.

Calcaneocuboid Joint

Dorsal and Plantar Glide (Fig. 14-65)

Restriction. General hypomobility.

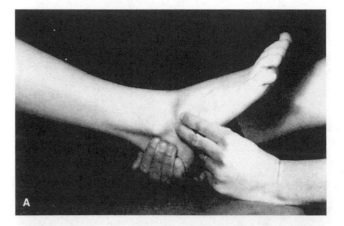

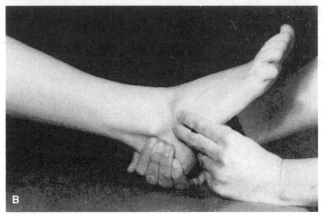

▲ **Figure 14.65** (**A**) Posterior and (**B**) plantar glide of the cuboid.

Open-Packed Position. Anatomical position.

Positioning. The subject may be either supine or long sitting, with the knee joint flexed. The examiner grasps the calcaneus with one hand to provide stabilization. The thumb and index finger of the mobilizing hand are placed on the plantar and dorsal surfaces of the cuboid.

Movement. The examiner applies a dorsal-plantar force to the cuboid in the direction of hypomobility.

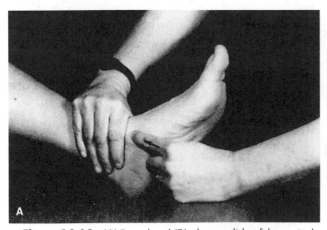

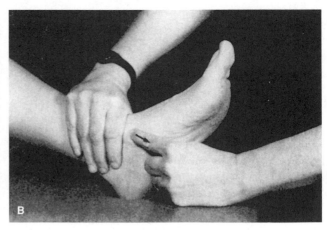

▲ **Figure 14.64** (**A**) Dorsal and (**B**) plantar glide of the navicular.

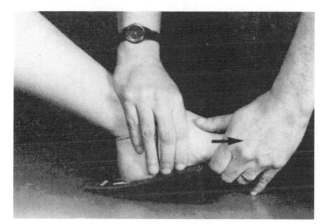

▲ **Figure 14.66** Distraction of the tarsometatarsal joints.

Tarsometatarsal Joints

Distraction (Fig. 14-66)

Restriction. General hypomobility.

Open-Packed Position. Anatomical position.

Positioning. The subject's foot is placed on a stabilizing wedge so that the tarsal bone that articulates with the metatarsal being examined is stabilized. The examiner places one hand over the dorsum of the tarsal bone on the wedge to provide additional support. The mobilizing hand is placed with the thumb and fingers gripping the metatarsal on the dorsal and plantar surfaces.

Movement. The examiner applies a distraction force to the metatarsal.

Plantar Glide (Fig. 14-67)

Restriction. General hypomobility.

Positioning. The subject lies supine or sits. The metatarsal adjacent to the one being treated is placed on the stabilizing wedge. The examiner places one hand on the dorsum of the foot over the metatarsal on the wedge to provide additional support. The thenar eminence of the other hand is placed on the dorsal surface of the metatarsal being treated.

Movement. The examiner applies a plantar force through the metatarsal. This mobilization is not only for tarsometatarsal restrictions, but also is effective for intermetatarsal mobility.

First Metatarsophalangeal Joint

Distraction (Fig. 14-68)

Restriction. General hypomobility.

Open-Packed Position. From 5 to 10 degrees of metacarpophalangeal extension.

Positioning. The subject may be either supine or sitting. The examiner stabilizes the first metatarsal by grasping it between the thenar eminence and the four fingers. The thumb and index finger of the mobilizing hand grip the dorsal and plantar surfaces of the proximal phalanx.

Movement. The examiner applies a distraction force to the proximal phalanx.

Plantar Glide (Fig. 14-69)

Restriction. Flexion.

Positioning. The subject is sitting or supine. A stabilizing wedge is placed beneath the first metatarsal. The examiner puts one hand around the subject's foot on the wedge to provide additional stabilization. The thumb and index finger of the mobilizing hand are placed on the dorsal and plantar surfaces of the proximal phalanx.

Movement. The examiner applies a force to the proximal phalanx in the plantar direction.

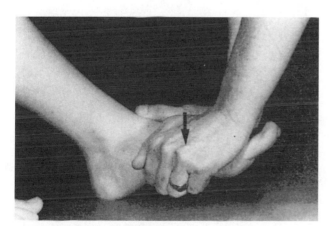

▲ **Figure 14.67** Plantar glide of the tarsal bones.

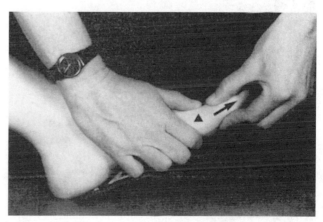

▲ **Figure 14.68** Distraction of the first metatarsophalangeal joint.

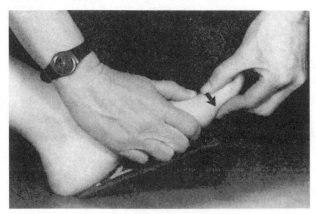

▲ **Figure 14.69** Plantar glide of the proximal phalanx of the great toe.

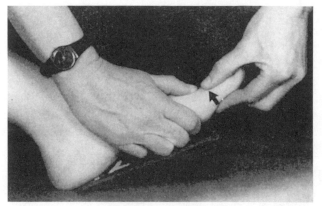

▲ **Figure 14.70** Dorsal glide of the proximal phalanx of the great toe.

Dorsal Glide (Fig. 14-70)

Restriction. Extension.

Positioning. The subject lies prone. A stabilizing wedge is placed beneath the first metatarsal. The examiner puts one hand around the subject's foot on the wedge to provide additional stabilization. The thumb and index finger of the mobilizing hand are placed on the dorsal and plantar surfaces of the proximal phalanx.

Movement. The examiner applies a force to the proximal phalanx in the dorsal direction.

Second to Fifth Metatarsophalangeal Joints and All Interphalangeal Joints

Distraction and Plantar and Dorsal Glide (Fig. 14-71)

Restriction. General hypomobility, flexion, extension.

Open-Packed Position. Slight flexion.

Positioning. The subject lies supine. The examiner stabilizes the proximal articulating bone with one

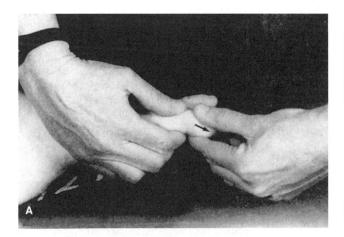

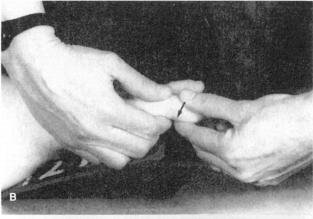

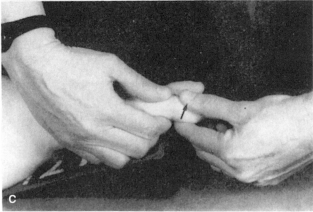

▲ **Figure 14.71** **(A)** Distraction of interphalangeal joints. **(B)** Plantar and **(C)** dorsal glide of the distal phalanx.

hand. The other mobilizing hand is placed on the distal articulating bone as close to the joint line as possible.

Movement. The examiner applies a distraction force to the distal articulating bone for general hypomobility. A plantar force is given for restrictions in flexion and a dorsal force for limitations in extension.

Tarsal Bone Mobility Testing

Kaltenborn has described a sequential method of assessing the mobility of the individual carpal bones. The approach to examination of the tarsal area is as follows (Fig. 14-72):

1. Stabilize the second and third cuneiforms and mobilize the third metatarsal.
2. Stabilize the second and third cuneiforms and mobilize the second metatarsal.
3. Stabilize the first cuneiform and mobilize the first metatarsal.
4. Stabilize the navicular and mobilize the first, second, and third cuneiforms.
5. Stabilize the talus and mobilize the navicular.
6. Stabilize the cuboid and mobilize the fourth and fifth metatarsals.
7. Stabilize the navicular and cuneiform and mobilize the cuboid.
8. Stabilize the calcaneus and mobilize the cuboid.
9. Stabilize the talus and mobilize the calcaneus.
10. Stabilize the talus and mobilize the tibia and fibula.

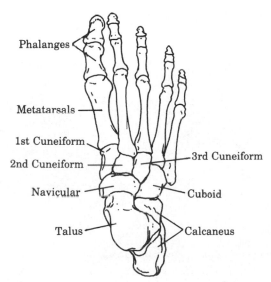

▲ **Figure 14.72** Dorsal view of the anatomical relationships of the tarsal bones.

Phalanges

Metatarsals

1st Cuneiform

2nd Cuneiform

3rd Cuneiform

Navicular

Cuboid

Talus

Calcaneus

Summary of Joint Play of Ankle and Foot

Table 14-1 provides a summary of joint play in the ankle and foot.

BIOMECHANICAL EXAMINATION OF THE FOOT AND ANKLE

The examiner's ability to perform an accurate biomechanical examination of the foot and ankle complex is the key to successful management of pathologies involving the lower quarter. Because of the biomechanical intimacy of the structures that comprise the lower quarter, the examination process involves not only the foot and ankle, but also the pelvis, hip, femur, knee, tibia, and fibula in weight-bearing and non–weight-bearing positions.

The examination of the foot at rest, or in the non–weight-bearing position, is performed to determine structural or functional ability and prevent any compensation of the foot. The stance phase or weight-bearing portion of the examination indicates the amount of compensation that occurs for structural abnormalities. The examination process may be organized effectively by grouping the assessment procedures according to the subject's position, as follows:

SUPINE EXAMINATION

1. *Hip rotation:* Hip rotation should be tested in various positions of hip and knee flexion to determine whether restriction of motion is due to soft-tissue tightness or to a bony deformity. If the available range of motion changes with the alteration of hip and knee position, the limitation is a result of soft-tissue tightness. If the amount of hip rotation remains consistent regardless of hip and knee position, the limitation is secondary to a bony restriction.
2. *Hip and knee flexion:* The ranges of hip and knee flexion are assessed and recorded.
3. *Flexibility testing:* Flexibility testing should be performed for the hip flexor musculature (Thomas' test), hamstring musculature (straight leg raise), and the tensor muscle and iliotibial band (Ober's test).
4. *Leg-length discrepancy:* Measurement of leg length should be performed in weight-bearing and non–weight-bearing positions to determine whether a discrepancy exists. Testing should be done for true and apparent leg-length discrepancy.
5. *Torsional relationships:* Determination of femoral anteversion-retroversion is performed

TABLE 14.1	**Summary of Joint Play of the Ankle and Foot Complex**		
GLIDE	RESTRICTION	FIXED BONE	MOVING BONE
Talocrural Joint			
Distraction	General hypomobility	Tibia	Talus
Ventral	Plantar flexion	Tibia	Talus
Dorsal	Dorsiflexion	Tibia	Talus
Subtalar Joint			
Distraction	General hypomobility	Talus	Calcaneus
Distal	General hypomobility	Talus	Calcaneus
Midtarsal Joint: Talonavicular			
Ventral	General hypomobility	Talus	Navicular
Dorsal	General hypomobility	Talus	Navicular
Midtarsal Joint: Calcaneocuboid			
Ventral	General hypomobility	Calcaneus	Cuboid
Dorsal	General hypomobility	Calcaneus	Cuboid
Metatarsophalangeal Joints			
Distraction	General hypomobility	Respective metatarsal	Respective proximal phalanx
Plantar	Flexion	Respective metatarsal	Respective proximal phalanx
Dorsal	Extension	Respective metatarsal	Respective proximal phalanx
Interphalangeal Joints			
Distraction	General hypomobility	Respective proximal phalanx	Respective distal phalanx
Plantar	Flexion	Respective proximal phalanx	Respective distal phalanx
Dorsal	Extension	Respective proximal phalanx	Respective distal phalanx

by palpating the greater trochanter and then rotating the hip until the greater trochanter is in its most lateral position. In this position, the femoral condyles are examined, and a conclusion is drawn. Normally, with the greater trochanter located in its most lateral position, the femoral condyles should lie completely in the frontal plane. If the lateral femoral condyle lies anterior to the medial femoral condyle, femoral anteversion exists. Femoral retroversion is assessed when the medial condyle lies anterior to the lateral one.

An alternate method of assessment is to place the femoral condyles flat on the examining table in the frontal plane and, with the thigh in this position, to palpate the greater trochanter. Femoral anteversion is present when the greater trochanter is located posterior to its most lateral position. Femoral retroversion is identified when the greater trochanter is palpated anterior to its most lateral position.

Malleolar torsion, a transverse plane measurement, ranges from 13 to 18 degrees of external tibial rotation in normal people. Measurement of malleolar torsion is performed with the subject supine and the femoral condyles in the frontal plane. An angle made by an imaginary line connecting the apices of the malleoli and a line parallel to the floor rep-

resents the amount of malleolar torsion (Fig. 14-73). Malleolar torsion greater than 18 degrees results in a toe-out gait, while a value less than 13 degrees produces a toe-in gait. Both of these deformities cause abnormal pronation.

6. *Foot motion:* Assess calcaneal inversion-eversion and note the amount of forefoot motion with the calcaneus both inverted and everted.
7. *First ray and fifth ray mobility:* The first and fifth metatarsals normally should lie in the same plane as the other metatarsals. If the first or fifth metatarsal lies in a plane superior

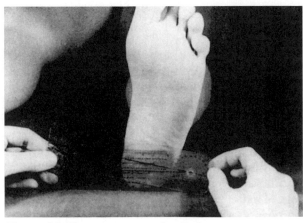

▲ **Figure 14.73** Measurement of malleolar torsion.

to the other metatarsals, a dorsiflexed first ray is evident. Conversely, a plantar flexed first or fifth ray is identified when the respective metatarsal lies in a plane inferior to the rest of the metatarsals.

Measurement of the range of motion of the first or fifth ray is considered normal when there is as much movement of the ray into dorsiflexion as there is into plantar flexion from its neutral position. A ray with more dorsiflexion than plantar flexion from the neutral position is termed a dorsiflexed ray, while one with more plantar flexion than dorsiflexion is called a plantar flexed ray.

8. *Hallux dorsiflexion:* From 60 to 70 degrees of hallux dorsiflexion is necessary for normal push-off during gait; therefore, assessment of the available motion is important. Goniometry should be performed in both non–weight-bearing and weight-bearing positions.

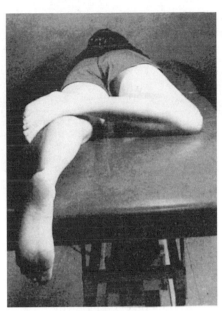

▲ **Figure 14.74** Prone position for examining foot biomechanics.

PRONE EXAMINATION

1. *Ankle dorsiflexion and plantar flexion:* The range of ankle dorsiflexion and plantar flexion should be assessed with the knee flexed and extended. Normal gait requires 10 degrees of talocrural dorsiflexion with the knee in both flexion and extension. If the available amount of dorsiflexion is less than 10 degrees as measured from the neutral position, the deformity is recognized as ankle equinus and is compensated by pronation at the subtalar joint. The normal range of plantar flexion is 0 to 45 degrees, but this is not significant in the biomechanical examination.

2. *Measurement of rearfoot and forefoot motion:* The examination and assessment of the rearfoot and forefoot should be done with the limb in the frontal plane. The frontal plane position is achieved by having the subject flex, abduct, and externally rotate the opposite hip and by placing the foot on the dorsal surface of the limb being examined (Fig. 14-74).

Before beginning actual examination of the foot, one must identify certain osseous landmarks. These landmarks include the distal third of the leg, the vertical borders of the calcaneus, and the plantar calcaneal border. After these landmarks have been identified, markings are made on the subject with a skin pencil. One line bisecting the distal third of the leg is drawn on the subject. It is important not to use the Achilles' tendon as the midline, because this structure usually does not lie cen-

trally. Another line is made representing the bisection of the calcaneus (Fig. 14-75).

3. *Subtalar joint neutral:* The examiner holds the fourth and fifth metatarsal heads with one hand and palpates the talar heads with the other hand. While palpating the talar heads, the examiner gently dorsiflexes the fourth and fifth metatarsal heads to the point of slight resistance. This bending ensures locking of the forefoot when the subtalar joint is in the neutral position. As dorsiflexion of the metatarsal heads is maintained, the foot is moved medi-

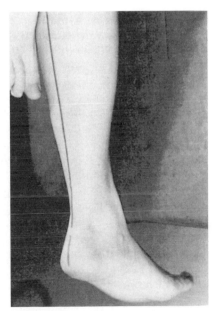

▲ **Figure 14.75** Bisection of leg and calcaneus.

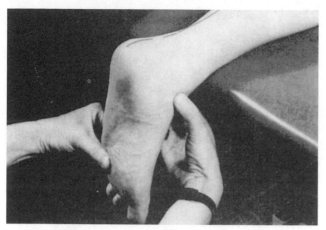

▲ **Figure 14.76** Subtalar neutral position.

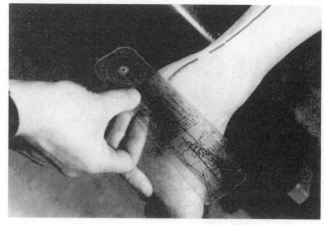

▲ **Figure 14.77** Forefoot to rearfoot measurement.

ally and laterally until congruence of the talar heads is apparent or neither head is prominent (Fig. 14-76). This position is identified as the subtalar joint neutral position of the foot.

Another method of distinguishing subtalar joint neutral position is to observe the concavities superior and inferior to the lateral malleolus. When both concavities appear symmetrical and equal in size, the subtalar joint is in the neutral position. Subtalar neutral is the position in which the foot is neither pronated nor supinated and in which maximal function can occur.

Objective assessment of subtalar neutral is performed with one arm of a goniometer aligned with the bisection of the distal third of the leg and the other arm aligned with the bisection of the calcaneus. A normal rearfoot position is one in which the angle created by these two goniometric alignments is 0 to 4 degrees of varus. If the calcaneus is inverted greater than 4 degrees relative to the tibia in the subtalar joint neutral position, the condition is defined as rearfoot varus. If the calcaneus is everted relative to the tibia in the subtalar joint neutral position, the condition is termed rearfoot valgus.

Objective assessment of maximal rearfoot pronation and supination should also be performed, because measurement will provide an indication of the subject's ability to compensate for rearfoot and forefoot problems. Measuring from the subtalar joint neutral position, the normal subtalar range of motion should demonstrate a 2:1 ratio of calcaneal inversion to eversion.

4. *Forefoot to rearfoot assessment:* While maintaining the rearfoot in a subtalar joint neutral

position, the examiner compares the relationship of the forefoot to the rearfoot. Normally, the metatarsal heads lie in the same plane as the plantar calcaneal border. Goniometric measurement is performed with one arm of the goniometer aligned parallel to the plane of the metatarsal heads and the other arm parallel to the plane of the bisected plantar border of the calcaneus (Fig. 14-77). Ideally, the forefoot and rearfoot should lie in the same plane, thereby providing an angular measurement of 0 degrees. Inversion of the forefoot with respect to the rearfoot is termed a forefoot varus; eversion of the forefoot with respect to the rearfoot is identified as a forefoot valgus.

STATIC STANDING EXAMINATION

1. *Posture:* A postural examination should be carried out with the subject standing and the feet maintained in subtalar joint neutral and in the compensated, or relaxed, posture, to assess the influence of extrinsic factors causing abnormal foot mechanics (see Chapter 4).
2. *Tibia varum:* The subject stands with the subtalar joints of the feet maintained in subtalar neutral. One arm of the goniometer is aligned with the bisection of the lower third of the leg. The other arm is parallel to the table or floor (Fig. 14-78). Normal tibia varum falls in the range of 0 to 2 degrees. Tibia varum should also be assessed with the feet in the relaxed, comfortable, compensated posture.
3. *Hallux dorsiflexion:* Hallux dorsiflexion is assessed in the standing position by maximally lifting the heel off the table while keeping the first MTP joint and great toe on the table. Normally, 90 or more degrees of hallux dorsiflex-

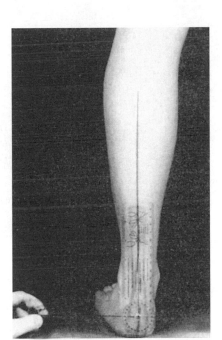

▲ **Figure 14.78** Measurement of tibia varum.

ion is available in this position as a result of plantar flexion of the first ray.

DYNAMIC EVALUATION

The subject is observed walking, while gait is evaluated. Particular attention should be given to calcaneal motion (especially at heel strike), forefoot abduction or adduction, weight transfer between limbs, and tibial position throughout stance.

REFERENCES

1. Jass MH: Disorders of the Foot. Philadelphia, WB Saunders, 1982
2. Kelikian H, Kelikian AS: Disorders of the Ankle. Philadelphia, WB Saunders, 1985
3. Rasmussen O, Tovborg-Jensen I: Anterolateral rotational instability in the ankle joint. Acta Orthop Scand 52:99–102, 1981
4. Thompson T, Doherty J: Spontaneous rupture of the tendon of achilles. A new clinical diagnostic test. Anat Res 158:126, 1967

List of Suggested Readings

American Society for Surgery of the Hand: The Hand: Examination and Diagnosis. Aurora, CO, 1978

Anderson TE: Anatomy and physical examination of the elbow. In Nicholas JA and Hershman EB (eds): The Upper Extremity in Sports Medicine. St. Louis, CV Mosby, 1990

Aspinall W: Clinical testing for cervical mechanical disorders which produce ischemic vertigo. J Orthoped Sports Phys Ther 11:176–182, 1989

Aulcino PL and DuPuy TE: Clinical examination of the hand. In Hunter J, et al (eds): Rehabilitation of the Hand: Surgery and Therapy. St. Louis, CV Mosby, 1990

Backhouse KM and Hutchings RT: Color Atlas of Surface Anatomy. Baltimore, Williams and Wilkins, 1986

Bateman J and Trott A (eds): The Foot and Ankle. New York, Theime-Stratton, 1980

Bowling RW and Rockar PA: The elbow complex. In Gould JA (ed): Orthopedic and Sports Physical Therapy. St. Louis, CV Mosby, 1990

Campbell SK: Measurement and technical skills: neglected aspect of research education. Phys Ther 61:523, 1981

Cipriano JJ: Photographic Manual of Regional Orthopedic Tests. Baltimore, Williams and Wilkins, 1985

Corrigan B and Maitland GD: Practical Orthopedic Medicine. Boston, Butterworth, 1983

Cross MJ and Crichton KJ: Clinical Examination of the Injured Knee. Baltimore, Williams and Wilkins, 1987

Feagin JA: The Crucial Ligaments. Edinburgh, Churchill Livingstone, 1988

Fisk JW and Balgent ML: Clinical and radio assessment of leg length. N.Z. Med J 81:477, 1975

Friedman MH and Weisberg J: Application of orthopedic principles in evaluation of the temporomandibular joint. Phys Ther 62:597, 1982

Friedman MH and Weisberg J: Screening procedures for temporomandibular joint dysfunction. Am Fam Physical 25:157, 1982

Garrick JG and Webb DR: Sports Injuries: Diagnosis and Management. Philadelphia, WB Saunders, 1990

Gelb H: Patient evaluation. In Gelb H (ed): Clinical Management of Head, Neck, and TMJ Pain and Dysfunction. Philadelphia, WB Saunders, 1977

Gould JA and Davies GJ: Orthopedic and Sports Physical Therapy. St. Louis, CV Mosby, 1985

Grieve GP: Common Vertebral Joint Problems. New York, Churchill Livingstone, 1981

Grieve GP: Mobilization of the Spine, 4th ed. New York, Churchill Livingstone, 1984

Grieve GP (ed): Modern Manual Therapy of the Vertebral Column. New York, Churchill Livingstone, 1986

Grimsby O: Manual Therapy of the Spine, 2nd ed. New York, Sorlandets Sysikalase Institutt AS, 1980

Gruebel Lee DM: Disorders of the Hip. Philadelphia, JB Lippincott, 1983

Helland NM: Anatomy and function of the temporomandibular joint. J Orthoped Sports Phys Ther 1:145, 1980

Hislop HJ and Montgomery J: Daniels and Worthingham's Muscle Testing: Techniques of Manual Examination. Philadelphia, WB Saunders, 1995

Hollinshead WH and Jenkins DB: Functional Anatomy of the Limbs and Back. Philadelphia, WB Saunders, 1981

Hoppenfeld S: Physical Examination of the Spine and Extremities. New York, Appleton-Century-Croft, 1976

Jackson DW and Drez D Jr: The Anterior Cruciate Deficient Knee: New Concepts in Ligament Repair. St. Louis, CV Mosby, 1987

Kaltenborn M: Mobilization of the Extremity Joints, Oslo, Bygdoy Alle, 1980

Kapanji IA: The Physiology of Joints, Vol. 3. Edinburgh, Churchill Livingstone, 1974

Kendall FP, McCreary EK and Provance PG: Muscles Testing and Function. Baltimore, Williams and Wilkins, 1993

Kessler RM and Hertling D: The hip. In Hertling D and Kessler RM (eds): Management of Common Musculoskeletal Disorders, 3rd ed. Philadelphia, Lippincott-Raven Publishers, 1996

Kisner C and Colby LA: Therapeutic Exercise: Foundations and Techniques. Philadelphia, FA Davis, 1986

Losee RE: Diagnosis of chronic injury to the anterior cruciate ligament. Orthop Clin North Am 16:1, 1985

Magee DJ: Orthopedic Physical Assessment. Philadelphia, WB Saunders, 1992

Maitland GD: The Peripheral Joints: Examination and Recording Guide. Adelaide, Australia, Virgo Press, 1973

Malone TR, McPoil T and Nitz AJ: Orthopedic and Sport Physical Therapy, St. Louis, CV Mosby, 1997

McGann WA: History and physical examination. In Steinberg ME (ed): The Hip and Its Disorders. Philadelphia, WB Saunders, 1991

McKensie RA: The Lumbar Spine. Lower Hutt, New Zealand, Spinal Publications, 1981

McPoil TG and Brocato RS: The foot and ankle: Biomechanical evaluation and treatment. In Gould JA (ed): Orthopedic and Sports Physical Therapy. St. Louis, CV Mosby, 1990

Mellion B: Sports Injuries and Athletic Problems. Philadelphia, Hanley and Belfus, 1988

Moore K: Clinically Oriented Anatomy. Baltimore, Williams and Wilkins, 1992

Mueller W: The Knee: Form, Function and Ligament Reconstruction. New York, Springer-Verlag, 1983

Norkin C and Levangie P: Joint Structure and Function: A Comprehensive Analysis. Philadelphia, FA Davis, 1995

Norkin CC and White DJ: Measurement of Joint Motion: A Guide to Goniometry. Philadelphia, FA Davis, 1985

Paris SV: The Spine (course notes). Atlanta, Institute Press, 1979

Porterfield JA and DeRosa C: Mechanical Low Back Pain: Perspectives in Functional Anatomy. Philadelphia, WB Saunders, 1991

Reid DC and Kushner S: The elbow region. In Donatelli R and Wooden MJ (eds): Orthopedic Physical Therapy. Edinburgh, Churchill Livingstone, 1989

Riddle DL, Rothstein JM and Lamb RL: The reliability of shoulder joint range of motion measurements in a clinical setting. Presented at the annual meeting of the American Physical Therapy Association, Chicago, 1980

Root ML, Orien WP and Weed JH: Normal and Abnormal Function of the Foot. Los Angeles, Clinical Biomechanics Corp, 1977

Sahrmann SA: Program for Correction of Muscle Imbalance: Concepts and Principles. Boston, Continuing Education Workshop, 1986

Saudek, CE: The hip. In Gould JA (ed): Orthopedic and Sports Physical Therapy. St. Louis, CV Mosby, 1990

Saunders HD: Evaluation and Treatment of Musculoskeletal Disorders. Minneapolis, HD Saunders, 1985

Schneider RD, Kennedy JC and Plant ML: Sports Injuries: Mechanisms, Prevention and Treatment. Baltimore, Williams and Wilkins, 1985

Slocum DB, James SL, Larson RL and Singer KM: A clinical test for anterolateral rotary instability of the knee. Clin Orthop Relat Res 118:63, 1976

Smith LK, Weiss EL and Lehmkuhl LD: Brunnstrom's Clinical Kinesiology. Philadelphia, FA Davis, 1996

Spengler DM: Low Back Pain: Assessment and Management. Orlando, Grune & Stratton, 1982

Strobel M and Stedtfeld HW: Diagnostic Evaluation of the Knee. Berlin, Springer-Verlag, 1990

Subotnick S: Pediatric Sports Medicine. Mount Kisco, NY, Futura Publishing, 1975

Travell J: Temporomandibular joint pain referred muscles of the head and neck. J Prosthet Dent 10:745, 1960

Tubiana R: The Hand. Philadelphia, WB Saunders, 1981

Weinstein SL and Buckwalter JA: Turck's Orthopaedics: Principles and Their Application, 5th ed. Philadelphia, Lippincott-Raven Publishers, 1995

Appendix A: Recording Forms for Use in Physical Therapy Assessment Procedures

RANGE-OF-MOTION RECORD

UPPER LIMBS

Name: _____

LEFT								RIGHT				
					EXAMINER							
					DATE							
					SHOULDER							
					Flexion	0–180						
					Extension	180–0						
					Hyperextension	0–45						
					Abduction	0–180						
					Medial rotation	0–65						
					Lateral rotation	0–90						
					Horizontal adduction	0–120						
					Horizontal abduction	0–30						
					SCAPULA							
					Upward rotation							
					Downward rotation							
					Abduction							
					Adduction							
					ELBOW							
					Flexion	0–145						
					Extension	145–0						
					RADIOULNAR							
					Supination	0–90						
					Pronation	0–90						
					WRIST							
					Flexion	0–90						
					Extension	90–0						
					Hyperextension	0–70						
					Abduction	0–25						
					Adduction	0–35						

RANGE-OF-MOTION RECORD (continued)

UPPER LIMBS

Name: _____

LEFT								RIGHT				
					EXAMINER							
					DATE							
					THUMB							
					Flexion MP	0–50						
					Extension MP	50–0						
					Flexion IP	0–80						
					Extension IP	80–0						
					Hyperextension IP	0–90						
					Flexion CMC	30–15						
					Extension CMC	0–70						
					Opposition CMC							
					Abduction CMC	0–60						
					Adduction CMC	60–0						
					Hyperextension MP	0–10						
					SECOND DIGIT							
					Flexion MP	0–90						
					Extension MP	90–0						
					Hyperextension MP	0–30						
					Flexion PIP	0–120						
					Extension PIP	120–0						
					Flexion DIP	0–80						
					Extension DIP	80–120						
					Abduction MCP	0–20						
					Adduction MCP	20–0						
					Hyperextension DIP	0–10						
					THIRD DIGIT							
					Flexion MP	0–90						
					Extension MP	90–0						
					Hyperextension MP	0–30						
					Flexion PIP	0–120						
					Extension PIP	120–0						
					Flexion DIP	0–80						
					Extension DIP	80–0						
					Abduction MCP	0–20						
					Adduction MCP	20–0						
					Hyperextension DIP	0—10						

UPPER LIMBS

Name: _____

		LEFT			EXAMINER			RIGHT		
					DATE					
					FOURTH DIGIT					
					Flexion MP	0–90				
					Extension MP	90–0				
					Hyperextension MP	0–30				
					Flexion PIP	0–120				
					Extension PIP	120–0				
					Flexion DIP	0–80				
					Extension DIP	80–0				
					Abduction MCP	0–20				
					Adduction MCP	20–0				
					Hyperextension DIP	0–10				
					FIFTH DIGIT					
					Flexion MP	0–90				
					Extension MP	90–0				
					Hyperextension MP	0–30				
					Flexion PIP	0–120				
					Extension PIP	120–0				
					Flexion DIP	0–80				
					Extension DIP	80–0				
					Abduction MCP	0–20				
					Adduction MCP	20–0				
					Hyperextension DIP	0–10				

REMARKS:

Key: The anatomical position is considered zero and is the starting position for all measurements with the exception of rotation at the shoulder (shoulder is abducted 90 degrees).

Passive motion is recorded unless notation of active motion is made.

Use black pen to record patient's normal range.
Use red pen to record limited range.

RANGE-OF-MOTION RECORD (continued)

LOWER LIMBS

Name: _____

		LEFT					RIGHT			
					EXAMINER					
					DATE					
					HIP					
					Flexion	0–125				
					Extension	125–0				
					Hyperextension	0–10				
					Abduction	0–45				
					Adduction	0–20				
					Medial rotation	0–45				
					Lateral rotation	0–45				
					KNEE					
					Flexion	0–130				
					Extension	130–0				
					ANKLE					
					Dorsiflexion	0–20				
					Plantar flexion	0–45				
					Inversion	0–30				
					Eversion	0–25				
					FIRST DIGIT					
					Flexion MP	0–45				
					Extension MP	45–0				
					Hyperextension	0–90				
					Flexion IP	0–90				
					Extension IP	90–0				
					LATERAL DIGITS					
					Flexion MP	0–40				
					Extension MP	40–0				
					Hyperextension MP	0–45				
					Flexion PIP	0–35				
					Extension PIP	35–0				
					Flexion DIP	0–60				
					Extension DIP	60–0				

MANUAL MUSCLE TESTING RECORD

UPPER LIMBS

Name:							
LEFT				RIGHT			
			EXAMINER				
			DATE				
			Upper Limb				
			CN XI—Upper trapezius	Spinal accessory			
			C3–5—Levator scapulae	Dorsal scapular			
			CN XI—Middle trapezius	Spinal accessory			
			CN XI—Lower trapezius	Spinal accessory			
			C4 & 6—Rhomboid major & minor	Dorsal scapular			
			C5–7—Serratus anterior	Long thoracic			
			C7—Pectoralis minor	Medial & lateral pectoral			
			C5—Anterior deltoid	Axillary			
			C6—Coracobrachialis	Musculocutaneous			
			C6 & 7—Latissimus dorsi	Thoracodorsal			
			C6—Teres major	Lower subscapular			
			C5—Supraspinatus	Suprascapular			
			C5—Middle deltoid	Axillary			
			C5—Posterior deltoid	Axillary			
			C6—Pectoralis major (clavicular) C7 & 8—(sternal)	Lateral & medial pectoral			
			C5—Infraspinatus & teres minor	Axillary			
			C6—Subscapularis	Upper and lower subscapular			

MANUAL MUSCLE TESTING RECORD *(continued)*

UPPER LIMBS

			Name: _____						
	LEFT						RIGHT		
			EXAMINER						
			DATE						
			Upper Limb						
			C7—Pronator teres		Median				
			C6—Supinator		Radial				
			C6—Biceps brachii		Musculocutaneous				
			C6—Brachialis		Musculocutaneous & radial				
			C6—Brachioradialis		Radial				
			C7 & 8—Triceps		Radial				
			C8—Palmaris longus		Median				
			C8—Flexor carpi ulnaris		Ulnar				
			C7—Flexor carpi radialis		Median				
			C8—1 Flexor digitorum profundus	1	Median				
			2	2	Median				
			3	3	Ulnar				
			4	4	Ulnar				
			C8—1 Flexor digitorum superficialis	1	Median				
			2	2	Median				
			3	3	Median				
			4	4	Median				
			C8—Extensor carpi ulnaris		Radial				
			C6 & 7—Extensor carpi radialis longus (brevis)		Radial				
			C8—Extensor pollicis longus		Radial				
			C8—Extensor pollicis brevis		Radial				
			C8—Abductor pollicis longus		Radial				
			C8—Abductor pollicis brevis		Median				
			C8—Flexor pollicis brevis		Median & ulnar				
			C8—Opponens pollicis		Median				
			C8—Abductor pollicis		Ulnar				
			C8—Flexor pollicis longus		Median				
			C8—Extensor indicis		Radial				
			C7—1 Extensor digitorum	1	Radial				
			2	2	Radial				
			3	3	Radial				
			4	4	Radial				

Name:													
		LEFT								RIGHT			
					EXAMINER								
					DATE								
					Upper Limb								
					T1—1 Lumbricals	1	Median						
					2	2	Median						
					T1– 3	3	Ulnar						
					4	4	Ulnar						
					T1—1 Dorsal interossei	1	Ulnar						
					2	2	Ulnar						
					3	3	Ulnar						
					4	4	Ulnar						
					T1—1 Palmar interossei	1	Ulnar						
					2	2	Ulnar						
					3	3	Ulnar						
					T1—Opponens digiti minimi		Ulnar						
					T1—Flexor digiti minimi		Ulnar						
					T1—Abductor digiti minimi		Ulnar						

MANUAL MUSCLE TESTING RECORD *(continued)*

UPPER LIMBS

				LEFT								RIGHT		
			EXAMINER											
			DATE											
			Upper Limb C7—Extensor digiti minimi					Radial						

LOWER LIMBS

Name: _____							
LEFT						RIGHT	
			EXAMINER				
			DATE				
			Lower Limb				
			L1–2—Iliopsoas	Spinal nerve			
			L3–4—Rectus femoris	Femoral			
			L2–3—Sartorius	Femoral			
			S1 & S2—Gluteus maximus	Inferior gluteal			
			L5—Gluteus medius	Superior gluteal			
			L5—Gluteus minimus	Superior gluteal			
			L4–5—Tensor fasciae latae	Superior gluteal			
			L3—Adductor longus	Obturator			
			L3—Adductor brevis	Obturator			
			L3–4—Adductor magnus	Obturator and tibial			
			L2—Gracilis	Obturator			
			L4–S2—Lateral rotators				
			S1—Biceps femoris				
			Long head	Tibial			
			Short head	Peroneal			
			L5–S1—Semitendinosus	Tibial			
			L5–S1—Semimembranosus	Tibial			
			L3 & L4—Quadriceps	Femoral			
			L5–S2—Gastrocnemius	Tibial			
			L5–S2—Soleus	Tibial			
			L5–S2—Soleus	Tibial			

MANUAL MUSCLE TESTING RECORD *(continued)*

LOWER LIMBS

Name: _____

LEFT   RIGHT

			EXAMINER			
			DATE			
			Lower Limb			
			St. L4—Tibialis anterior Deep peroneal			
			L4 & L5—Tibialis posterior Tibial			
			L5–S1—Peroneus longus Superficial peroneal L5–S1—Peroneus brevis Superficial peroneal			
			S1–2—Lumbricals Tibial			
			S3—Flexor hallucis brevis Medial plantar			
			S2—Flexor hallucis longus Tibial			
			S3—Flexor digitorum brevis Medial and lateral plantar			
			S2—Flexor digitorum longus Tibial			
			S1 & S2—Extensor hallucis brevis Deep peroneal L5–S1—Extensor hallucis longus Deep peroneal			
			S1 & S2—Extensor digitorum brevis Deep peroneal L5–S1—Extensor digitorum longus Deep peroneal			
			L5–S1—Abductor hallucis Medial plantar			
			L5–S2—1st Lumbrical Medial plantar			
			L5–S2—2nd, 3rd & 4th lumbricals Lateral plantar			
			S1–S2—Adductor hallucis Medial plantar			
			S1–S2—Abductor digiti minimi Lateral plantar			
			S1–S2—Dorsal interossei Lateral plantar			
			S1–S2—Plantar interossei Lateral plantar			

COMMENTS: _____

_____

_____

POSTURAL ASSESSMENT RECORD

STANDING—POSTERIOR VIEW

NAME _____

AGE _____ HANDEDNESS _____

LEFT				RIGHT		
			EXAMINER			
			DATE			
			Head and Neck Head tilt			
			Head rotated			
			Shoulder Dropped			
			Elevated			
			Medially rotated			
			Abduction (valgum)			
			Scapula Adducted			
			Abducted			
			Winged			
			Trunk Scoliosis			
			Pelvis Lateral tilt			
			Rotated			
			Hip Abduction (valgum)			
			Adduction (varum)			
			Knee Genu varum			
			Genu valgum			
			Ankle and Foot Pes planus			
			Pes cavus			

COMMENTS: _____

_____

_____

_____

Check (✔) each box where a postural fault exists.

POSTURAL ASSESSMENT RECORD *(continued)*

STANDING—ANTERIOR VIEW

NAME _____

AGE _____ HANDEDNESS _____

LEFT				RIGHT		
			EXAMINER			
			DATE			
			Head and Neck Lateral tilt			
			Rotated			
			Mandibular asymmetry			
			Shoulder Dropped			
			Elevated			
			Elbow Cubitus valgus			
			Cubitus varus			
			Hip Laterally rotated			
			Medially rotated			
			Knee External tibial torsion			
			Internal tibial torsion			
			Ankle and Foot Hallux valgus			
			Claw toes			
			Hammer toes			

COMMENTS: _____

_____

_____

_____

Check (✔) each box where a postural fault exists.

STANDING—LATERAL VIEW

NAME _____						
AGE _____ HANDEDNESS _____						
LEFT					RIGHT	

			EXAMINER			
			DATE			
			Head and Neck Forward head			
			Flattened lordosis			
			Excessive lordosis			
			Shoulder Forward			
			Tight thoracolumbar fascia			
			Thorax and Chest Kyphosis			
			Pectus excavatum			
			Barrel			
			Pectus cavinatum			
			Lumbar Lordosis			
			Sway back			
			Flat back			
			Pelvis and Hip Anterior tilt			
			Posterior tilt			
			Knee Genu recurvatum			
			Flexed			
			Ankle Forward posture			

COMMENTS: _____

_____

_____

_____

Check (✔) each box where a postural fault exists.

POSTURAL ASSESSMENT RECORD (continued)

SITTING AND HANDS AND KNEES

NAME _____

AGE _____ HANDEDNESS _____

LEFT				RIGHT		
			EXAMINER			
			DATE			
			Sitting Posterior pelvic tilt			
			Anterior pelvic tilt			
			Hands and Knees Winged scapula			
			Trunk Lumbar lordosis			
			Thoracic kyphosis			
			Rotated			
			Laterally flexed			
			Hip Decreased flexion			
			Increased flexion			
			Rotated			
			External tibial torsion			
			Ankle and Foot Dorsiflexed			
			Inverted			
			Everted			

COMMENTS: _____

_____

_____

_____

_____

Check (✔) each box where a postural fault exists.

POSTURAL ASSESSMENT RECORD *(continued)*

STANDING ON ONE FOOT

NAME _____						
AGE _____			HANDEDNESS _____			

LEFT				RIGHT		
			EXAMINER			
			DATE			
			Hip Lateral tilt			
			Trunk Excessive lateral shift			
			Ankle/Foot Pronation/supination			

COMMENTS: _____

_____

_____

_____

_____

Check (✔) each box where a postural fault exists.

GAIT ASSESSMENT RECORD

NAME _____ AGE _____

EXAMINER _____

EVALUATE WITH SUBJECT WALKING

	LEFT				RIGHT	
			DATE			
			Stride Unequal length			
			Slow cadence			
			Short stance			
			Head Forward flexed			
			Deviated laterally			
			Shoulders Nonreciprocal arm swing			
			Unequal arm swing			
			Trunk Forward flexed			
			Deviated laterally			
			Pelvis Excessive rotation			
			Excessive lateral tilt			
			Excessive posterior tilt			
			Excessive anterior tilt			
			Hips Medially rotated			
			Laterally rotated			
			Abducted			
			Adducted			
			Flexed			

			Knees Hyperextended				
			Restricted extension				
			Exaggerated flexion				
			Genu valgum				
			Genu varum				
			Ankles Exaggerated preswing				
			Decreased preswing				
			Foot slap				
			Foot drop				
			Excessive dorsiflexion				
			Feet Pes planus				
			Pes cavus				

SUMMARY OF GAIT DEVIATIONS: _____

_____

_____

_____

Check (✔) each box where a gait deviation exists.

Choose the one best answer to each question.

▲ Chapter 2

1. Three criteria are essential for an accurate muscle test. One of these, validity, requires that "you test what you claim to be testing." How can you best ensure that your muscle test is valid?

   a. Follow the standard procedure for test positions.
   b. Compare the involved side with the normal side.
   c. Repeat the test several times.
   d. Be aware of substitutions and prevent them.

2. Maximal strength of a muscle at a given joint is greater when the muscle contraction is _____ .

   a. isometric.
   b. concentric.
   c. eccentric.
   d. isotonic.

3. Resistance applied to a muscle containing predominantly type I muscle fibers is:

   a. greater than that applied to type II muscle.
   b. less than that applied to type II muscle.
   c. the same as that applied to type II muscle.
   d. generally not applied.

4. The force of gravity has the greatest leverage and therefore is able to produce the greatest torque on the body segment when the segment is:

   a. at a 90-degree angle to the joint.
   b. horizontal.
   c. in the anatomical position.
   d. at a 45-degree angle to the joint.

5. Which position of the hip would produce active insufficiency of the hamstrings?

   a. Flexion.
   b. Extension.
   c. Abduction.
   d. Lateral rotation.

6. Muscles that are able to retain a favorable length through a large range allowing the rate of shortening to be less are:

   a. one-joint muscles.
   b. two-joint muscles.
   c. fusiform muscles.
   d. penniform muscles.

7. A person is sitting with the knee flexed 60 degrees. When the knee is extended to 0 degrees, the rotatory component of the force of gravity on the leg _____ .

   a. increases.
   b. decreases.
   c. remains the same.

8. A therapist begins testing a subject who is lying supine. The subject can abduct the hip several times without difficulty. What should the therapist do next?

   a. Apply resistance to the distal end of the femur.
   b. Assign a grade of 2 (Poor).
   c. Repeat the test with the patient in the side-lying position.
   d. Apply resistance above the lateral malleolus.

9. When utilizing the break test in muscle testing, resistance should be applied _____ .

   a. at the beginning of the range.
   b. at the end of the range.
   c. at the strongest point in the range.
   d. anywhere within the range.

10. Which of the following must be true of a subject before a manual muscle test can be performed?

   a. The subject has voluntary control of the muscles and can understand the therapist's instructions.
   b. The subject has normal range of motion and is free of pain.
   c. The subject has normal strength on one side for comparison with the involved side.
   d. If the subject has partial nerve or muscle trauma, the pattern of injury can be anticipated.

11. Which of the following grades is assigned to a muscle that is able to hold against the resistance of the examiner?

    a. Fair +.
    b. Fair.
    c. Fair −.
    d. Poor +.

12. When is a gross muscle test preferable to a specific muscle test?

    a. When the subject's muscles are too weak to take resistance.
    b. When the subject cannot be positioned correctly for a specific test.
    c. When a surgeon wants to know the strength of a muscle prior to a muscle transfer.
    d. When the therapist does not remember how to perform a specific test.

13. Which of the following statements are true? Goniometric measurements should be taken at the end of the range of motion because _____.

    1. external landmarks for the axis of motion may change as the joint is moved.
    2. accurate alignment of the goniometer is accomplished with greater ease when the parts are stationary.
    3. accurate alignment of the lever arms with skeletal segments localizes the axis of motion.

    a. 1 only is correct.
    b. 1 and 3 are correct.
    c. 1, 2, and 3 are correct.
    d. 1 and 2 are correct.

14. Which of the following statements are true? In order to measure joint range of motion, the goniometer must be aligned with the _____.
    1. axis of the joint.
    2. skeletal segments on either side of the joint.
    3. midline of the body part on either side of the joint.

    a. 1 only is correct.
    b. 1 and 3 are correct.
    c. 1, 2 and 3 are correct.
    d. 1 and 2 are correct.

15. The preferred position of the subject when taking goniometric measurements is supine in the anatomical position because _____.

    a. the end range is assisted by gravity.
    b. a concentric contraction is easily performed.
    c. the joint is in a closed-packed position.
    d. the two joint muscles are relaxed.

16. All of the following are inert structures *except* _____.

    a. nerves.
    b. cartilage.
    c. tendon.
    d. capsule.

17. Passive range of motion testing for assessment of inert structures will be positive for contractile involvement only when _____.

    a. contractile elements are being shortened passively.
    b. contractile elements are being lengthened passively.
    c. the lesion is located at the periosteal attachment of the tendon.
    d. Passive testing assesses only inert structures.

18. From most to least restricted, the capsular pattern of the shoulder is _____.

    a. external rotation, abduction, internal rotation.
    b. abduction, internal rotation, external rotation.
    c. abduction, external rotation, internal rotation.
    d. external rotation, internal rotation, abduction.

19. What position would one place the hip to produce passive insufficiency of the hamstrings muscles?

    a. medial rotation.
    b. adduction.
    c. extension.
    d. flexion.

20. Which one-joint muscles may produce active insufficiency compared to a two-joint muscle?

    a. rectus femoris.
    b. soleus.
    c. gastrocmenius.
    d. biceps brachii.

21. Which of the following is an example of active insufficiency of a multi-joint muscle?

    a. The grip strength is less when the wrist is flexed than when it is extended.
    b. The degree of dorsiflexion of the ankle is less when the knee is extended than when it is flexed.

c. Pain is felt in the back of the knee when a person flexes over to touch the toes while keeping the knees extended.

d. The strength of the biceps brachii is greater when the elbow is flexed 90 degrees than when it is fully extended.

▲ Chapter 4

1. Which postural faults are examined from a lateral view with the subject standing?

   a. Forward shoulders, lumbar lordosis, and anterior pelvic tilt.
   b. Lumbar lordosis, dropped shoulder, and coxa vara.
   c. Anterior pelvic tilt, coxa vara, and genu recurvatum.
   d. Genu recurvatum, pes planus, and external tibial torsion.

2. Tightness of the iliotibial band may cause _____.

   a. genu varum.
   b. coxa valga.
   c. external tibial torsion.
   d. lateral pelvic tilt.

3. Excessive pelvic rotation during ambulation may be caused by _____.

   a. tightness in the hamstring muscles.
   b. decrease in ankle dorsiflexion.
   c. tightness of the hip flexor muscles.
   d. weakness of the trunk flexors.

4. Femoral anteversion may lead to _____.

   a. hip lateral rotation.
   b. hip abduction.
   c. limited knee extension.
   d. genu valgum.

▲ Chapter 5

1. When testing the lower trapezius muscle, a grade of 2 (Poor) should be given when a subject _____.

   a. lifts the affected limb through partial range of motion and takes minimal resistance.
   b. lifts the affected limb through full range of motion but is unable to take resistance.
   c. is unable to lift the affected limb, but palpation reveals contraction of the muscle and scapular movement.

d. raises the affected limb through full range of motion and takes minimal resistance.

2. What shoulder motion is the best to use to test the anterior deltoid muscle?

   a. Medial rotation.
   b. Horizontal abduction.
   c. Shoulder abduction.
   d. Shoulder flexion.

3. All of the following may be tested in a gravity-minimized sitting position *except* the _____.

   a. upper trapezius.
   b. serratus anterior.
   c. rhomboids.
   d. posterior deltoid.

4. Where is the best place to palpate the teres major muscle?

   a. Posterior border of the axilla.
   b. Deep in the axilla.
   c. Immediately inferior to the spine of the scapula.
   d. The midaxillary line on the thorax.

5. Both the rhomboids and the middle trapezius muscles are tested as adductors of the scapula and may easily be confused. When testing the rhomboids how should you position the subject's shoulder to give the rhomboids an advantage over the middle trapezius?

   a. In 90 degrees of abduction.
   b. In adduction.
   c. In 90 degrees of flexion with the elbow flexed.
   d. In medial rotation.

6. Where is resistance applied when testing the rhomboid muscles?

   a. On the vertebral border of the scapula, pushing the scapula into abduction and upward rotation.
   b. On the spine of the scapula, pushing the scapula into abduction and elevation.
   c. On the axillary border of the scapula, pushing the scapula into adduction and downward rotation.
   d. On the flexor surface of the wrist, pushing downward.

7. Which of the following shoulder muscles can be tested against gravity with the subject in the supine position?

   a. Serratus anterior, upper trapezius, anterior deltoid.
   b. Serratus anterior, anterior deltoid, pectoralis major.
   c. Pectoralis major, teres major, middle deltoid.
   d. Anterior deltoid, middle deltoid, serratus anterior.

8. What muscle is being tested when the subject lies prone with the shoulder abducted 135 degrees and raises the upper limb?

   a. Lower trapezius.
   b. Middle trapezius.
   c. Latissimus dorsi.
   d. Posterior deltoid.

9. What muscles are being evaluated when the strength of lateral rotation is tested?

   a. Posterior deltoid and teres major.
   b. Infraspinatus and teres minor.
   c. Subscapularis and supraspinatus.
   d. Latissimus dorsi and pectoralis major.

10. Hawkins test at the shoulder is an impingement test for assessing the _____.

    a. long head of the biceps tendon.
    b. short head of the biceps tendon.
    c. infraspinatus muscle.
    d. supraspinatus muscle.

11. All of the following are clinical tests for shoulder subluxation *except* _____.

    a. Yergason's test.
    b. the posterior apprehension test.
    c. the anterior apprehension test.

12. Contractile testing of shoulder flexion assesses _____.

    a. the biceps brachii.
    b. the anterior deltoid.
    c. the supraspinatus.
    d. a and b.
    e. All of the above.

13. Contraction of the pectoralis major muscle, as a medial rotator of the shoulder joint, decreases when the shoulder joint increases in flexion from 0 degree to 90 degrees because it:

    a. becomes passively insufficient.
    b. becomes actively insufficient.
    c. decreases the distance of muscle insertion.
    d. decreases in cross sectional area.

14. What is the preferred position for evaluating tightness of the pectoralis minor muscle?

    a. sitting with arms behind the head, shoulder horizontally abducted.
    b. prone with upper limbs overhead in the sagittal plane.
    c. supine with upper limbs in the anatomical position.
    d. standing facing wall with hands on the wall at shoulder height.

▲ Chapter 6

1. To obtain maximal contraction of the brachioradialis muscle as an elbow flexor, the best position for the forearm is _____.

   a. supinated.
   b. pronated.
   c. in mid-position.
   d. in any position.

2. The most common substitution for pronation of the forearm is _____.

   a. lateral flexion of the trunk to the same side.
   b. lateral flexion of the trunk to the opposite side.
   c. abduction and lateral rotation of the shoulder.
   d. adduction and medial rotation of the shoulder.

3. If the subject is capable of 70 degrees of pronation and 85 degrees of supination, the total range of motion is _____.

   a. 15 degrees.
   b. 25 degrees.
   c. 75 degrees.
   d. 155 degrees.

4. Which muscle could flex the elbow if the three elbow flexors were *not* palpable?

   a. The pronator teres.
   b. The flexor pollicis longus.
   c. The supinator.
   d. The pronator quadratus.

5. Tinel's sign at the elbow is a clinical test for assessment of _____.

   a. median nerve involvement.
   b. ulnar nerve involvement.
   c. musculocutaneous nerve involvement.
   d. radial nerve involvement.

6. What tests other than flexion, extension, pronation, and supination should be performed as part of the assessment of inert structures around the elbow?

   a. Tinel's sign.
   b. The valgus stress test.
   c. The varus stress test.
   d. All of the above.

7. Denervation of the musculocutaneous nerve would result in the following contractile finding when assessing elbow flexion:

   a. Strong and painful.
   b. Weak and painful.
   c. Weak and pain-free.
   d. Strong and pain-free.

▲ Chapter 7

1. When testing the strength of the wrist extensors, the subject's fingers must be relaxed to prevent _____.

   a. active insufficiency of the long finger extensors.
   b. substitution by the tenodesis action of the extensor digitorum.
   c. passive insufficiency of the flexor digitorum profundus.
   d. substitution by the extensor digitorum.

2. A subject who lacks an opponens pollicis and an abductor pollicis brevis muscle is nevertheless able to touch the tip of the thumb to the tip of the little finger. What muscle is substituting for them?

   a. Opponens digiti minimi.
   b. Abductor pollicis longus.
   c. Adductor pollicis.
   d. Flexor pollicis brevis.

3. Which of the following is true of goniometry for wrist radial deviation?

   a. The axis of the goniometer is placed over the pisiform bone.

b. The stationary arm of the goniometer is placed along the midline of the dorsum of the forearm.
   c. The moving arm of the goniometer is placed along the midline of the dorsum of the third finger.
   d. Radial deviation at the wrist is also referred to as adduction of the wrist.

4. What is the best way to prevent the flexor digitorum profundus muscle from substituting for the flexor digitorum superficialis muscle?

   a. Allow motion to occur only at the distal interphalangeal joint.
   b. Stabilize the metacarpophalangeal joint of the finger being tested in extension.
   c. Stabilize in full extension the fingers not being tested.
   d. Palpate the tendon of the flexor digitorum superficialis on the palmar surface of the proximal phalanx.

5. Which combination of symptoms indicates injury to the median nerve?

   a. The middle and index fingers lose the ability to flex and the thumb cannot adduct or extend.
   b. The ring and little fingers lose the ability to flex, and the little finger cannot abduct or oppose.
   c. The inability of the wrist and fingers to extend interferes with grasp.
   d. The middle and index fingers lose their ability to flex, and the thumb cannot oppose.

6. Finkelstein's test is designed to assess involvement of which of the following contractile structures?

   a. Extensor pollicis longus and abductor pollicis brevis muscles.
   b. Extensor pollicis brevis and abductor pollicis longus muscles.
   c. Extensor pollicis longus and abductor pollicis longus muscles.
   d. Extensor pollicis brevis and abductor pollicis brevis muscles.

7. All of the following are tests used in the diagnosis of carpal tunnel *except* _____.

   a. Tinel's sign.
   b. Phalen's test.
   c. the three-jaw chuck test.
   d. Allen test.

8. The Brunnell–Littler test is a test of _____.

   a. all hand intrinsics.
   b. the interossei.
   c. the lumbricals.
   d. the flexor retinaculum.

9. Stretching or lengthing would be most evident in which one of the following muscles if the elbow, wrist and fingers were extended:

   a. flexor digitorum profundus.
   b. flexor digitorum superficialis.
   c. extensor digitorum.
   d. extensor pollicus longus.

10. What would be the ideal position to stretch the finger flexors with the wrist:

    a. extended, MP's and IP's flexed.
    b. flexed, MP's and IP's flexed.
    c. extended, MP's and IP's extended.
    d. flexed, MP's and IP's extended.

▲ Chapter 8

1. The facial nerve supplies all of the following muscles *except* the _____.

   a. buccinator.
   b. masseter.
   c. zygomaticus major.
   d. frontalis.

2. An examiner palpating the side of the nose would be feeling for contraction of the _____.

   a. corrugator.
   b. orbicularis oculi.
   c. orbicularis oris.
   d. procerus.

3. What nerve innervates the muscle for winking?

   a. facial.
   b. oculomotor.
   c. abducens.
   d. trigeminal.

4. What grades are generally used when testing the muscles of facial expression?

   a. zero, good, normal.
   b. zero, trace, fair, normal.

   c. weak and normal.
   d. zero, trace, poor, fair, good, and normal.

5. Inability to move the eyeball laterally by contraction of the lateral rectus muscle might indicate damage to which one of the following cranial nerves:

   a. I—optic.
   b. III—oculomotor.
   c. IV—trochlear.
   d. VI—abducens.

▲ Chapter 9

1. Which motion can best be measured with a gravity or bubble goniometer?

   a. Neck rotation.
   b. Trunk flexion.
   c. Trunk rotation.
   d. Neck flexion.

2. A normal range of motion for neck flexion measured with a bubble goniometer is approximately _____.

   a. 40 degrees.
   b. 70 degrees.
   c. 100 degrees.
   d. 140 degrees.

3. The alar ligament test assesses stability of the _____.

   a. atlas.
   b. axis.
   c. C3 spinal segment.
   d. occiput on the atlas.

4. What is the position of the head and neck for the vertebral artery test?

   a. Flexion and rotation.
   b. Flexion and sidebend.
   c. Extension and rotation.
   d. Uniplanar extension.

5. Palpating on the anterior and lateral side of the neck as the head is rotating, one feels which muscle:

   a. levator scapula.
   b. sternocleidomastoid.
   c. trapezius.
   d. serratus anterior.

▲ Chapter 10

1. Which one of the following muscles does NOT insert into the linea alba?

    a. rectus abdominus.
    b. external abdominal oblique.
    c. internal abdominal oblique.
    d. transverse abdominus.

2. Name a true or intrinsic back muscle?

    a. trapezius.
    b. longissimus.
    c. latissimus dorsi.
    d. rhomboid major.

3. When performing manual muscle testing for the upper rectus abdominus muscle, a grade of F+ (3+) would be given if:

    a. a contraction was felt and full depression of the thorax occurred.
    b. the arms were at the side and the trunk begins motion against gravity.
    c. the arms were held straight in front of the patient and the inferior angles of the scapula cleared the table.
    d. the hands were behind the head with elbows forward and the inferior angle of the scapula clears the table.

4. The femoral nerve stretch primarily assesses the _____.

    a. L3 nerve.
    b. L5 nerve.
    c. L4 nerve.
    d. L2 nerve.

▲ Chapter 11

1. A common site of referred pain by the sacroiliac joint is the:

    a. coccyx.
    b. ischial tuberosity.
    c. posterior superior iliac spine.
    d. anterior superior iliac spine.

2. In the supine to sit test, the leg of the affected side with a posterior iliac rotation will be:

    a. longer supine and shorter sitting.
    b. shorter supine and longer sitting.
    c. shorter supine and shorter sitting.
    d. longer supine and longer sitting.

3. In a patient with a left anterior S1 rotation, a standing postural exam will reveal:

    a. a lower ASIS on the left and a higher PSIS on the left as compared to the right.
    b. a higher ASIS on the left and a lower PSIS on the left as compared to the right.
    c. symmetrical ASIS and PSIS heights compared to the right.
    d. higher left ASIS and PSIS heights compared to the right.

▲ Chapter 12

1. Where do you apply resistance when testing the hip adductor muscles?

    a. Distal to the knee medially.
    b. Proximal to the ankle medially.
    c. Distal to the knee laterally.
    d. Proximal to the knee medially.

2. In what position would you place a subject to evaluate Fair+ (3+) strength of the gluteus maximus muscle if there is a 30-degree hip flexion contracture?

    a. Sidelying, hip flexed 90 degrees.
    b. Prone, leaning over the edge of the table with the hips flexed.
    c. Prone, hip extended.
    d. Sitting, hips flexed 90 degrees.

3. Using a full-circle goniometer to measure the hip may produce an inaccurate measurement because _____.

    a. the scale on the full-circle goniometer is smaller and more difficult to read than that on other types.
    b. the scale on a full-circle goniometer requires the subtraction of the measured degrees of motion from 360 to obtain the correct measurement.
    c. the 360-degree goniometer does not allow accurate alignment of the axis because the treatment table is in the way.
    d. None of the above.

4. While you are muscle testing hip flexion in the sagittal plane, the subject moves the hip into abduction and lateral rotation. What muscle is the subject using?

    a. Tensor fascia lata.
    b. Sartorius.
    c. Gluteus medius.
    d. Gluteus maximus.

5. When testing the rectus femoris muscle as a hip flexor, the best place to palpate is between which two muscles?

    a. Tensor fascia lata and iliopsoas.
    b. Tensor fascia lata and sartorius.
    c. Gluteus medius and sartorius.
    d. Sartorius and adductor longus.

6. When muscle testing for hip flexion, the pelvis is in _____.

    a. extension.
    b. anterior tilt.
    c. neutral position.
    d. posterior tilt.

7. The examiner evaluating joint range of motion must be aware that a common substitution for medial rotation of the hip is _____.

    a. inversion of the foot on the test side.
    b. elevation of the buttocks on the "nontest" side.
    c. elevation of the buttocks on the test side.
    d. adduction of the hip on the test side.

8. In goniometry of the hip, for which measurement does the axis of the goniometer *not* fall in the vicinity of the greater trochanter?

    a. Flexion.
    b. Extension.
    c. Medial rotation.
    d. Hyperextension.

9. Thomas' test can be modified to test all the following *except* _____.

    a. rectus femoris muscle.
    b. iliopsoas muscle.
    c. tensor muscle.
    d. gluteus medius muscle.

10. A positive contractile test found in assessment of abduction may implicate all *except* the _____.

    a. tensor muscle.
    b. sartorius muscle.
    c. iliopsoas muscle.
    d. gluteus medius muscle.

11. Which of these ranges of straight leg raising is considered within normal limits?

    a. Greater than 90 degrees.
    b. Greater than 80 degrees.
    c. Greater than 70 degrees.
    d. 60 to 70 degrees.

12. In the sitting position, tightness of the hamstrings is evident when the knee joint is extended and the:

    a. pelvis remains in an anterior pelvic tilt.
    b. low back maintains a lordosis.
    c. fingers do not touch the toes.
    d. pelvis remains in a posterior pelvic tilt.

13. The hamstring muscles could substitute for hip adduction if the hip is _____.

    a. medially rotated.
    b. flexed.
    c. laterally rotated.
    d. extended.

▲ Chapter 13

1. Hip flexion may result when resistance is applied to the hamstring muscles during knee flexion because of _____.

    a. passive insufficiency of the hamstrings.
    b. active insufficiency of the hamstrings.
    c. imbalance of strength between hamstrings and quadriceps.
    d. tightness of the hip flexor musculature.

2. The starting position for muscle testing knee extension is with the hip _____.

    a. in a neutral position.
    b. flexed 45 degrees.
    c. flexed 90 degrees.
    d. extended.

3. Normal range of the Q angle in males is _____.

    a. 10 to 15 degrees.
    b. 15 to 20 degrees.
    c. 0 to 5 degrees.
    d. 5 to 10 degrees.

4. A finding of intense pain during contractile testing of knee extension may indicate _____.

    a. rupture of the quadriceps muscle.
    b. femoral nerve injury.
    c. patellar tendinitis.
    d. iliotibial band syndrome.

5. The most reliable test for anterior cruciate insufficiency is _____.

   a. Lachman's test.
   b. the anterior drawer test.
   c. the Slocum's test.
   d. the pivot shift.

▲ Chapter 14

1. A substitution in muscle testing for ankle dorsiflexion and inversion is _____.

   a. action of the extensor digitorum longus and peroneus tertius muscles.
   b. quick dorsiflexion then relaxation.
   c. active contraction of the tibialis posterior muscle.
   d. active contraction of the tibialis posterior and extensor hallucis longus muscles.

2. Where would you palpate the tibialis posterior muscle?

   a. Anterior to the lateral malleolus.
   b. Anterior to the navicular.
   c. Posterior to the medial malleolus.
   d. Distal to the cuboid bone.

3. What would you evaluate to substantiate a deep peroneal nerve lesion if ankle dorsiflexion was not evident?

   a. Weakness of the peroneal muscles.
   b. Contraction of the extensor digitorum brevis.
   c. Sensory deficit medially on the leg.
   d. Decreased Achilles tendon reflex.

4. The most common substitution for ankle plantar flexion during goniometric measurement is

   _____.

   a. forefoot flexion.
   b. inversion.
   c. eversion.
   d. supination.

5. In measuring ankle dorsiflexion, the moving arm of the goniometer is placed parallel to the

   _____.

   a. midline of the first metatarsal.
   b. bottom of the heel on the plantar side.
   c. dorsal midline of the second metatarsal.
   d. lateral midline of the fifth metatarsal.

Answers to Examination Questions

▲ Chapter 2

1. D
2. C
3. A
4. B
5. B
6. B
7. A
8. C
9. B
10. A
11. A
12. B
13. C
14. D
15. A
16. A
17. B
18. A
19. D
20. B
21. A

▲ Chapter 4

1. A
2. B
3. C
4. D

▲ Chapter 5

1. C
2. D

3. A
4. A
5. D
6. A
7. B
8. A
9. B
10. A
11. A
12. D
13. B
14. C

▲ Chapter 6

1. B
2. B
3. D
4. A
5. B
6. D
7. C

▲ Chapter 7

1. D
2. D
3. B
4. D
5. D
6. B
7. D
8. C

9. B
10. C

▲ Chapter 8

1. B
2. D
3. A
4. B
5. D

▲ Chapter 9

1. D
2. B
3. B
4. C
5. B

▲ Chapter 10

1. A
2. B
3. C
4. B

▲ Chapter 11

1. C
2. B
3. A

▲ Chapter 12

1. D
2. B

3. C
4. B
5. B
6. D
7. C
8. D
9. D
10. C
11. B
12. D
13. C

▲ Chapter 13

1. B
2. B
3. A
4. C
5. A

▲ Chapter 14

1. D
2. C
3. D
4. A
5. D

Page numbers followed by *f* refer to figures; page numbers followed by *t* refer to tables.